SHOCKS TO THE SYSTEM

By the same author

Psychotherapy of the Brain-Injured Patient: Reclaiming the Shattered Self
Freud's Brain: Neuropsychodynamic Foundations of Psychoanalysis
Inner Natures: Brain, Self, and Personality

A NORTON PROFESSIONAL BOOK

SHOCKS
TO THE
SYSTEM

Psychotherapy of
Traumatic Disability Syndromes

Laurence Miller, Ph.D.

W. W. NORTON & COMPANY
New York • London

Copyright © 1998 by Laurence Miller

Composition by PRD Group
Manufacturing by Haddon Craftsmen

Library of Congress Cataloging-in-Publication Data

Miller, Laurence, 1951–
    Shocks to the system : psychotherapy of traumatic disability
syndromes / Laurence Miller.
        p.   cm.
    "A Norton professional book"--Prelim. p.
    Includes bibliographical references and index.
    ISBN 0-393-70256-1
    1. Psychic trauma--Treatment.   2. Psychotherapy.   3. Post
-traumatic stress disorder--Treatment.   4. Stress (Psychology)-
-Treatment.   I. Title.
    [DNLM: 1. Stress Disorders, Post-Traumatic--therapy.   2. Stress
Disorders, Post-Traumatic--psychology.   3. Stress, Psychological-
-therapy.   4. Psychotherapy--methods.   WM 170 M648s 1998]
RC552.P67M55   1998
616.85'210651--dc21
DNLM/DLC
for Library of Congress   98-14545   CIP

W. W. Norton & Company, Inc., 500 Fifth Avenue, New York, N.Y. 10110
http://www.wwnorton.com
W. W. Norton & Company, Ltd., 10 Coptic Street, London WC1A 1PU

1   2   3   4   5   6   7   8   9   0

For those who reach for the courage
to transcend their pain.

And for those who help them find it.

FOREWORD

A century ago, two Austrian physicians, Sigmund Freud and Josef Breuer, began treating patients who had failed to respond to the treatments available at the time. These patients presented an array of bewildering physical and emotional symptoms that could not be adequately explained in exclusively medical terms. Out of this work two broad causes of psychopathology were identified: intrapsychic conflict and environmental trauma. It was left to others to elaborate further on the traumatic underpinnings of mental suffering and symptoms. In *Shocks to the System*, Laurence Miller elegantly and accessibly integrates a vast body of empirical studies and infuses it with the clinical wisdom he has gleaned from treating patients exposed to traumatic environmental events. He brings together, for the first time in one volume, a way to make sense of and treat a range of traumas, both physical and psychic, arising from both intentional and accidental as well as both natural and man-made violence to the system.

None of us wants to believe we will ever fall victim to assault, damaging industrial or motor vehicle accidents, or horrific natural disasters that threaten to shatter our bodies, our lives, and our fundamental relationships. Yet, statistics indicate that the *majority* of us will have such an experience in our lifetimes. When our tragedies are met with understanding and compassionate responses from others, our suffering is alleviated or even entirely eliminated, and some few of us will even grow from the experience. There is potential truth in the Chinese character so often pointed to by those of us working in the field of crisis intervention: within crisis there is both danger and opportunity. In this sense, Nietzsche was right in saying that whatever doesn't kill me makes me stronger.

What if, instead of empathic understanding, we go from doctor to doctor, agency to agency, friend to friend, attorney to attorney in the hopes of finding help and justice and are met with bewilderment, dismissal, and suspicion of malingering or of being weak or neurotic? These responses are often as damaging as the original trauma and can propel us into a downward spiral of dysfunction and despair the author terms "traumatic disability syndrome." Or what if we are not ourselves the victim of trauma but work so recurrently with those who are broken and anguished by trauma that we develop compassion fatigue or vicarious traumatization? To whom does the helper turn for help? The answers to these questions are the work of this volume.

This book is written mainly for practicing psychotherapists. In it therapists will find coherent ways of understanding and current modalities for treating the increasing numbers of trauma victims who are finding their way to the consulting room. It is also explicitly intended for attorneys and case managers. Yet, because the author writes in a characteristically plain-speaking, highly evocative style, this book will also be welcomed by the entire range of individuals who have been traumatized or who come in regular contract with victims of trauma. The knowledge imparted will make the pivotal difference in whether one is able to contribute to the alleviation of suffering or unwittingly contribute to its perpetuation.

Lisa Lewis, Ph.D.
Director of Neuropsychological Services
Menninger Clinic
Topeka, Kansas

CONTENTS

INTRODUCTION

Are we becoming a traumatized society? Paradoxically, twentieth-century America is overall a safer, healthier, and more pleasant place to live than most people have enjoyed throughout human history. Nevertheless, accidents, assaults, and injuries are a regular part of modern life. Workers are hurt on the job, motorists crash into one another, buildings collapse, trains derail, toxic chemicals spill into our air and water, fires and electrical charges sear and shock us, strangers assault us, mother nature overwhelms us. Sometimes, the body is left with physical pains, deformities, deficits, and malfunctions; other times no outer scars are visible, but the mind has been shattered by stress and horror. In all such cases, we say that *trauma* has occurred.

Much has been written and spoken about trauma recently; indeed, "trauma" has become the self-help buzzword of our time. Books, professional journals and popular magazines, conferences and seminars, talk shows, tabloid shockumentaries, and movies of the week have all covered the sometimes lurid family and sexual traumas that create clinical and political grist for the mills of countless special interest agendas. After repeated exposure, a kind of intellectual and emotional desensitization occurs, a form of "compassion fatigue," if not outright cynicism, on the part of professionals and the general public alike. Inevitably, this is creating a clinical, legal, and political backlash, with the risk that the legitimate traumas and injuries of everyday life will be downplayed or ignored.

Till now, both professional clinicians and pop psychology panderers have focused on two main areas of stress and trauma: wartime posttraumatic stress disorder, largely from the Vietnam era, and sexual abuse, either in childhood or in the context of rape or marital conflict. Largely ignored have been the millions of people who are injured and traumatized in seemingly more mundane incidents, such as auto accidents, workplace injuries, criminal assaults, and toxic exposures.

These are real injuries that are often not taken seriously because they exist in the shadow world between medicine and psychology. They include the persistent mental confusion caused by a "mild" concussion; chronic pain following a back or neck injury that never seems to go away; impaired thinking and emotional functioning after inhaling or ingesting a toxic substance; nightmares, jumpiness, and marital friction that follow a terrifying car crash or mugging.

The affected individuals travel from doctor to doctor, agency to agency, lawyer to lawyer, groping for some explanation, some help, some justice. They may be ignored, maligned, or abused by the health care, insurance, and legal systems, further compounding their trauma. After months or years of this runaround, they frequently end up bitter, depressed, paranoid, rejected by doctors, alienated from friends and family, doubting their own sanity.

As these patients are shunted into the mental health system in increasing numbers, psychotherapists can expect to see more and more of these types of cases. Indeed, the coming decade will see a growing need for skillful and knowledgable trauma therapists, a call that will come from physicians, attorneys, insurance companies, law enforcement and emergency services, the government and military, and the corporate and business sectors. The present volume offers a guide to the evaluation and treatment of these challenging cases.

The content of this book is based on two primary sources: first, a review of the scientific literature on stress, pain, and trauma; and second, my own clinical experience in working within this sometimes uncharted field. I first became intrigued with the impact of trauma through my work with brain-injured patients who had sustained concussions, usually in auto or workplace accidents. In addition to the effects on memory, reasoning, and coordination, many of these patients seemed to have been emotionally scarred by the injuring event, far beyond what one would expect from the nature of their physical injuries alone. As months dragged on into years, their continuing mental and social disability often took an increasing toll on their lives and those of their families. These experiences led me to record my clinical observations and treatment recommendations in *Psychotherapy of the Brain-Injured Patient*.

But traumatic injuries rarely affect only one somatic or psychological system. During the time when my clinical and forensic brain injury caseload was growing, I started getting increasing numbers of referrals of treatment-resistant chronic pain patients, the disabling syndromes sometimes having persisted for years following the original injury. Many of these patients just didn't seem to "get better," so naturally they were classified as hysterical, malingering, or some other pejorative clinical label, and duly referred to the shrink.

Other patients I worked with had been exposed to toxic substances or electric shocks. Here again, their failure to respond briskly to traditional medical treatment—to "snap out of it"—was seen as a sign of either weak-willed neuroticism or cunning deception, and so they ended up at my door. These referrals were often expressed in terms of a "last resort" by doctors, lawyers, or insurance companies who wanted to "close the case."

Along with these patients, an increasing number of criminal assault and workplace violence victims began to be referred for psychotherapy, and many of these patients seemed to suffer disturbances in their daily functioning that far outlasted what was supposed to be a "normal" recovery period. All too often, a bad situation was made far worse by these patients' ungracious treatment within the criminal justice system, which—with some glowing exceptions—typically regards the rights and feelings of the crime victim as incidental to solving and prosecuting the case (I'm happy to report that this is beginning to change under the influence of a number of enlightened investigators, prosecutors, and judges).

Only recently has the need to address the traumatic stress reactions in the professional helpers themselves—police officers, firefighters, paramedics, and other rescue and crisis personnel—been recognized. My work with these skilled and dedicated "tough guys" has provided valuable insights into the nature of the human coping response. Finally, unlike the common stereotype of making a living by sitting on their butts, today's crisis intervention and trauma psychotherapists frequently find themselves immersed in an active, demanding, stressful, and at times dangerous occupation that can lead to premature burnout if they neglect their own needs. These courageous front-line professionals also have much to teach about coping and giving.

In working with all of these patients and colleagues, I began to see how injury, stress, pain, and trauma often mutually reinforce one another in a vicious cycle of disability and despair. While individual premorbid personality and coping styles must always be taken into account, traumatically disabled patients' ongoing fruitless struggles with the medicolegal system can turn even once happy, healthy, and productive human beings into deteriorated shells of their former selves. Part of this is the nature of the syndrome, part the result of ignorance and maltreatment delivered by many of those who are supposed to help.

The all-too-frequent end result of this downward spiral is the development of what I term a *traumatic disability syndrome:* a persistent impairment
in adaptive functioning, caused or triggered by a traumatic injury or
incident, that is resistant to conventional medical and psychological treatment, appears "out of proportion" to the precipitating event, and affects
the person's thought, mood, behavior, work role, family relations, and
social interactions.

In an effort to understand and aid these patients, I began to research
the clinical and scientific literature on stress, pain, and trauma, to see
what insights others had to come up with that I could combine with my
own observations and experiences. It soon became apparent that many
clinicians are treating the proverbial trees while missing the forest. That
is, they are addressing chronic pain, or postconcussion syndrome, or
posttraumatic stress disorder, as an individual, discrete clinical entity,
without recognizing how each of these procrustian diagnostic categories
relates to the larger issue of psychic wounding and traumatic disability.

All too often, even well-meaning and conscientious clinicians who may
be skilled therapists in their own areas of specialization simply don't have
adequate knowledge of, or experience with, these traumatic disability
syndromes. With nothing to guide them, they fall back on standard
diagnoses and treatments. Therefore, one goal of this book is to make
the necessary information accessible to those in the helping professions
who are charged with the task of caring for trauma survivors.

This book provides down-to-earth, practical treatment strategies for
psychotherapists who see these patients in the real clinical world, in the
"trenches." But it also develops a broader view of how traumatic disability
syndromes develop in response to a wide range of adversities, an overarching philosophy of trauma therapy, if you will. This perspective can also
be valuable for attorneys and case managers who deal with traumatic
disability cases. Overall, my guiding principle in writing this book has
been to "tell it straight." This means being scientifically accurate in
describing causes, treatments, and theories, and also being realistic about
recovery and outcomes.

But realism doesn't have to mean therapeutic nihilism. True, traumatic
injury is a nasty business. It causes great pain and warps lives. These
patients may be extraordinarily demanding and difficult to work with,
and a good number will never fully recover. But many do overcome their
ordeal and get on with living, if—and here's the important point—*if*
they receive effective treatment by skilled and knowledgeable clinicians.
And a few do more than survive: they surpass, they transcend, they forge
from the strip-mined ores of their psyche a new alloy of resilient strength
that bestows a quantum advantage in handling future adversities and

passing their healing wisdom on to others. That's why the final chapter of this book explores how the lessons learned from the deepest depths of human horror and despair can be applied to the understanding of human fortitude and resilience—how the lessons learned from pain and trauma can be usefully applied to the practice of psychotherapy as a whole.

One of the challenges in organizing the material for this volume was how to divide the chapters, as there is obviously a lot of overlap between many of the topic areas. However, the plan of the book is as follows. Chapter 1 introduces the concept of traumatic disability syndromes arising from diverse types of physical and psychological injuries. It traces the history of trauma syndromes from antiquity, through the extensive work at the turn of the century, to modern conceptualizations and misconceptions. Using its most frequently recognized prototype—posttraumatic stress disorder—the chapter describes the common symptoms of the trauma response that may lead to a traumatic disability syndrome. The emphasis is on the continuities and commonalities of the psychological reactions to different types of injuries and traumas, so that psychotherapists may create meaningful diagnostic formulations and realistic treatment plans.

Chapter 2 describes the basic principles of psychotherapy for traumatic disability syndromes. Once again, most of the literature on this topic has addressed posttraumatic stress disorder, and the chapter reflects this emphasis. Much culling had to be done to include material that I believe will be most useful to clinicians treating traumatic disability syndromes, since the general therapeutic principles of this chapter guide and inform the more focused treatment efforts described for the individual syndromes in later chapters.

Chapters 3, 4, and 5 cover the traumatic disability syndromes most likely to begin with physical ravages to brain or body: the postconcussion syndrome, chronic pain, and toxic trauma. Typically, these are the patients who don't "read the textbooks" and so fail to recover within the normal six-to-twelve month window expected by their physicians or employers. These patients' misunderstanding and rejection by the medical, legal, and compensation systems all too often accelerate their descent into debilitating invalidism and despair.

Chapters 6 and 7 deal with the potentially traumatizing effects of nature and technology: transportation accidents as well as natural and man-made disasters. These chapters emphasize the necessity of prioritizing treatment, from the most basic provision of food, shelter, and medical care, to the most complex and delicate therapeutic ministrations, in order to restore normal everyday functioning and build the patient's emotional strength to cope with learning to drive again or rebuilding his or her community.

Chapters 8 and 9 address the malign acts of our fellow human beings. The topics of crime victimization and workplace violence remind us that no one is completely safe from the ill will of our workmates or fellow citizens, and attacks by other persons are often the most psychologically destabilizing and faith-destroying of all traumas. Workplace violence is dealt with in considerable detail, because this is one of the most *preventable* of everyday traumatic events and yet, paradoxically, one of the most blindly ignored by workers, managers, and therapists alike. After reading this chapter, there will be no excuse for ignorance or inaction.

Chapters 10 and 11 salute the helpers and healers—police, firefighters, paramedics, rescuers, support personnel, and trauma therapists—who regularly put their lives and sanity on the line to mitigate the tragedies visited upon us by technology, nature, or our fellow creatures. Not an easy bunch to work with, true, but I've been impressed by the willingness of a new generation of law enforcement and emergency service managers to recognize the value of mental health services for the men and women under their command. Now it's our turn as clinicians to rise to the challenge—not to mention the responsibility of taking care of our own wounded, so that a decade from now the best and brightest among us aren't burnt out, sold out, or forced out of the clinical and helping professions.

Chapter 12 asks, What about the small but important group of trauma survivors who never see us, don't need us, don't want us, and can cope and move on quite well without us? Clinicians need to pay more attention to the developmental psychodynamics and cognitive styles of those who independently and adaptively cope with, and in a few cases, even grow from, their traumas. That way, we can hopefully apply these lessons to the less fortunate souls under our care.

Because, as cold-bloodedly realistic as this book urges trauma therapists to be, our work is, after all, about hope. Traumas, recent and past, hold a hallowed place in the history of psychology and psychotherapy, but most of the emphasis has been on trauma's downside, since that's what we get paid to treat. However, in applying the lessons learned from successfully coping traumatized persons to the understanding of human strength and resilience more generally, we expand exponentially our clinical and social contribution by tackling the issues that may ultimately make for a more stable, safe, and healthy society.

God bless the English language, but we *still* don't have a convenient gender-neutral pronoun. Therefore, based on a combination of editorial advice and my own good conscience, here's how this book handles the matter: Specific patients will be referred to by their own gender. When referring to patients generally, "he" or "she" will be used in alternate chapters. Exceptions to this rule will occur in chapters or chapter sections where the patient population by nature demographically favors one sex over another. Since I personally identify with the "psychotherapist" in this book, and I'm male, "he" will be used to refer generally to therapists. I know this jerry-built linguistic schema is not a perfect solution to the gender-language problem, but if anyone has a better idea, let me know.

ACKNOWLEDGMENTS

I'll take both credit and critique for the basic content and format of this book, but of course, endeavors of this scope can never be solo projects. The support, encouragement, and professionalism of literary agent John Ware are once again responsible for my work finding its audience. It's been a pleasure to cook up another volume with Norton editor Susan Barrows Munro, whose simmering redaction has once more helped separate the steak of my message from the sizzle. My appreciation goes to the editorial staff of *Psychotherapy* and the *Journal of Cognitive Rehabilitation*, in whose pages many of this book's ideas were first developed.

I've learned much from my patients, students, support group members, and colleagues. It continues to be my privilege to work with the Palm Beach County Critical Incident Stress Management Team; the members' selfless dedication to their traumatized peers exemplifies the true meaning of service and honor. The clinicians and staff at the South Florida Pain and Rehabilitation Center and at Associates in Neurology of Hollywood have provided much professional stimulation in my work with traumatic disability patients.

My participation in the activities of support and advocacy groups continues to inspire my faith in the power of the few to strengthen and heal the spirit of the one or the many. Special thanks to the South Florida Brain Tumor Association, the Palm Beach County Chapter of the Brain Injury Association of Florida, the Epilepsy Association of Eastern Florida, and Palm Beach County Victim Services for the opportunity to work with their staff, members, and families. My students at Florida Atlantic University have kept me on my toes and reminded me that knowledge is never static but must adaptively evolve in the face of new scientific and clinical challenges.

And finally, my gratitude goes to my family, Joan and Halle, because very little of this work could happen without their love and support. Crisis intervention and trauma therapy are, by their nature, frequently unscheduled and unpredictable. For all the disturbing calls in the middle of the night, for all my sudden rushings-off to conduct critical incident debriefings or deal with accident or crime emergencies, for all the last-minute court appearances that forced us to change family plans, for all the times you've asked me when I'll be home and I had to answer "I don't know," and, on top of that, for all the additional hours I've stolen to *write* about this stuff—for all these accommodations, allowances, and indulgences, thank you for enabling me to do the work I've chosen and for providing a home to come back to.

Chapter 1

THE WOUNDED SOUL

Posttraumatic Stress Disorder and the Trauma Syndrome

Wounds heal and become scars.
But scars grow with us.

—Stanislaw Lec

"The worst part about the whole thing," Gail told me tearfully, "is that I saw it coming, I knew it was going to happen and there was nothing I could do about it."

Gail was returning home from a huge pre-holiday shopping expedition, the car stuffed with groceries plus her seven-year-old son, Kevin, whom she'd just picked up from school. Stopped at an intersection near her home, she chatted with her son while waiting for the light to change. The light turned green just as the last car at the crossroad passed in front of her. She began to move forward, when she noticed out of the corner of her eye that a pickup truck was zooming toward the intersection.

"I just assumed he would stop, since his stoplight was already red, but I guess he was trying to beat the light," she related. By the time Gail realized the pickup wasn't slowing down, she was already into the intersection, unable to back up because of the cars behind her. "I froze. I saw the truck coming right at me, I was staring at it, my mind went blank. Then he hit us."

The impact knocked Gail's car out of the road and onto a nearby grassy knoll. The car overturned once and bounced into an upright position. "It's crazy, it's like I was sitting in this rolling car, calmly thinking of what kind of Christmas my family was going to have without

1

me." A few seconds later, "all I could think about was getting Kevin out of the car." With a cool deliberativeness that surprised even her, she was able to reach past the broken glass bottles and strewn groceries, carefully free her son from his seatbelt, and find a door that would open wide enough for both of them to get out. Miraculously, they walked away from the wreck—actually Gail walked, carrying a frightened, but unhurt Kevin.

The police and paramedics arrived quickly. A few bruises, a gash on the leg, and several days of muscle soreness comprised the extent of Gail's injuries. Belted in and cushioned by huge grocery bags, Kevin was apparently unscathed. The pickup's driver turned out to be drunk and was arrested at the scene. "Why didn't I just wait?" Gail sobbed in my office. "I could have lost my boy." And the worst part? "Everybody keeps telling me how lucky I am. Do I look 'lucky' to you?"

The word *trauma* comes from the Greek word for "wound." Each year, millions of people suffer psychological trauma that may or may not accompany a bodily physical injury. While it often leaves no visible physical scar, the psychological trauma may subject them to months or years of disability and demoralization. Research and clinical experience show that prompt, effective, and compassionate treatment for what has come to be known as *posttraumatic stress disorder,* or PTSD, typically leads to good recovery in the majority of cases. Yet these patients are often dismissed by doctors, employers, and insurance companies, and undergo the gratuitous "secondary wounding" of being misdiagnosed and inappropriately treated for their trauma. The result is often a chronic disorder that produces disabling symptoms, subjects its sufferers to mis-understanding, contempt, and ridicule, and may finally leave the victims doubting their very sanity.

This book begins with a discussion of PTSD because it is prototypical of most of the other traumatic disability syndromes in the nature and form of psychological traumatization it produces. It is also representative of the misunderstanding and mistreatment that traumatically disabled patients so often encounter.

HISTORY OF THE TRAUMA CONCEPT

Historically, the pendulum of interest in posttraumatic stress syndromes has swung back and forth between military and civilian traumas (Evans, 1992; Rosen, 1975; Trimble, 1981; Wilson, 1994). During warfare, rulers and generals have always had a stake in knowing as much as possible about any factors that might adversely affect their fighting forces. To this end, doctors have been pressed into service to diagnose and treat soldiers with the aim of getting them back to the front lines as soon as possible. In times of peace, attention turns to the everyday accidents and individual acts of mayhem that can produce stress, pain, and trauma in the lives of ordinary civilians.

The effect of *physical* trauma—a shattered limb, a bashed-in brain—on a person's ability to fight, work, love, or raise a family is fairly obvious. More mystifying is why an event that seems to shatter only the senses, that bashes in one's heretofore safe and comfortable view of the world, should in so many cases produce pervasive and catastrophic disability. And so explanations have been sought, theories advanced.

One of the first modern conceptualizations of posttraumatic stress was proferred in 1678 by the army surgeon Hoffer (in Rosen, 1975). Not satisfied with merely dressing wounds and amputating mutilated appendages, Hoffer was also concerned with the morale of his men in battle. He developed the concept of *nostalgia*, which he defined as a deterioration in the physical and mental health of homesick soldiers. The cause of this malady was attributed to the formation of abnormally vivid images in the affected soldier's brain by battle-induced overexcitation of the "vital spirits." Here, in effect, was one of the first attempts to explain how a psychological event could affect brain functioning and, in turn, influence health and behavior.

With the eighteenth and nineteenth centuries came the mechanized progress of the Industrial Revolution, bringing with it new and monstrous machines to crush, grind, and flay the scores of workers who tended them too carelessly or toiled too close by. At about the same time, a new form of high-speed transportation, the railroad, began to reveal a disturbing propensity to rattle and strew its passengers about in derailments and collisions.

All too often, it was noticed, long after the physical scars had healed, or even when injury to the body was minor or nonexistent, many accident victims showed lasting disturbances in thought, feeling, and action that could not readily be explained by the conventional medical knowledge of the day. Some patients were afflicted by strange paralyses or neurasthenic fatigues, while others trembled continuously, twitched and postured bizarrely, jumped at the slightest sound, or holed up for weeks or months, refusing all human contact.

As the number of psychologically impaired train wreck and industrial accident cases swelled the patient loads of hospitals and sent formerly productive workers to their beds, physicians strained for some medically comprehensible explanation. In 1882, Erichson introduced the concept of *railway spine*, which he believed could be traced to as-yet unobservable perturbations in the structure of the central nervous system caused by blows to the body—no matter that in many cases there was no evidence at all that such bodily concussions actually occurred. Others among Erichson's colleagues considered that the strange disorders of sensation and movement might be due to disruptions in the blood flow to the spinal cord, or even to small hemorrhages.

While these organically-minded physicians were squinting to discern structural microtraumas in nervous tissue, others expanded their gaze to view the origin of posttraumatic impairment syndromes as a *psychological* phenomenon—albeit, straying none too far from the home base of neurophysiology. This was reflected in the theory of *nervous shock*, introduced by Page in 1895, which posited that a state of overwhelming fright or terror—not physical bangs and jolts—was the primary cause of traumatic impairment syndromes in railway and industrial accidents. Similarly, at around the same time, Oppenheim (1890) theorized that a stimulus perceived through the senses alone, if strong enough, might actually jar the nervous system into a state of disequilibrium.

For his part, the famous Charcot (1887) regarded the effects of psychical trauma as a form of hysteria, the symptoms arising as a consequence of disordered brain physiology caused by the terrifying memory of the traumatic event. In postulating the impact of a psychological force on the physical functioning of the brain, these late nineteenth century theories were reminiscent of Hoffer's conceptualization, two centuries earlier, except that electrophysiological impulses now had replaced vital spirits as the underlying mechanism of the disorder.

Attention, however, soon shifted back to the fields of battle. Advances in weapons technology during the First World War produced an alarming accumulation of horrid battlefield casualties from the newly invented machine guns, poison gas, and long-range artillery. This led to the widely applied concept of *shell shock*, a form of psychological incapacitation at first thought to be produced by the brain-concussing effects of exploding shells. This wartime stress theory was, after all, not too different from the earlier civilian concept of railway spine. In both cases, undocumentable effects on the nervous system were postulated on the basis of observed disorders in behavior.

In the meantime, the organic determinists continued to push for a biological explanation of traumatic stress syndromes, now marshalling new findings about the role of the autonomic nervous system in regulating states of arousal and bodily homeostasis. For example, Wilson and his colleagues (Frazier & Wilson, 1918; Mearburg & Wilson, 1918) described a syndrome called *irritable heart* found in traumatized soldiers, which they attributed to overstimulation of the sympathetic—"fight-or-flight"—branch of the autonomic nervous system.

Even Sigmund Freud got into the act. No stranger to neuroscientific theory and practice himself (see Miller, 1991), Freud (1920) regarded the tendency to remain "fixated" on traumatic events as having a biological basis. But recurring recollections and nightmares of a frightening nature seemed to fly in the face of Freud's theory of the pleasure principle. Consequently, he was forced to consider a psychogenic cause—that traumatic dreams and other symptoms served the function of helping the traumatized person master the terrifying event by working it over and over in the victim's mind. Unfortunately, this line of theorizing took Freud into some rather morbid metaphysical speculations about the death instinct and organic dissolution that had the effect of keeping his ideas on the fringes of trauma theory even to the present day.

Meanwhile, soldiers were still being scared out their wits on the battlefield and the civilian railway and industrial accident cases continued to pile up. The persistently annoying failure of medical science to discover any down-to-earth organic basis for these debilitating stress syndromes led to a gradual, if grudging, acceptance of psychodynamic explanations, as the Freudian influence began to be felt more generally throughout psychiatry. This contributed to the replacement of shell shock by the more psychological-sounding concept of *war neurosis*.

Apparently making a theoretical virtue of empirical necessity, doctors now no longer felt compelled to tether their diagnoses and treatments to ephemeral defects of nervous tissue. Accordingly, Ferenczi, Abraham, and Simmel (1921) elaborated the basic model of traumatic neurosis that is still largely accepted today among psychodynamic theorists. They described the central role of anxiety, the persistence of morbid apprehension, regression of the ego, the attempted reparative function of recurring nightmares, and the therapeutic use of catharsis.

For the most part, then, physicians had put their neurophysiological theorizing on the back burner and had begun to concentrate on trying to treat these wounded souls by any means that worked. All the sophisticated biological theories didn't, after all, seem to yield commensurately effective biological treatments. In fact, the patients themselves seemed to do best with the kinds of psychologically cathartic and supportive approaches that were provided by caring counselors, ministers, nurses—and even the occasional psychiatrist.

Continuing research seemed to bear this out. After surveying over a thousand reports in world literature published during the First World War, Southard (1919) concluded that shell shock, war neurosis, and similar syndromes were true psychoneuroses. Kardiner (1941) followed a group of patients with war neuroses for more than a decade and concluded that severe war trauma produced a kind of centripetal contraction or collapse of the ego that prevented these patients from adapting to and mastering life's subsequent challenges. Kardiner elaborated a conceptualization of trauma he called *physioneurosis* that is startlingly close to the modern concept of posttraumatic stress disorder. The features in Kardiner's description included (1) persistence of a startle response or irritability; (2) a proclivity to explosive behavior; (3) fixation on the trauma; (4) an overall constriction of the personality; and (5) a disturbed dream life, including vivid nightmares.

The experiences of the Second World War contributed suprisingly little to the development of new theories and treatments for wartime trauma, now redubbed *battle fatigue*. In fact, resistance to the concept of battle fatigue, with its implications of mental weakness and lack of moral resolve, was widespread in both medical and military circles. There was a war on, plenty of guys were getting killed or wounded, and the army had little sympathy for the pusillanimous whinings of a few slackers and nervous nellies who couldn't buck up and pull their weight. This went as far as General George Patton's infamous slap-heard-'round-the-world of a traumatized enlisted man in a World War II field hospital. No doubt, less well publicized incidents at somewhat lower levels of command took place regularly to keep soldiers in line. Not inconsequentially, the same contemptuous attitude toward civilian psychological trauma—perhaps minus only the slapping—is expressed by many medical doctors today.

But it was becoming apparent that wartime psychological trauma could take place in circumstances other than the actual battlefield. In World War II, then Korea and Vietnam, and most recently in the Persian Gulf, clinicians began to learn about disabling stress syndromes associated with large-scale bombings of civilian populations, prisoner of war and concentration camps, "brainwashing" of P.O.W.'s, civilian atrocities, and terrorism.

With sad predictability, today's daily newspapers continue to churn out more than ample case material from every imaginable species of human tragedy: war crimes, industrial injuries, plane crashes, auto accidents, rapes, assaults, domestic violence, child abuse, earthquakes, hurricanes, fires, floods, toxic spills, terrorist bombings—the list goes on. Stress syndromes were finally codified as an identifiable type of psychopathological syndrome—*posttraumatic stress disorder* (PTSD)—in the American Psychiatric Association's official *Diagnostic and Statistical Manual of Mental Disorders* (APA, 1980, 1987, 1994), although debate continues as to whether this response constitutes a distinct "disorder" or merely an extreme reaction pattern to different kinds of stresses.

THE TRAUMA SYNDROME:
BASIC FEATURES

As I emphasize repeatedly throughout this book, the first step toward true healing is knowledge and understanding. For this reason, I typically spend a lot of time explaining to my patients the nature of the symptoms and syndromes they're experiencing—postconcussion syndrome, chronic pain, neurotoxic trauma, PTSD, and so on—and the factors that cause and sustain it. Giving the clinical syndrome a context, a meaning, a name, is almost always an essential first step toward effective treatment and recovery.

Posttraumatic Stress Disorder: The Clinical Syndrome

In clinical science, a *syndrome* is defined as a set of symptoms and signs that occur in a fairly regular pattern from patient to patient, under a given set of circumstances, and with a specific set of causes (even though individual variations may be seen). In this definition, PTSD is a syndrome of emotional and behavioral disturbance that follows exposure to a traumatic stressor or set of traumaticially stressful experiences that is typically outside the range of normal, everyday experience for that person. As a result, there develops a characteristic set of symptoms (APA, 1994; Meek, 1990; Merskey, 1992; Miller, 1993b, 1994; Modlin, 1983, Parker, 1990; Weiner, 1992).

ANXIETY. The patient describes a continual state of free-floating anxiety or "nervousness." There is a constant gnawing apprehension that something terrible is about to happen. He maintains an intensive hypervigilance, scanning the environment for the least hint of impending threat or danger. Panic attacks may be occasional or frequent.

PHYSIOLOGICAL AROUSAL. The patient's autonomic nervous system is always at least on yellow alert, often on red alert. He experiences increased bodily tension in the form of muscle tightness or "knots," tremors or shakiness, restlessness, fatigue, heart palpitations, breathing difficulties, dizziness, headaches, stomach and bowel disturbances, urinary frequency, or menstrual disturbances. About one-half of PTSD patients show a classic startle reaction: surprised by an unexpected door slam, telephone ring, sneeze, or even just hearing their name called, the patient will literally "jump" out of his seat and then spend the next few minutes trembling with fear and anxiety.

IRRITABILITY.   There is a pervasive chip-on-the-shoulder edginess, impatience, loss of humor, and quick anger over seemingly trivial matters. Friends get ticked off, coworkers shun the patient, and family members may be abused and alienated. A particularly common complaint is the patient's increased sensitivity to children's "noisiness" or the family's "bothering" questions.

AVOIDANCE/DENIAL.   The patient tries to blot out the event from his mind. He avoids thinking about the traumatic event, shuns news articles, radio programs, or TV shows that remind him of the incident. "I just don't want to talk about it" is the standard response, and the patient may claim to have "forgotten" important aspects of the event. Some of this is a deliberate, conscious effort to avoid trauma-reminders; part of it also involves an involuntary psychic numbing that blunts most incoming threatening stimuli. The emotional coloring of this denial may range from blasé indifference to nail-biting anxiety.

INTRUSION.   This is the flip-side of avoidance and denial. Despite the patient's best efforts to keep the traumatic event out of mind, the horrifying incident pushes its way into his consciousness, often rudely and abruptly in the form of intrusive images of the event by day and frightening dreams at night. In the most extreme cases, patients may experience flashbacks or reliving experiences in which they seem to be mentally transported back to the traumatic scene in all its sensory and emotional vividness, sometimes losing touch with current reality. More commonly, the intrusive recollection is described as a persistent psychological demon that "won't let me forget" the trauma and the terrifying events surrounding it.

REPETITIVE NIGHTMARES.   Even sleep offers no respite. Sometimes the patient's nightmares replay the actual traumatic event; more commonly, the dreams echo the general theme of the trauma, but miss the mark in terms of specific content. For example, a patient traumatized in an auto accident may dream of falling off a cliff or having a wall collapse on him. Or a mugging victim may dream of being attacked by vicious dogs or standing frozen in front of an oncoming train. The emotional intensity of the original traumatic experience is retained, but the dream partially disguises the event itself. It's as though the dreaming mind tries to work through the terrifying material, while at the same time trying to protect the sleeper from the full remembered details of the event.

IMPAIRED CONCENTRATION AND MEMORY.   Patients complain of having gotten "spacy," "fuzzy," or "ditzy." They have trouble remembering names, tend to misplace objects, lose the train of conversations, or can't keep their mind focused on reading material. They may worry that they have brain damage or that "I'm losing my mind."

SEXUAL INHIBITION. Over 90 percent of PTSD patients report decreased sexual activity and interest; this may further strain an already stressed-out marital relationship. In some cases, complete impotence or frigidity occurs.

WITHDRAWAL/ISOLATION. The patient shuns friends, neighbors, and family members. "Leave me alone," is the standard refrain. The trauma survivor has no patience for the petty, trivial concerns of everyday life— bills, gossip, news events—and gets annoyed at being bothered with these piddles. The hurt feelings this engenders in those he rebuffs may spur retaliatory avoidance, leading to a vicious cycle of rejection and recrimination.

IMPULSIVITY AND INSTABILITY. More rarely, trauma survivors may take sudden trips, move from city to city, walk off their jobs, disappear from their families for prolonged periods, uncharacteristically engage in drunken binges, gambling sprees, or romantic trysts, make garish purchases, or take dangerous physical or legal risks. It's as if the trauma has goaded the survivor into a "what the hell" attitude that overcomes his usual good judgment and common sense. Obviously, not every instance of irresponsible behavior can be blamed on trauma, but when this kind of activity follows an identifiable traumatic event and is definitely out of character for that person, then some relationship is suspected. Far from taking such walks on the wild side, however, the majority of PTSD patients continue to suffer in numbed and shattered silence.

Characteristics of the Trauma Response

Seemingly resolved or dormant PTSD may be triggered by such heightened stresses as returning to work, increased responsibilities, or resuming curtailed activities. In addition, PTSD and other stress-related disorders may be exacerbated by concurrent traumas or by stressors occurring in late life or in the aging process. The more chronic the symptoms, the longer they last. Additionally, the more serious and complicated the loss or injury, the worse the prognosis for recovery or the more prolonged the reaction.

PTSD responses may occur in people who have not been directly injured or threatened but have been secondarily affected as bystanders or witnesses. These types of traumatizing events include learning about danger or harm to loved ones, losing one's home or community, or seeing something horrible happen to someone else, even a stranger. Rescuers or treatment personnel may also suffer PTSD (see Chapters 10 and 11). Traumatic events may happen to isolated individuals, as in muggings, car crashes, or workplace accidents, or they may occur to groups or even to whole populations, such as in shipwrecks, building fires, hurricanes, or toxic spills.

Overlapping Syndromes and Differential Diagnosis

A wide variety of psychological reactions may occur in the aftermath of trauma, and PTSD may overlap with a number of other posttraumatic disorders, including postconcussion syndrome, depression, phobia, generalized anxiety disorder, panic disorder, chronic pain, somatization disorder, and neurotoxic trauma (Green, 1995; Kuch, 1989; Miller, 1993a, 1993b, 1994, 1995; Modlin, 1983; Muran & Motta, 1993; Simon, 1995).

Subsyndromal or "partial" forms of PTSD may also occur, in which fewer than the requisite number of symptoms in the various categories of numbing/avoidance or increased arousal are diagnostically tabulated. While the severity of disability may be less in the partial syndrome than in full-blown PTSD, significant impairment in family, vocational, and psychosocial functioning neverthess occurs in the sybsyndromal form (Stein, Walker, Hazen, & Forde, 1997). It's thus possible to have a different degrees of PTSD, with varying levels of distress and disability.

To account for the different species of trauma response that are often observed in clinical practice, a further typology of PTSD has been proposed by Alarcon, Deering, Glover, Ready, and Eddleman (1997). This typology includes:

1. A *depressive* subtype, which presents with psychomotor retardation, social withdrawal, inability to deal with everyday occurrences, loss of interest, low self-esteem, self-criticism, guilt feelings, and suicidality.
2. A *dissociative* subtype, in which there is a predominance of flashbacks, pseudo-hallucinatory experiences, depersonalization, fugue-like behavior, derealization, and symptoms of multiple personality disorder.
3. A *somatomorphic* subtype whose primary manifestation is chronic pain or other physical symptomatology, typically without clear localization or identifiable cause (see Chapter 4).
4. A *psychotic-like* subtype, in which the patient shows distortions of consciousness, fantasizing, staring, inattentiveness, impaired motivation and activity, paranoia, and behavioral regression.

5. An *organic-like* subtype, which presents with impaired attention, concentration, learning, memory, and cognition, along with confusion, slowness in thought, speech, and behavior, and in some cases, a dementia-like appearance (see Chapter 3).
6. A *neurotic-like* subtype, characterized by anxiety, phobic avoidance, restlessness, hypersensitivity, obsessionalism, and panic episodes.

Whatever reasonable diagnostic and classificatory scheme the therapist employs, it is obvious that adequate evaluation, differential diagnosis, and case conceptualization are vitally important for developing and implementing an effective treatment plan.

EVOLUTION OF THE TRAUMA RESPONSE

Surprisingly, during the traumatic event itself, most people don't become overwhelmed or paralyzed by intense fear or shock—in the breach, many behave quite adaptively (Aldwin, 1994; Weiner, 1992). Assault victims may calculate their avenues of escape and many car occupants purposefully unstrap themselves from their seats and climb out the window of their burning or sinking vehicle. The entire organism seems to go "on automatic" and is directed toward survival. A certain degree of depersonalization takes place, an unnatural mental detachment from the surrounding events that enables the person to deal with the practical survival needs of the situation; this is often described in retrospect as "like being in a dream" or "happening in slow motion." Indeed, Hollywood portrayals to the contrary, wild-eyed, screaming panic is a remarkably rare phenomenon during the acute threat.

After the event, the numbing depersonalization may continue for some time, the survivor feeling confused, bewildered, and alienated. It's as if the psychoanesthetic freeze elicited during the trauma incident needs time to thaw out in the more temperate affective climate of real life. Unfortunately, though, "real life" doesn't last very long, as the intrusive recollective and emotional gale rushes in at the weak chinks that begin to form in the crumbling psychic armor. Thus begins the wrenching emotional seesaw of painful intrusion alternating with numbing denial, along with many of the other posttraumatic stress symptoms described above.

In the best cases, the major symptoms and disturbances diminish in the course of weeks to months as the event becomes integrated into the life narrative and personal history of the individual. A more realistic awareness of individual vulnerability is built up, so that basic feelings of security and confidence are restored. However, in some cases, a number of mental roadblocks may stand in the way of the trauma survivor's making peace with himself and the world (Everstine & Everstine, 1993; Matsakis, 1994; McCann & Pearlman, 1990; Miller, 1994).

One of these involves guilt and stigma. Many trauma survivors believe that they could have somehow prevented the traumatic event from occurring. Others interpret the event as a kind of "hard-knocks" wake-up call for their poor judgment or as cosmic punishment for past misdeeds. Many survivors feel "marked by fate," especially if this is not their first traumatic experience. Still others experience a violation of their bodily and territorial integrity. They feel fragmented and scattered, and the slightest upset makes them irritable and isolative. They may literally wince when touched or when others encroach upon their personal space, and they become panicky in rooms or in crowds where they are unable to negotiate a clear route of escape.

The traumatic event and its aftermath comprise a shattering existential experience. The trauma survivor is starkly confronted by his own vulnerability, his own mortality, in a way most of us manage to avoid by using the normal, adaptive denials of everyday life, of "business as usual." The victim's existential violation may be all the more painful if the trauma took place at the hands of another person; worse still if the action of the malfeasor was maliciously intentional or uncaringly negligent. And even more devastating may be traumas perpetrated by a known and heretofore trusted person, such as a family member, friend, workmate, neighbor, or doctor.

Being in a trauma mode is difficult to stop, hard to let go of. Many trauma survivors generalize the helplessness of the cognitive survival state to other aspects of their lives, now feeling powerless to control even their own behavior or to influence the actions of others. Or they may impute domineering or retaliatory motives to anyone who tries to exert even the normal, socially appropriate influence or control over them, e.g., bosses, doctors, parents, or spouses. In some cases, outright paranoia and hostility may develop.

Even after things seem to have calmed down, when the trauma survivor has achieved some measure of delicate equilibrium, the stresses of returning to the normal routines of work or family life may trigger PTSD reactions. Also, delayed PTSD reactions may crop up years or even decades after the event as illness or the aging process begin to deplete the individual's adaptive reserves.

In general, the more severe the trauma and the longer the trauma response persists, the more pessimistic the outcome. That's why it's important for trauma survivors to get quick, effective treatment. And even after a delay, the proper treatment can still have a significant impact, so no situation should ever be considered categorically hopeless.

Trauma leaves a wide wake. While it's easy to identify the primary victim of a convenience store holdup, traffic accident, or worksite injury, we may forget the bystanders who witnessed the shooting, the helpers who pulled the bleeding passengers out of the car, the family of the worker who was crippled. Only recently have mental health clinicians officially recognized the possibility of stress reactions or full-blown PTSD in persons who have been secondarily traumatized by seeing something terrible happen to another person, or hearing of injury to a loved one (APA, 1994).

PSYCHOLOGICAL THEORIES OF THE TRAUMA RESPONSE

Etiological hypotheses for the different species of traumatic disability syndromes will be considered in the respective individual chapters. Here we will discuss the general nature of the trauma response and some of the explanations that have been offered to explain it.

Kretschmer (1926) described two classes of behavioral responses that organisms throughout the animal kingdom use to ward off attack or the threat of attack. The first he characterized as the *violent motor reaction*, exemplified by the wild flailing response many animals show when trying to escape injury or confinement. The counterpart to this in human clinical conditions would occur in the form of dissociative fugue states, convulsive paroxysms, and violent emotional attacks with subsequent amnesia and tremors.

Kretschmer's (1926) second kind of reaction was called the *sham death*, or *immobilization reflex*, in which inaction and seemingly stuporous features predominate. Many animals "freeze" when confronted with a threat; this immobilization serves to obscure the identity or whereabouts of the threatened party or conveys a message of innocuous nonchallenge that will hopefully deflect the confrontation. Human analogs to this second pattern might include dreamy hypnoid states, hysterical sensory or motor impairment, speechlessness, or "spells" of many kinds, reminiscent of the posttraumatic reactions to threat and injury.

Ludwig (1972) has revived and expanded Kretschmer's (1926) formulation by positing a pervasive natural tendency for animals and humans to react in progressively more primitive ways when confronted with potentially dangerous and inescapable situations. Under such conditions, organisms readily and automatically resort to behaviors appropriate at earlier stages of development, behaviors that appear regressive or "imma-ture." These include babbling, rocking, crying, vivid fantasizing, mute withdrawal, incontinence, and so on—the kinds of reaction often associ-ated with "shell shock" or other kinds of acute traumatic states.

Modlin (1983) has succinctly characterized the psychodynamic expla-nation of PTSD as follows. Facing definable external danger, the human organism mobilizes for action. If, however, the protective fight-flight mechanism is prevented or inhibited from going into action, then the mental apparatus is suffused with an excessive amount of stimulation. On the psychological level, the alarm devices of the ego keep pace with the psychological alerting. The normal ego has stored energy available to bind or discharge excessive amounts of excitation, but if the discharge is blocked and homeostatic balance is disrupted, free-floating anxiety and continuing tension result.

In other cases, such as posttraumatic amnesia produced by a closed head injury, the victim may first become aware that the accident occurred when consciousness is later regained. Realistic external danger no longer exists to be met or handled in the present. The fight-flight mechanism is temporarily mobilized, but finds no substantial target to act against or escape from. Action is not actually blocked, but is rather simply "too late" and therefore irrelevant. One immediate task the ego must accomplish in this kind of situation is to regain its suddenly disrupted contact with reality and to grasp and justify what has occurred. The bewildered ego is flooded with alarm and anxiety because it has failed in its self-preservative duty. When this psychohomeostatic task fails, panic may result.

The process of coping with traumatic stress through alternation be-tween intrusive reexperiencing and denial is seen by some authorities (Brom & Kleber, 1989) as a normal, adaptive process. The individual is, in effect, self-titrating the "dose" of the traumatic recollections so that he is not overwhelmed by the intensity of emotions and other reactions that the memories evoke. The intrusive reexperiencing may offer the opportunity to assimilate the experience—to mentally "digest" it—as well as to revise the expectations and general worldview of the individual.

Almost always, the response to significant trauma involves a strong existential component. Coping, virtually by definition, involves a search for meaning. Brom and Kleber (1989) point out that people ordinarily prefer to perceive the world as organized, predictable, and comprehensi-ble. A serious traumatic life event shatters one's assumptions and beliefs about the world and oneself, prompting the typical reaction of "Why me?" One way to overcome the perceived chaos and create some order in the situation is to attribute an active role to the self in circumstances where the victim was actually powerless; this is often referred to as *cognitive* or *interpretive control* (Thompson, 1981). In this way, the victim tries to preserve at least the illusion of control and thereby diminish the threat of recurrence. Many people would rather blame themselves than feel helpless.

NEUROPSYCHOLOGY AND PSYCHOBIOLOGY OF PTSD

Cognitive Impairment in PTSD

As noted above, one reason that many trauma survivors feel they're "going crazy" is that their mental faculties seem to have been dumbed down and blunted since the trauma, and many such patients complain of deficits in attention, concentration, memory, judgment, and decision-making. Many traumatizing experiences occur in the context of other injuries, including traumatic brain injury, toxic exposure, electric shock, and so on; these will be discussed in subsequent chapters. Apparently, however, severe emotional trauma, even in the absence of documentable brain or nervous system injury, may impair cognitive functioning, sometimes permanently and to a degree that is difficult to distinguish from organic brain damage (Knight, 1997; Miller, 1993b, 1993c; Parker, 1990; Weiner, 1992). This ubiquitous clinical observation is corroborated by several field studies and research reports.

Weiner (1992) has reviewd the earlier literature on the relationship of traumatic stress to cognitive impairment. This includes studies of Norwegian merchant mariners who manned cargo ships that were repeatedly attacked by German war planes and submarines during World War II. Some ships were sunk and many sailors floundered for hours in the icy waters of the North Atlantic before being rescued. Most of these sailors sustained no serious physical injuries, yet after the war many of the survivors suffered persisting cognitive impairment, in some cases comparable to frank dementia. Cognitive disturbances were also reported in almost 90 percent of Norwegian survivors of Nazi concentration camps, a third of whom had not suffered any serious physical injury. The presence of severe cognitive disturbance in psychologically traumatized individuals without concomitant neurological or other physical injury led these early researchers to appreciate the role of psychological stress on human cognition (Eitinger, 1965, 1971).

More recently, Everly and Horton (1989) administered a memory test to a group of patients diagnosed with PTSD. Twelve of the 14 patients in the study scored below the cut-off for cognitive impairment. Gill, Calev, Greenberg, Kugelmas, and Lerer (1990) compared the performance of patients with PTSD to that of psychiatric patients and normal controls on a comprehensive neuropsychological test battery. The PTSD patients had been involved in traumatic military battles, terrorist attacks, or auto accidents, but had not been physically injured and were free of alcohol and drug abuse. Both the PTSD and psychiatric groups reported feeling subjectively more impaired than the controls. Performance on measures of intelligence, verbal fluency, memory, and attention was significantly poorer in both the PTSD and psychiatric patients than in the normal controls. The premorbid intelligence of both the PTSD patients and the psychiatric patients was judged to be average and to have deteriorated significantly by the time of the current testing.

The issue of concomitant diagnoses was further examined by Barrett, Green, Morris, Giles, and Croft (1996), who administered a neuropsychological test battery to four groups of Vietnam veterans: those with no psychiatric diagnosis; those with a PTSD-only diagnosis; those with a diagnosis of anxiety, depression, or substance abuse; and those with both a PTSD diagnosis and another psychiatric diagnosis. Results showed that veterans with both PTSD and concurrent diagnoses exhibited greater cognitive impairment than the other groups. The study concluded that cognitive deficits seen among PTSD groups may have as much or more to do with concomitant diagnoses than with the PTSD itself.

This question of what actually accounts for impaired cognitive functioning in PTSD patients—the PTSD itself, concurrent disorders, hidden organic brain damage, or preexisting vulnerability—probably will have its own answer in each individual case. However, therapists working with these groups should be sensitive to the "concreteness" or rigidity of defense mechanisms that characterize many of these cases, and should gear their therapeutic approach accordingly. This will be discussed further in Chapter 2.

Neuropsychology of PTSD

Recently, several theoretical models have been put forth to describe the brain mechanisms that may account for the trauma response and the symptoms of PTSD. Kolb's (1987) theory of PTSD takes as its point of departure the concept, first articulated by Freud (1920), of a *cortical stimulus barrier* that serves to protect the individual from being overwhelmed by excessive traumatic stimulation. Massive psychic trauma may overcome this stimulus barrier and, according to Kolb's hypothesis, produce synaptic changes by way of neurophysiological sensitization. If continued at high intensity and repeated frequently over time, those neural processes mediating discriminative perception and learning may be impaired, including the possibility of actual neuronal death. Kolb cites Sapolsky, Krey, and McEwen's (1984) report of cellular death in the brain's hippocampus, which has a high number of stress-responsive glucocorticoid hormone receptors.

Parker (1990) points out that multiple afferent stress signals through sensory and emotional brain pathways lead to the adrenal gland's secretion of glucocorticoid hormones such as cortisol—the classic "stress hormone." High levels of cortisol appear to depress brain cell functioning, especially in the hippocampus, which plays an important role in memory as well as an important feedback role in the modulation of the stress response. Oscillations in the brain's stress-memory system may account for the cycles of intrusion and avoidance seen in PTSD.

Kolb (1987) identifies another limbic system structure, the amygdala, as interacting with the hippocampal system in mediating stress effects. The amygdala functions as sort of a rapid-decision "good or bad" emotional evaluator of environmental stimuli. Stress overload in this system may force the individual into a state of hair-trigger hypersensitivity, in which a multitude of internal and external stimuli lead to continued heightened arousal. Recurrent intense emotional arousal further sensitizes and simultaneously disrupts those processes related to habituation and learning, leading to an exacerbation of PTSD symptoms.

With excessive limbic sensitization and diminished capacity for adaptive information-processing by the cortical stimulus barrier, subcortical and brainstem structures escape from inhibitory cortical control and repeatedly reactivate the perceptual, cognitive, affective, and somatic clinical expressions related to the original trauma. These abnormally reactivated memory loops are projected into daytime consciousness as intrusive thoughts and images, and into sleep as traumatic nightmares.

Cortical neuronal changes are responsible for impairment of perceptual discrimination, reduced impulse control, and affective blunting. Excessive activation or release of subcortical systems results in conditioned startle reactions, irritability, hyperalertness, intrusive thoughts, repetitive fearful nightmares, and psychophysiological symptoms such as heart palpitations, panic attacks, musculoskeletal pain, headache, and gastrointestinal disturbances. The repeated reminders of the traumatic event associated with somatic symptoms disrupt the patient's body-image and self-concept and are responsible for numbing and avoidance behaviors such as social withdrawal, alcohol and drug abuse, and compulsive risk-taking, as well as emotional disturbances that include depression, survivor guilt, shame, and suicidality.

Deitz's (1992) neuropsychological theory attempts to extend Kolb's (1987) formulation by conceptualizing a dual pathway of traumatic information-processing by the brain. The first system links perceptual evaluation and emotional tone with the cognitive and language regions of the brain, allowing the individual to "make sense" of the experience, no matter how frightening or painful. A second, independent limbic system pathway bypasses the conscious evaluative system and feeds directly into the emotion-memory complex of the hypothalamus, hippocampus, and amygdala.

For survival purposes, it is critical that the amygdala-processed positive/negative, good/bad discrimination be made as fast as possible to allow time for the appropriate fight-or-flight or approach-avoidance response. However, in order to link the affective tone to neocortical processing—the conscious feelings and meanings connected to language and abstract thought—the second, phylogenetically newer pathway is needed. Where these two systems are "out of sync," as in the case of severe trauma, the conscious cognitive-linguistic memory of the trauma may be "repressed," while the emotional reaction persists in response to stimuli the patient may not even recognize.

Charney, Deutsch, Krystal, Southwick, and Davis (1993) have proposed that stress-induced impairment of long-term neural potentiation in the amygdala and locus coeruleus may be responsible for the development of learning and memory impairment in PTSD. Because extinction appears to involve an active learning process—an idea that goes back to Pavlov (1927)—deficits in learning may impair normal extinction in patients with PTSD, leading to the abnormal persistence of emotional memories. At the same time, locus coeruleus activation of the amygdala enhances traumatic memory retrieval. By this mechanism, some of the acute neurobiological responses to trauma may facilitate the enhanced encoding of traumatic memories. This may partially explain the "paradox" of learning and memory deficits coexisting with abnormally intense intrusive recollections in PTSD.

Thus, in patients with PTSD, specific sensory phenomena, such as sights, sounds, and smell that are circumstantially related to the traumatic event, persistently reactivate traumatic memories and flashbacks. Neutral situations or environments become "guilty by association" with the intense reaction elicited from the limbic system emotional and memory mechanisms. Like the proverbial "broken record," the PTSD program continues to play again and again, affecting wider and wider areas of the patient's life (Miller, 1997).

The lesson of this chapter is that PTSD comes in many shapes and forms and that its symptoms may persist indefinitely unless and until proper therapeutic intervention breaks the vicious mind-brain-body cycle of traumatic disability. As clinicians, we must be vigilant and knowledgeable in assessing our patients, defining the limits and extent of the disorder, separating the various threads of etiology, recent and remote, and then using this information to devise the best treatment or combination of treatments for the patient in question. It is to this that we now turn.

Chapter 2

REAL HEALING

Psychotherapy of
Posttraumatic Stress Disorder

A thousand ills require a thousand cures.

—Ovid

Wounds cannot be cured without searching.

—Francis Bacon

Just as the PTSD syndrome is emblematic of many of the traumatic disability syndromes (TDSs) discussed in this book, the psychotherapeutic treatment of PTSD can also serve as a model for the treatment methods to be discussed later for the individual TDSs. Thus, the specialized treatment techniques for these particular syndromes build upon and extend many of the principles of psychotherapy discussed in this chapter. The following guidelines and recommendations are based on a selective review of the literature and my own clinical experience in treating trauma patients of different types. The general therapeutic guidelines presented here will be fleshed out in their applications to individual TDSs in the chapters that follow.

GENERAL CONSIDERATIONS
OF TREATMENT

A number of authors (Brom, Kleber, & Defares, 1989; Everstine & Everstine, 1993; Shalev, Galai, & Eth, 1993a) have stressed the need to consider the trauma response, and its corresponding treatment, in terms of a series of *stages* that may vary in length and severity from patient to patient, depending on such factors as premorbid personality, past experience, prior trauma, and the response of others to the patient. Another expression of this idea appears in Everly's (1990, 1993, 1995) *two-factor* conceptualization of PTSD and its treatment, consisting of (1) a *neurobiological hypersensitivity* involving heightened nervous system and endocrine responsivity in the wake of trauma, and (2) a *psychological hypersensitivity* involving disruptions and transfigurations in the individual's worldview and self-concept.

In virtually no other field of clinical practice, with the possible exception of treating terminally ill patients, does the psychotherapist so starkly confront his own vulnerability and mortality as with severely traumatized patients. The clinician must negotiate carefully between entering the traumatized reality of the patient and avoiding enmeshment, which can compromise clinical judgment and objective treatment planning (Brom & Kleber, 1989; Everstine & Everstine, 1993; McCann & Pearlman, 1990).

Another clinician variable concerns the issue of therapeutic "techniques." Everly (1995) uses the term *metatherapy* to refer to an overarching, guiding therapeutic approach, a strategic therapy formulation as opposed to a rigid tactical set of cookbook therapeutic guidelines. In line with the concept of patient individuality, the specific therapeutic interventions may vary from patient to patient, depending on the idiosyncratic needs of the patient and the orientation and style of the therapist. This does not mean that there are "no rules" of trauma psychotherapy or that "anything goes"—far from it. In a field rife with crackpot theories and dubious remedies, it's especially important that responsible intervention be grounded in both solid research and clinical experience and judgment. But not every aspect of treatment can be codified and manualized, and the best therapists seem to be those who are able to productively meld empirical technique, practiced knowledge, and insightful clinical intuition (Miller, 1993a).

It's important that the trauma patient be oriented to psychotherapy as part of an overall program of trauma care, not as a clinical afterthought or "last resort" pursued because there is something abnormal or weak about the way the patient is handling her ordeal. Many trauma survivors will talk freely, even obsessively, to a friend, relative, spouse, clergyman, lawyer, or physician, but clam up in the psychotherapy session, because seeing a "shrink" constitutes an unwelcome indignity, linked with cowardice, malingering, or craziness. Other patients fear losing emotional control or "falling apart" if they talk about the trauma or their reaction to it (Everstine & Everstine, 1993; Modlin, 1983; Shalev et al., 1993a).

Thus, effective treatment begins with a tactful and sensitive referral. In the best case, psychotherapy maintains a seamless continuity with the medical aspects of treatment, an ideal that unfortunately approaches reality only in some enlightened interdisciplinary treatment settings. In the real world, the trauma therapist may need to preface treatment per se with a period of education and orientation as to the nature of the trauma response and the type of treatment the patient can expect.

EDUCATIVE AND
SUPPORTIVE MEASURES

Trauma often produces a curious reciprocal relationship between physical and psychological damage (Modlin, 1983). While significant physical injury produces heightened stress in some patients, for others it seems to bind or neutralize the reactive anxiety or depression, since the patient now has a "real" injury to cope with instead of something as intangible as psychological "stress." In this model, far from coddling patients into permanent invalidism, solicitous medical and nursing administrations in the acute phase of the trauma, as well as an acceptable period of legitimate convalescence, can actually prevent the development of subsequent, persistent traumatic disability. Indeed, immediate rest, sedation, isolation, enforced quiet, and special attention under empathic clinical authority were routinely applied to traumatized soldiers in Korea and Vietnam, resulting in an impressively low incidence of acute psychiatric casualties.

Conversely, a sudden frightening accident with little or no physical injury is a more common precipitant of PTSD, since the shattered psyche is typically not given the same consideration as the battered body, and the patient's natural desire to temporarily retreat and lick his emotional wounds is often disapproved of, clinically and socially. In most civilian settings, a PTSD patient's first referral for psychological care often occurs months or years after the accident, and then usually only when the psychological disturbances have become blatantly overwhelming for the patient, the family, and the health care system. Another large group of late referrals comes from attorneys who are seeking to document psychological impairment and disability for insurance and personal injury cases.

In the present model, early, focused treatment offers the best chance for long-term recovery. PTSD resulting from a single, short-onset, frightening experience is probably most amenable to treatment, and Modlin (1983) claims that approximately one-half of his cases are cured in three to four sessions. The approach used involves the therapist first demonstrating his understanding by asking questions that elicit the nature of the common PTSD symptoms, then offering a comprehensible explanatory model that emphasizes the universality and normality of the stress response and its manifestations.

This formula is then repeated in each session. The patient may not completely grasp the psychological explanation, but what she does hear is that the therapist understands what she has gone through, believes she has a legitimate clinical syndrome with a name and a cause, and knows what to do about it. With such early and unambiguous clinical support, the probability of chronic secondary gain becomes less likely and the outlook more favorable. The key, then, is for the clinician to show *respect* both for the syndrome, by demonstrating his knowledge and experience surrounding these disorders, and for the patient, by assertively evaluating and treating the trauma syndrome up front.

Therapists accustomed to nondirective forms of treatment with relatively high-functioning, reasonably insightful patients may have to get used to a more down-to-earth, directive approach with traumatized patients, at least in the early stages. The importance of providing such concrete, practical help is often underestimated (Brom & Kleber, 1989). Immediately after the trauma there may be a need for referrals to shelters and soup kitchens, advice on specific procedures to follow, medical recommendations and other basic support.

Some patients may refuse medical treatment for fear of having to face the reality of their disfigurement or disability; others may overemphasize physical complaints to bind or deflect posttraumatic anxiety. While patients cannot be forced to seek medical care, gently and supportively exploring the issues behind the resistance and providing concrete reassurance about even minor matters over which the patient can exert some control sometimes helps whittle down the resistance, enabling the patient to get needed basic care as a first step to more comprehensive treatment (Matsakis, 1994).

As noted above, general information about the natural processes of coping and expectable symptoms can be very reassuring to the trauma patient, as long as it is given in close connection with her actual experiences. This information enables the patient to place her own reactions into the framework of normal coping.

In the acute trauma stage, the patient's concept of reality is profoundly altered. Accordingly, in the first phase of contact the therapist should try to bring structure to the experiences of the trauma patient in an adaptive, reality-oriented manner. This is done by first following the narrative of the patient and then labeling the emotions as they are expressed. During this initial stage, the therapist encourages the patient in only a limited way to explore her feelings further or deeper, as a prematurely intense discussion of emotions may increase confusion and evoke an atmosphere of crisis. As time passes and the patient begins to recapture a sense of fundamental safety and control, she will need this structuring form of support less and less. The therapist can then adopt a more probing and challenging approach that incorporates confrontation and reality-testing, although the atmosphere of understanding and trust remains the most important basis of the therapeutic relationship (Brom & Kleber, 1989; Everstine & Everstine, 1993; Shalev, Schreiber, Galai, & Melmed, 1993b).

TREATING POSTTRAUMATIC SYMPTOMS

For many patients the most disturbing aspect of the PTSD syndrome is the presence of intrusive symptoms, such as flashbacks, nightmares, phobias, dissociative states, emotional numbing, flashpoint anger, and hair-trigger jumpiness. These make many trauma patients feel like they're losing control of their own minds and going crazy. While therapeutic working-through of the traumatic experience and regaining a sense of mastery and safety often have long-term ameliorating effects on these symptoms, in many cases early treatment must address these disturbances on their own terms. In such circumstances adequate symptom control is a prerequisite to more integrative psychotherapeutic approaches.

The Importance of Symptoms

For PTSD patients, control and mastery issues—of the body, thoughts, emotions, reactions—are paramount, and learning to control a symptom sometimes plants the crucial therapeutic seed that sprouts into the message of "hey, everything *isn't* all shot to hell," that some tendril of control can still be extended and perhaps nurtured into a growing organism of self-mastery.

On the other hand, at some point patients need to understand that, while symptoms may be managed and controlled, they may never entirely disappear. As with residual chronic back pain or postconcussive forgetfulness, often the goal is for the symptoms to fade into the background of the patient's life, rather than occupy the foreground of consciousness, to eventually become episodically annoying but philosophically tolerated, like an occasional headache that one ignores until it goes away or that the patient distracts by engaging in some activity that "takes my mind off it" (Everstine & Everstine, 1993; Matsakis, 1994).

Relaxation and Desensitization

Most symptom-oriented treatments for posttraumatic disturbances employ a *behavioral* or *cognitive-behavioral* approach. Thompson (1992) points out that posttraumatic stress symptoms may be particularly appropriate for graded exposure therapies in which patients gradually learn to confront the stimuli they would otherwise avoid. These kinds of therapies are derived from *systematic desensitization*, originally used to treat phobias and now well integrated into behavioral medicine. With PTSD, the aim is to reduce posttraumatic reactions such as flashbacks, intrusive memories, and startle responses through habituation, thereby bringing about the extinction of the conditioned aversive response.

Exposure therapy for desensitization is typically carried out either in imagination during a relaxation exercise or in real-life situations, when it is called *in vivo desensitization*. Both methods may be used in combination, the imagination exercise paving the way for the in vivo training. In Thompson's (1992) review, the results of desensitization treatment studies with PTSD patients are encouraging. For example, anxiety and intrusive memories were significantly reduced in 14 to 16 90-minute sessions, a treatment effect that was maintained at six-month follow-up (Keane, Fairbank, Caddell, & Zimmerling, 1989). Exposure desensitization therapy was significantly more effective than supportive counseling in reducing nightmares, arousal, and hypersensitivity to sounds (Cooper & Clum, 1989).

My own experience in applying this type of approach has been mixed. Many patients, most of whom were involved in auto or worksite accidents, seem to "get with the program," learn the relaxation technique, and desensitize themselves effectively to the traumatic situation. However, the most successful cases are typically the ones with the least distressing traumatic experiences, as discerned from the patients' self-reports. A few of the more severely traumatized patients resist all attempts at desensitization, fearing that "letting down their guard" during relaxation will render them vulnerable to overwhelming emotional arousal, a problem that has been noted for relaxation therapies in general (Lazarus & Mayne, 1990; Miller, 1994a). In such cases, a supportive-expressive cognitive therapy approach is often successful in helping patients work through the traumatic fear and pain of the injuring event in a more "rational" manner—trying, in effect, to turn the posttraumatic vigilance and rumination to constructive therapeutic advantage.

Interestingly, prior to reviewing this literature, my experience with desensitization of posttraumatic stress emerged as a side-effect of using relaxation and other behavioral medicine approaches in the treatment of headache and other chronic pain syndromes associated with closed head injury (Bennett, 1988; Miller, 1990, 1993b). Many of the patients who were able to learn the relaxation exercises and achieve some pain control also reported self-applications of the relaxation technique to controlling their arousal responses triggered by frightening recollections of the injury event. Since then, I have found that beginning with circumscribed physical symptom control—headache or back pain, for example—using relaxation, hypnosis, imagery, or any other effective behavioral medicine modality, often gives patients the confidence to deal with posttraumatic stress reactions that they have heretofore been reluctant to face for fear of "losing control."

Flashbacks

Waking flashbacks may occur in any sensory modality. In extreme cases, there may be flooding of visual, auditory, tactile, olfactory, and gustatory modalities simultaneously. These terrifying flashbacks and intrusive images or feelings are often what make patients feel they are "going crazy." The therapist should normalize the processes as much as possible for the patient, helping her to understand that this is a natural and expectable part of the recovery process, that the flashbacks will eventually fade, and that there are learnable ways to manage intrusive symptoms. The patient doesn't have to "fight" the flashback—it's possible to "ride out" many episodes without being overwhelmed, once she understands what she's dealing with. Patients who are severely traumatized may be afraid to reveal or even think about particularly horrifying or personally painful flashbacks. In such cases, they should be given the option of deferring such revelations or expressing only as much of their experiences as they can presently tolerate (Everstine & Everstine, 1993; Matsakis, 1994; Modlin, 1983).

Many flashbacks and other PTSD symptoms are triggered by stimuli in the environment, and sometimes internal stimuli; these may not always be conscious. Anniversary dates, people, places, objects, and even emotional situations that remind the survivor of the original trauma can serve as triggers. Current stressors, even if they are dissimilar to the original trauma—e.g., a health crisis, financial reversal, job stress, bereavement—can trigger flashbacks related to the original trauma. Media coverage of the traumatic event or meeting people associated with or resembling individuals involved in the traumatic event may trigger flashbacks. Essentially, any stimulus may serve as an idiosyncratic trigger for a particular patient. The first step in helping patients cope with triggers is to help them identify those triggers (Matsakis, 1994).

Some patients come to therapy all too painfully aware of what stimuli trigger their posttraumatic symptoms. If anything, they are paralyzed into inactivity by their constant vigilance against exposing themselves to trigger situations. Other patients may recognize some triggers but fail to see the connection with equally important ones. Matsakis (1994) recommends having patients chart their triggers, if possible, with the aid of trusted family and friends. I find this works for some patients, especially those who need something tangible to "get a handle on" right away; in fact, this may offer the initial control hook. For other patients, however, having to focus so systematically on triggers and symptoms acts as a form of retraumatization or taxes an already overloaded cognitive system. In such cases it is preferable to allow these clinical data to emerge at their own pace, while other therapeutic issues, such as safety and normalization, are tackled first.

Once triggers are identified, several techniques may be useful in dealing with them (Matsakis, 1994). A staple of low-arousal behavioral medicine approaches for a wide range of disorders is some form of deep breathing, often combined with progressive muscle relaxation and/or imagery; this is often subsumed under the heading of "meditation." Again, some patients may react to relaxation with a panicky sense of vulnerability, as the induced expansive mental state invites a flood of traumatic memories in patients who have hitherto used intense ruminative focusing to blot out such disturbing thoughts. Therefore such meditative applications should be carefully titrated, with the therapist closely monitoring the patient's reaction as the therapy proceeds. As the patient learns to control the physiological hyperresponsiveness of her own body, a sense of mastery develops, which can be utilized in further psychotherapeutic endeavors.

More cognitively based approaches involve planning ahead for anticipated trigger situations. Matsakis (1994) recommends training the patient to ask herself the following questions when faced with a potential trigger situation:

- What will I have to do?
- How have I reacted to similar situations in the past?
- Did anything terrible happen?
- What are the chances of something bad happening again?
- If the worst occurs, what could I do?
- What are my worst fantasies?
- What are the actual chances of these terrible things occurring?
- How can I ask others to help me?
- Who would I ask for help?

Just the act of going through this kind of list often builds a cognitive firewall between the spark of the triggering stimulus and the tinderbox of traumatic memories that can flare into a full-scale emotional conflagration. Additionally, taking the time to "think it through" gives the patient experience in using her own brain to solve problems, thus increasing the sense of control. Similar socratic questioning techniques may be used by therapists themselves in crisis intervention with suicidal or decompensating patients (Gilliland & James, 1993). With symptomatic PTSD patients, the therapist may first model these adaptive coping questions and statements, and then teach the patient to self-utilize them in trigger situations.

Matsakis (1994) recommends having the patient do her own research on the statistical probabilities of worst-case scenarios occurring, e.g., how many shootings actually take place in shopping malls, or how many passenger cars are actually struck by large tractor-trailers. Be careful, however, that this doesn't lead to the patient's morbid preoccupation and increased rumination about the "likelihood" of new traumas occurring. Also important is normalizing and legitimizing the residual psychophysiological reactions the patient may continue to experience in trigger situations. The goal is not to waft the patient into a perpetual bliss-out: painful situations will occasionally arise and she must learn to deal with them. If the patient gets a little anxious and queasy but is able to self-moderate her arousal level and successfully follow through with the task at hand, that is a therapeutic victory to be applauded.

Matsakis (1994) recommends beginning with the least threatening situations and gradually working up to the more difficult ones, a stimulus-hierarchy concept familiar to behavior therapists who treat phobias. I would recommend saving a few easy items for "boosters" later on, just in case things start to slip or an intervening trauma forces a setback. Having a couple of "guaranteed successes" in one's therapeutic pocket can provide a much-needed dose of morale when the going gets tough.

Dreams and Nightmares

As noted in Chapter 1, traumatic dreams are seldom rote replications of the traumatic incident itself. Instead, they tend to recapitulate the emotional terror of the event or symbolically represent important issues related to the event, such as survival, betrayal, or loss. Often there is a hiatus in the dream process between anxiety dreams in the early recovery stages and angry dreams of a later stage. During this interval, the patient may have few or no dreams that relate directly to the event. Then, suddenly, she begins having violent, sometimes horribly graphic nightmares that seem to come out of nowhere. In other cases, there is a slower progression through the fear and anxiety dreams to the angry ones. Everstine and Everstine (1993) recommend that, rather than letting the traumatic dreams catch the patient by surprise, the therapist should prepare her for the possible appearance of these disturbing dreams. Again, I suggest this be done carefully, to avoid "setting up" already-sensitized patients for additional symptoms. With some patients it is better to simply provide a therapeutic atmosphere that encourages verbalization of disturbing symptoms and to be there to explain and normalize symptoms when the patient reveals them.

Matsakis (1994) offers several suggestions for coping with traumatic dreams and nightmares. One technique is to have the patient "rewrite" her nightmares, incorporating empowering themes and outcomes into the revised versions. However, some patients may view this as a trivializing of their dream experiences and of the trauma itself, so therapists should use caution. I find that incorporating such revisions during therapeutic imagery exercises is generally more acceptable to patients because it suggests more of a reintrepretation of alternatives, rather than "changing the script," and also is less burdensome from the point of view of additional therapeutic homework in the early stages.

Matsakis (1994) also recommends "beating the dreams to death" through constant exposure and repetition, thereby stripping them of their intimidating power. This is actually an extension of the technique of repeated ventilation, exploration, and working-through of traumatic material in general, and again, my only caveat here is that the reexposure be truly dissipative, not retraumatizing. This involves the therapist's knowing when the patient is ready to handle the traumatic dream material and perhaps combining the repetition with other therapeutic techniques, such as relaxation or cognitive restructuring.

In addition, Matsakis (1994) calls attention to the importance of improving general sleep hygiene, which is often neglected in other therapeutic recommendations. Aside from nightmares per se, the generalized hypervigilance of the PTSD patient often makes falling asleep and staying asleep a nightly problem. The first step is to normalize the sleep difficulty, placing it in the context of other residual posttraumatic symptoms, which, while disturbing, are not necessarily dangerous and don't have to mean that the patient is "going crazy." Where practical, experimenting with different sleep locations, schedules, and bedtime activities may foster better quality of sleep. Relaxation exercises may aid in falling asleep and getting back to sleep when awakened.

Finally, although many nonmedical therapists are (often with good reason) circumspect about the overuse of psychotropic medication, chronically fatigued and frazzled patients do poorly in any kind of psychotherapy, so the judicious use of such medications under the direction of a competent physician often provides an important short-term jumpstart to the sleep recovery process. The same may be said of medications in general: used wisely, not cavalierly, they are often a vital adjunct to therapeutic process. A broken leg requires the use of a cast, crutches, and so on in the early stages of recovery and rehab, but the orthopedist and physical therapist know when it's time for the patient to walk on her own two feet. So with psychotropic medication: there is no point to the patient's suffering needlessly, especially in the early recovery stages, if a medication can take the edge off her pain and allow productive therapeutic work to proceed. Therapists doing trauma work should thus establish liaisons with responsible psychopharmacologists and refer appropriately.

Numbing and Dissociation

Intrusive symptoms constitute the proverbial "squeaky wheel that gets the grease" in posttraumatic therapy because they draw the most attention and seem to cause the most distress. For some patients, however, equal or greater disturbance is produced by the "zoning-out" numbing response of the posttraumatic syndrome. This should be carefully sought out by the therapist, as these kinds of symptoms are less likely to be reported by the patient or observed by others. Matsakis (1994) suggests asking the patient to let the therapist know when she goes numb in the sessions, and, if the therapist observes what he believes to be a numbing reaction, checking this against the patient's experience.

Some patients, especially those who have been multiply traumatized and/or traumatized from an early age, often with diagnoses of borderline personality disorder, respond to numbing by engaging in self-mutilation or substance abuse. In some cases, less harmful forms of self-stimulation or reality-grounding can be taught to the patient, such as taking a hot or cold shower, drinking a carbonated beverage, using a wrist-snapping rubber band, doing some vigorous exercise, or palpating a "safe object" such as a stuffed animal (Matsakis, 1994). Several of my patients have learned to substitute applying ice or the teeth of a comb to their skin in place of self-mutilating with a knife or lit cigarette.

Sometimes just making human contact with a family member, friend, or, if necessary, the therapist will pull the patient out of the numbed or dissociative state, if the therapist is mindful about forestalling excessive dependency (Matsakis, 1994). However, when guilt or other psychodynamic issues besides mere stimulus-grounding fuel the self-harm response, this behavior may prove quite refractory to simple stopgap measures, and more focused and intensive psychotherapy will be needed.

Eye Movement Desensitization and Reprocessing (EMDR)

In the last few years, much clinical attention has focused on the use of *eye movement desensitization and reprocessing*, or EMDR (Shapiro, 1995) in the treatment of posttraumatic and other disorders. The elements of the treatment technique include the following.

During the preparatory and evaluation phase, the clinician defines the problems to be addressed, takes a clinical history, and orients the patient to the technique and rationale of treatment. The patient is asked to identify a "target" traumatic event and to generate a key image of that event, along with a negative cognition that expresses in words the negative belief about the patient or traumatic event. Next, the patient is asked to provide a positive cognition that expresses some upside of the traumatic event, such as courage shown or a lesson learned. Along with the key image and negative cognition, the patient is then asked to evoke the emotions and the bodily sensations associated with the traumatic event.

The therapist next instructs the patient to evoke simultaneously the image, negative cognition, and body sensation associated with the target event, and then tells the patient to "follow my fingers with your eyes," leading the patient in several sets of bidirectional eye movements. Immediately thereafter, the patient is instructed to put the painful traumatic experience out of mind. Several repetitions of this sequence, perhaps over several sessions, are required to "desensitize" the negative images, cognitions, emotions, and bodily sensations associated with the traumatic experience.

Next, the therapist leads the patient through another sequence of eye movements designed to reinforce the positive cognitions about the traumatic event. The process is repeated to reinforce positive body sensations. Throughout the treatment, the standard techniques of stress management, therapeutic rapport and support, and homework assignments are utilized to consolidate the therapeutic gains.

Evidence for the clinical efficacy of EMDR has, to date, been largely anecdotal. Many such case studies report near-miraculous cures of PTSD-like syndromes caused by catastrophic injuries (McCann, 1992) or resulting from decades-old trauma (Shapiro, 1995). Critics point to its lack of a credible theoretical rationale, its self-touting as a paradigmatically novel and original form of treatment, the proprietary marketing of the tech-

nique, and the cultlike following and practice by often lightly creden-
tialed and poorly trained practitioners (Allen & Lewis, 1996; Cowley &
Biddle, 1994; Meichenbaum, 1994; Marano, 1994). Of course, the same
could be said of many of the myriad other "therapies" out there that
range from the sublime to the ridiculous.

My own take on EMDR is that it's old wine in a new bottle. That is,
to the extent that EMDR proves effective in treating some kinds of
traumatic disability syndromes in some kinds of patients, it really relies
on a combination of the old tried-and-true behavioral medicine modalities
of low arousal, suggestion, cognitive reappraisal, and interpersonal therapeutic rapport. More recently, empirical studies are beginning to be
carried out that attempt to factor-analyze the effective components of
the EMDR package and explore modifications and extentions of the
technique. I anticipate that after the polemical centrifuge comes to rest,
the important core strains of EMDR will have blended into the general
psychotherapeutic vintage, while the hyperbolic dregs quietly rinse away.

POSTTRAUMATIC
PSYCHODYNAMIC PSYCHOTHERAPY

As effective as they are, psychophysiological and cognitive-behavioral
strategies have their limitations in dealing with the full cognitive and
emotional range of posttraumatic stress reactions and bringing about a
reintegrative healing of the personality. Eventually, most authorities
agree, some form of constructive confrontation with the traumatic experience has to take place. The term *psychodynamic* is used broadly here to
include not just traditional psychoanalytic approaches (Horowitz, 1986),
but any therapeutic modality that addresses the effect of trauma on the
person's personality and the need to deal with worldview and existential
issues in the psychological healing process (Yalom, 1980).

General Psychotherapeutic Guidelines

It should go without saying that the efficacy of any therapeutic intervention—from the most objectively behavioristic to the most gnostically
psychodynamic—depends strongly on the quality of the therapeutic
alliance between clinician and patient. Without trust and collaboration
on mutual goals, all the brilliant therapeutic gimmicks and tricks in the
world can secure no healing purchase on the jaggedly scarred psyche of
the posttrauma survivor.

To this end, considerable effort and sensitivity are required by the therapist to stay in touch with the patient's frequently shifting needs and emotional states. Therapists must be tolerant of, and learn how to utilize, the often back-and-forth nature of therapeutic progress. Always, the most basic and fundamental intervention is to make it clear to the patient that the therapist is willing to listen to every detail of her experience, no matter how depressing, frightening, or gruesome, to systematically absorb, dilute, detoxify, and reprocess the concentrated psychic poisons that are initially squeezed full-strength from the patient's emotional wounds (Matsakis, 1994; McCann & Pearlman, 1990).

At some point in treatment, the therapist must take the trauma patient back to the event and have her discuss it in progressive degrees of detail. The goal is to counteract maladaptive avoidance tendencies and to diminish the chance that they will congeal into longstanding patterns of behavior. In the case of the avoidant victim who copes with trauma by downplaying its importance, the moment of graphic recapitulation may occur much later in the course of therapy, and its onset may catch the therapist by surprise. This late outpouring of emotion should not necessarily be confused with "regression," but may in fact represent a sign of progress. Sometimes sufficient therapeutic trust, ego-bolstering, and working-through of peripheral issues must take place to lay the groundwork for direct exploration of the traumatic event itself (Brom et al., 1989; Everstine & Everstine, 1993; McCann & Pearlman, 1990).

In this framework, then, treatment should facilitate the repair of the patient's adaptive defense mechanisms, while at the same time assisting her to reenter family, work, community, and other social roles. With these parallel therapeutic activities, both internal and external psychological integration can proceed. Bringing repressed thoughts to the surface or confronting disturbing or distorted memories should be handled with extreme care and sensitivity, to ensure that the experience is one of corrective mastery, not retraumatization.

Coping with emotional lability is an important part of posttraumatic therapy, as such mood swings can be confusing and disorienting, especially if they occur or recur late in the treatment process. The patient by this time has gotten a taste of psychological stability, feels pretty good for a while, and may think the ordeal is finally over. Then she hits some snag of frustration, stress, or disappointment and is yanked back into a state of anxiety and depression. During this unsettling process, patients will probably require even more therapeutic support than usual because they may feel they are backsliding and "losing it." Again, this phenomenon is not necessarily a sign of regression, and the temporarily increased amount of therapeutic contact that may be necessary at this stage should be viewed as an expectable response to these jarring bumps in the road to recovery (Everstine & Everstine, 1993; McCann & Pearlman, 1990).

Dealing with Anger

At some phase in the therapeutic process, mood swings may portend a stage of emerging anger, as patients begin to get in touch with the possibly malign or neglectful actions of others that have caused their trauma. Patients may be angry that the trauma occurred at all, that it happened to them, that they were injured, that loved ones died, that they have had to suffer secondary wounding and residual physical, psychological, and financial scars, that they may have been mistreated by the medical and legal systems, that they have forever been banished from a sense of rightness and goodness in the world, and that they are now forced to engage in a therapeutic process that is effortful, expensive, and emotionally painful and draining (Everstine & Everstine, 1993; Matsakis, 1994).

While this anger must eventually be faced and dealt with, pushing anger to the surface too quickly may impel the patient to act out in a dangerous way, to become paralyzed with helpless rage leading to depression, to develop a masochistic countertransference with the therapist and symbolically recreate the traumatic experience, or to flee the therapeutic setting entirely. Therefore, it is important that the therapist first help the patient to regain the requisite level of ego strength that will enable her to eventually express anger appropriately and constructively, in a manner that will not alienate those around her (Everstine & Everstine, 1993).

When a trauma patient engages in uncharacteristically risky or self-destructive behavior, anger and/or survivor guilt are often the driving factors, sometimes impelled by well-meaning comments by others about how "lucky" the patient was to have survived. The therapist must be careful that survivor guilt not be turned into a dependent form of masochistic transference in which the therapeutic relationship becomes yet another form of self-flagellatory abuse. Many trauma patients express intense anger at those persons or institutions they perceive to be "failed protectors"—employers, airline personnel, the police, doctors, product manufacturers, the government, and so on. Frustrated rage may also be displaced onto friends and family members who cannot understand why the trauma patient is "turning on them." Posttraumatic pain and rage may also be expressed through the filing of lawsuits and other legal actions, requiring direct and forthright therapeutic guidance in some cases (Brom & Kleber, 1989; Everstine & Everstine, 1993).

Trauma-related anger can color every aspect of a patient's life, including work, school, family functioning, daily habits, and especially her own self-image. Any seemingly trivial frustration will elicit an overblown reaction because of its additional charge of unresolved anger related to the trauma. Patients are often all too aware of their excessive hair-trigger responsiveness, and this feeling of being a "walking time bomb" further contributes to their sense of loss of control. Patients who deny or suppress anger, on the other hand, may spiral into self-harm, substance abuse, or disabling psychosomatic symptomatology, further eroding their self-esteem and stigmatizing themselves as weak, needy, or deficient (Matsakis, 1994). Suppressed anger may be especially difficult to work through, because, in a true avoidance paradigm, the patient recoils at any hint of anger recognition, fearing she will be overwhelmed and disintegrate. Other patients come to therapy virtually demanding that they be taught "how to control my anger," as if this will solve all of their problems.

Matsakis (1994) has developed an effective program of posttraumatic anger management, the main components of which I have found useful with many PTSD patients. This begins with validating the anger, inasmuch as in many cases, especially where the trauma occurred at the malicious hands of others, patients have very good reasons to be angry. But angry feelings need not be expressed in angry acts, because the latter are often ultimately self-defeating and good judgment in the service of avoiding further self-harm is always an important therapeutic goal.

Many patients carry lifelong assumptive baggage concerning the meaning of anger, justice, and vengeance, and the therapist needs to make it clear that managing one's anger does not mean minimizing or trivializing the extent of the pain and outrage the patient has endured, nor is it the same as "forgiving and forgetting" or "letting them win." Indeed, the ability to control and channel one's anger may actually help in formulating and pursuing practical justice, as in clearheadedly taking appropriate civil or criminal legal action. Even the Klingons say, "Revenge is a dish that is best served cold."

Much controversy surrounds the issue of whether overtly and forcefully venting anger is a legitimate therapeutic means of "letting off steam" or whether such emotional pyrotechnics only serve to reinforce and further entrench the rageful feelings. As in most areas of clinical judgment, the therapist must know his patient well enough to determine whether or not angry expressions will be productive and to tell how much is too much. Certainly, there should be nothing in terms of *content* that is off-limits for discussion, and, as noted above, therapists must be prepared to accept and absorb whatever feelings and reactions the patient may articulate. But unproductive spewing for spewing's sake should not be encouraged. Even here, there are exceptions, because sometimes the pain of recollection gets too great and patients really do just have to scream. The key is to allow such venting in an appropriate time and place and to follow it up with constructive therapeutic processing.

To this end, Matsakis (1994) recommends yelling while alone, for example, in one's car or into a pillow at home. Patients may bang pots and pans, tear up old phone books, make voodoo dolls, and so on. I hasten to point out that there is nothing inherently good or bad about any of these venting techniques; again, it depends on the patient. No doubt a paranoid patient with a crystallized revenge fantasy should be discouraged from endlessly tearing up pictures of a supposed nemesis and should be redirected into more contructive channels of justice-seeking, but what about a self-mutilating borderline who takes out her anger on the same picture instead of self-destructively cutting or burning herself? In cases like these, there is no substitute for knowing your patient and using informed clinical judgment.

Not that anger expression is all about teeth-gnashing and foaming at the mouth. There are other, less dramatic but often equally effective ways for patients to vent, such as talking to another person about their anger (obviously, much of this will occur in therapy), writing about their anger, speaking the anger into a tape recorder, drawing a picture about the anger, or telling God about the anger. Other techniques for managing anger include taking time-outs, keeping an "anger diary" and discussing the entries during therapy, and, most importantly, encouraging the patient to behave in self-empowering ways that give her a feeling of greater control (Matsakis, 1994). Anger feeds on helplessness, so any way that a patient's sense of control can be legitimately increased—getting a better handle on her emotions, improving relationships with supportive peers or family members, taking productive, realistic action—will go a long way toward reducing the need for defensive, reflexive anger. "Living well is the best revenge," as the saying goes, even though this ideal is rarely realized completely.

In these times, a special issue concerns guns. In many parts of the country, including the South Florida area where I practice, legal access to firearms is a fact of life. Many traumatized patients, men especially, if they weren't already doing so, now carry weapons "for protection." Obviously, there are different degrees of comfort level among therapists with regard to this issue. A few patients may hang up their guns because you tell them to, or because they're really scared of what they might do.

But the reality is that, in most cases, attempts to discourage otherwise lawful gun-toting will be, at best, blithely disregarded and, at worst, seen as one more psychic emasculating wound—and you can bid the therapeutic relationship goodbye.

What to do? Naturally, if you perceive the patient to be a clear and compelling danger to himself or others, take the necessary protective informative action, as you would for any other patient who is threatening harm, firearms or no. But, barring this extreme situation, one tactic I've found useful is to advise the patient that if he is going to carry a gun anyway, go ahead and apply for the state concealed weapons license and take the firearms training course.

This accomplishes two things. First, having a "carry license" gives the patient a feeling of being part of an elite fraternity, which often serves to boost the patient's overall sense of responsibility and care about firearms use. Second, it provides a state record of gun ownership that further serves to keep the bearer "honest." Paradoxically, this type of external constraint is just what many of these patients consciously or unconsciously are looking for. Even if not, the point is to provide the maximal forseeable protection against harm, while respecting reality so as to otherwise appropriately keep the patient in treatment if there is a credible chance for overall therapeutic improvement and normalization of life.

Existential Issues and Therapeutic Closure

In virtually every case of significant trauma, the patient struggles with shattered assumptions and fantasies about fairness, justice, security, and the meaning of life. It is part of the essential task of psychotherapy to help the trauma patient come to terms with these existential issues. Some patients obsess over what they did or should have done to avoid or escape more serious harm or help other people, and the therapeutic task becomes one of reorienting the patient to a more realistic state of self-acceptance. Many patients need to pass the anniversary date of the traumatic event, especially if their trauma was severe, before they can begin to bring the trauma response to closure. The process of simultaneously externalizing and integrating the trauma event allows the last stages of recovery to take place. As the trauma patient approaches closure, the therapist can help her form a newly realistic and adaptive self-image, which becomes the basis for a healthy future (Everstine & Everstine, 1993).

At one point, I assumed that direct assaults, such as muggings and beatings, would be inherently more "traumatic" than seemingly less personalized auto collisions or worksite accidents. In my experience, however, what has turned out to be a more important variable than the type or even the severity of injury is often the question of *responsibility*, and this seems to have two, seemingly paradoxical, expressions. Patients who feel that they were in some way responsible for the event that injured themselves or others, e.g., not taking sufficient safety precautions in a rough neighborhood or not paying enough attention while driving, may have especially severe posttraumatic stress reactions related to real or imagined guilt. Having had the opportunity to control or avoid the situation, and not taking advantage of it, puts an oppressive onus of responsibility and culpability on these patients.

Conversely, some patients are more overwhelmed by the idea that the injuring event was totally *out* of control. For example, a machine belt snaps, sending a piece of heavy equipment crashing down on a worker at just the moment he was passing underneath, or a drunk driver careens across the highway at just the moment a patient's car was driving by, or a patient is assaulted and robbed in what was supposed to be a "safe" parking lot. For these patients, the world has become a frighteningly unsure and dangerous place, the old rules and illusions don't apply, and any terrible thing can happen at any moment. Related to responsibility is "fault." Those patients whose injuries were caused by the uncaring negligence or willful malice of another may be immobilized into depression by their feeling of existential outrage and lack of justice in the world.

At some therapeutic juncture, it therefore becomes necessary to address what practical measures the patient can reasonably take to protect herself from future harm. This is part of the process of rebuilding the self-care aspect of healthy personality functioning. Having been forced rudely and abruptly to face her own mortality and vulnerability, the trauma patient comes to view both herself and the world differently from the "rest of the human race." Deftly handled in therapy, this can be a time when the patient looks over her values and reassesses what she truly wants from life and what life should mean. Through the stages of closure, the patient can find new meaning as a survivor and go on to choose a future path (Everstine & Everstine, 1993).

Similarly, Everly (1994, 1995) emphasizes the need to help traumatized patients reintegrate their sense of self, as well as their shattered worldview. This necessitates carefully paying attention to what the patient tells the therapist, in order for the latter to discern what specific aspects of the patient's self-schema and worldview have been most affected. Then, posttraumatic reintegration can be approached from one or more of three main perspectives, as follows.

First, the trauma can be integrated into the patient's existing worldview: these things happen, cars do get into accidents on the highway, people do get mugged, but there are certain precautions one can take to minimize the risk of this happening in the future.

Second, the trauma can be alternatively understood as a parallel aspect of the existing worldview, that is, "an exception to the rule": buildings are almost always safe and structural collapses almost never happen, so this tragedy, while certainly awful, is a one-shot deal that will most likely never happen to the same person again.

Third, the trauma can be used to demonstrate the invalidity of the patient's existing worldview and the need to create a new and modified outlook on life in which the trauma more readily fits: your mugging shows that the world is not all filled with good people, that justice doesn't always work out, that sometimes the innocent suffer and the guilty go free. But you can fashion a new way of looking at things that allows both realism and cautious optimism; you can learn to be realistic, even skeptical about human nature and motives, without becoming a complete, soul-shriveled cynic.

Everly (1995) believes that each of these approaches is successively less ego-syntonic and therefore successively more difficult to apply in therapeutic practice. However, I have found that much depends on the nature of the traumatic event and the type of patient. Predominantly externalizing patients seem to cleave to the once-in-a-lifetime, "lightning doesn't strike twice" type of explanation, putting their trust in fate or God or sheer statistical improbability. The "what can *I* do to keep this from happening again" reframe appeals more to patients who already possessed a degree of self-efficacy before the trauma and are therefore willing and able to try to solve problems by their own efforts once the therapist shows them the way.

In general, existential treatment strategies that focus on a quest for meaning, rather than an alleviation of symptoms, may productively channel the worldview conflicts generated by the trauma event, such as helping the patient to formulate an acceptable "survivor mission" (Shalev et al., 1993a). Indeed, in the best cases, the rift and subsequent reintegration of the personality leads to an expanded self-concept and even a new level of spiritual growth (Decker, 1993). Some trauma survivors are thus able to make positive personal or career changes out of a renewed sense of purpose and value in their lives. Of course, not all trauma victims are able to achieve this successful reintegration of the ordeal, and many struggle with at least some vestige of emotional damage for a long time, perhaps for life (Everstine & Everstine, 1993; Matsakis, 1994; McCann & Pearlman, 1990).

Therefore, my main caution about these transformational therapeutic conceptualizations is that they be presented as an opportunity, not an obligation. The extraction of meaning from adversity is something that must ultimately come from the patients themselves, not be foisted upon them by the therapist. Such existential conversions by the sword are usually motivated by a need to reinforce the therapist's own meaning system, or they may be part of a therapeutic "Clarence-the-angel fantasy" (Miller, 1993b, 1994b), wherein the enlightened therapist swoops down and, by dint of brilliantly insightful revisioning, rescues the patient from her darkest hour.

Realistically, we can hardly expect all or even most of our traumatized patients to miraculously transform their tragedy and thereby acquire a fresh, revitalized George Bailyean outlook on life—how many *therapists* would respond this well? But human beings do crave meaning (see also Chapter 12), and if a philosophical or religious orientation can nourish the patient in his or her journey back to the land of the living, then our therapeutic role must sometimes stretch to include some measure of guidance in affairs of the spirit.

POSTTRAUMATIC FAMILY THERAPY

One the primary tenets of this book is that traumatic disability syndromes virtually never occur in a vacuum; typically, the patient's family, friends, workmates, and other peers bear at least some of the brunt of the patient's posttraumatic adaptive struggles. Typically, friends, acquaintances, and distant relatives have the luxury of backing off, so in most cases the immediate family takes the biggest hit. In some cases, the whole family has been affected directly by the traumatic event, as in a car crash or disaster that strikes everyone at once. In other instances, the family is secondarily traumatized by the patient's dysfunctional behavior and may react with hostility and alienation, setting off a deteriorating vicious cycle.

Effect of Trauma on the Family

Whether trauma affects a whole family or a single member, the entire family endures the traumatic aftermath, and the primary parenting functions of protecting, loving, and teaching become disturbed. Trauma stops the developmental clock (Allen & Bloom, 1994), producing relational growth impasses in the traumatized family, just as it does in the individual. Trauma disrupts attachment bonds and severs important internal and external familial connections. Dangling without the support of its own members and blockaded from emotional nourishment from the outside, the family becomes unable to provide adequately the safety, affect modulation, and education that its members require.

Figley (1988) delineates four separate ways that families can be affected by trauma: (1) *simultaneous effects*, as when a catastrophe, such as a fire, natural disaster, or auto accident, directly strikes the entire family; (2) *vicarious effects*, as when a traumatic event strikes one family member, but the family is unable to make direct contact with the victimized member, such as in a foreign war or closed-off industrial accident site; (3) *chiasmal effects*, as when the traumatic stress appears to "infect" all the family members after making contact with the primary victim; and (4) *intrafamilial trauma*, as when a traumatizing experience comes from within the family, as in cases of incest, child abuse, or domestic violence. Each of these situations has its own treatment implications.

Family Treatment Strategies

Figley (1988, 1989) views the basic goal of family therapy as restoring the members to their pretrauma level of functioning, and divides the treatment of family PTSD into five phases.

Phase 1: Building commitment to the therapeutic objectives. Commitment and trust are crucial elements in all effective psychotherapy, and part of this involves the therapist's efforts, early on, to convey a sense of respect for the family members and an appreciation of the pain and struggles they're going through. Getting as many members of the family as possible to disclose their ordeal develops and reinforces commitment to the treatment program. Inculcating this feeling of empathy and support also requires that the therapist project an attitude of realistic confidence, authority, experience, and optimism about the treatment process.

Phase 2: Framing the problem. After building commitment to the treatment objectives, the family members must be allowed to disclose how they each view the problem, which necessitates gathering detailed information about their individual and collective reactions to the traumatic event. In this phase, the therapist must watch for blaming-the-victim responses, as the primary traumatized patient may be viewed by the rest of the family as weak, stupid, careless, or tainted by fate. This reaction typically represents the type of projective scapegoating whereby collaterals attempt to distance their own sense of vulnerability by "casting out"—literally, emotionally, or symbolically—the traumatized member. One of the goals of therapy is to enable family members to purge these feelings and eventually communicate, in words, actions, or attitude, a sense of forgiveness and acceptance of the primary trauma victim.

Phase 3: Reframing the problem. Eventually, it is the therapist's task to help the family develop a "healing theory" (see below) about the traumatic event and possible future traumas. This necessitates helping the family to reframe the individual members' experiences and insights in a form that is compatible with their evolving family healing theory. Often this can begin only when the main layers of family denial have been sufficiently excavated (Allen & Bloom, 1994). Hopefully, the family members will begin to reframe what they had originally regarded to be a tragic burden as more of a challenge that they can now work together to overcome. Moreover, they will come to realize that working through the present crisis together will make them better equipped as a mutually supportive, cohesive family unit to deal with future challenges and adversities.

Phase 4: Developing a family "healing theory." In a sense, this is a family version of the existential reformulation crafted by individual patients to provide some measure of meaning and purpose to their trauma experience. Developing such a healing theory, or *"whole family story"* (Allen & Bloom, 1994) that all family members can embrace is no easy task, especially in families characterized by poor pretrauma cohesion and unhealthy dynamics. It is not necessary for all family members to adopt the family theory with equal enthusiasm. What is important, however, is that the members accept the provisional family healing theory as a good working draft that will be serviceable until a better one can be formulated. The interim conceptualization will at least afford a respite of tranquility in the home—the first step toward getting the individual members accustomed to functioning like a whole family again.

Phase 5: Closure and preparedness. As the family members begin to craft their healing theory, the therapist begins to prepare them for the inevitable termination of treatment. This is done by reviewing the specific therapeutic objectives and encouraging a sense of accomplishment among all family members. While the family is basking in this glow of achievement, Figley (1988) recommends that the therapist pose one or more "practice" crisis situations for discussion. This allows the members to apply the insights and skills developed in the therapeutic process and to gain confidence in their ability to face and overcome future challenges.

Allen and Bloom (1994) emphasize the importance of the therapist's avoiding the trap of being caught between the primary trauma patient and her family as a surrogate rescuer, protector, or defender. Learning to self-protect is a necessary part of treatment for all family members. Family therapy should aim at turning the energy of the family from traumatogenic to supportive once the healthier members of the family join together to provide what the identified patient actually needs rather than playing auxiliary roles in the patient's traumatic reenactment.

Family members should be encouraged to contact the therapist as necessary, but to use the skills and insights they have developed in sessions to try to handle their own problems as they emerge. I usually schedule one to three follow-up sessions in order to formalize the follow-up process without stigmatizing the family for possible feelings of back-sliding in having to contact the therapist later on. Such "booster sessions" are a well-accepted component of follow-up psychotherapy in general.

As another method of reinforcing the gains made, the family should be encouraged to serve as a role model to other families seeking assistance (Figley, 1988). For example, mature and productive participation in support and advocacy groups is a powerful and important means for family members to forge meaning from adversity both for themselves and for others in distress. Finally, the sad truth is that some family members may be more willing than others to leave the grim past behind and move on; in such cases, family separations may be necessary for some members to leave the stifling emotional turmoil of unhealthy family enmeshment and misery in order to find their own way back into the world of living and loving.

Chapter 3

THE SHATTERED SELF

Traumatic Brain Injury and the Postconcussion Syndrome

If the human intellect functions,
it is actually in order to solve the problems
which man's inner destiny sets it.

—Jose Ortega Y Gasset

"Imagine waking up every day with a pounding headache, always feeling like you've got a hangover plus a bad flu after being up the last three nights in a row, and you're having trouble concentrating, remembering, and getting your thoughts together, and you're losing your temper and snapping at people for no reason, walking around jumpy and afraid of your own shadow, and on top of that nobody believes you or they tell you you're crazy, and maybe you'll understand what I've been going through since my accident."

This is how one patient described his situation approximately one year after a closed head injury in which he suffered no serious physical damage, was only momentarily dazed, was kept in the hospital for observation for only one night, and was told "you'll be better in a few days."

He wasn't. And so, like thousands of of such patients with so-called "mild" *traumatic brain injury* (TBI) or *head injury*, he began the long odyssey of doctor-shopping and lawyer-hopping, searching for some clinical or judicial validation, compensation, or just plain understanding. What he got, mostly, were dismissals by physicians, rejection of benefits by his insurance company, the alienation of his friends, former workmates, and family, a diagnosis of "malingering," and eventually a bout of psychiatric hospitalization for depression.

"MILD" HEAD INJURY AND THE POSTCONCUSSION SYNDROME

In the United States, an estimated 400,000 people are admitted to the hospital with traumatic brain injuries every year, and about one million people suffer from head injury effects at any given time (Slagle, 1990). In cases where there has been a prolonged period of unconsciousness after the injury, or where deficits in behavior are apparent on the neurological exam, there's usually no question that brain damage has occurred, and for the most part these patients are treated with sympathy and concern. However, where the "objective" medical tests are normal, but the patient continues to complain of disturbing, debilitating, and disabling symptoms, and where the nature of the head injury is judged to be "mild," suspicions of psychological overreaction, hysteria, hypochondriasis, lack of will, malingering, and outright deception begin to arise. "Quit complaining," these patients are told, "Snap out of it," "Don't be such a crybaby," and so on.

History and Concept of the Postconcussion Syndrome

The neurological versus psychiatric nature of the persisting impairment syndrome following supposedly mild head injury has been debated at least since the last century by such historical notables of neurology and psychiatry as Dupuytren, Strumpell, Oppenheim, and Charcot (see Levin, 1990, for an historical review). The malady was officially dubbed the *postconcussion syndrome* by Strauss and Savitsky in 1934, and many of the symptoms were described in that original report as being psychological in nature: irritability, poor concentration, loss of confidence, anxiety, depression, and intolerance of noise and bright lights. Physical symptoms included include fatigue, headache, dizziness, vertigo, and oversensitivity to alcohol.

Today, the term *postconcussion syndrome* (PCS) is used to describe a cluster of symptoms that occur following a closed head injury, that is, an injury where the skull has not been penetrated, but the brain has essentially been jostled and banged against the hard and rough inner surface of the skull (see below). The symptoms of postconcussion syndrome are often judged by clinicians to persist "inappropriately"—that is, beyond the point where the patient is supposed to have gotten better. The very term "postconcussion syndrome" is still often used pejoratively by unenlightened clinicians, but I will employ it descriptively in this chapter and throughout this book, as is the practice of most modern neuropsychologists.

Postconcussion Symptoms

Commonly reported postconcussion symptoms include headache, dizziness, fatigue, slowness and inefficiency of thought and action, diminished concentration, memory problems, irritability, anxiety, insomnia or poor sleep patterns, nightmares, heightened somatic concern, hypersensitivity to noise, hypersensitivity to light, blurred or double vision, problems in judgment, anxiety, depression, and altered sex drive (Gouvier, Cubic, Jones, Brantly, & Cutlip, 1992; Miller, 1993c, 1994b, 1997a; Parker, 1990; Slagle, 1990). The remainder of this section will consider these symptoms in more detail.

Cognitive Deficits

Cognition means "thinking" and problems in this area may involve any of the thinking functions that the brain performs, such as perceptual analysis, attention and concentration, language and communication, learning and memory, visual and spatial reasoning, and complex planning, judgment, and problem-solving. A common pattern after head injury is the presence of a general slowness or "fuzziness" of thinking, upon which may be superimposed a more severe focal deficit in one or more specific functions that reflect the parts of the brain most seriously damaged. In most cases of mild-to-moderate head injury, the symptoms largely clear up by six months to a year, but residual problems may remain after that, including the following.

DIFFICULTIES IN ATTENTION AND CONCENTRATION.   The patient has trouble following the train of conversations, keeping on track with reading material, or remembering why he got up to go into another room. He is slow to focus on tasks and to figure out what to do. A typical complaint is that "I'm not as sharp as I used to be." Others may notice that the patient seems distractible, that they have to repeat questions and statements for the patient to "get it," and that "Huh?" is a common response.

LEARNING AND MEMORY PROBLEMS.   These include difficulty retaining material heard or read, forgetting people's names or faces, confusing one person with another, having trouble recalling old information "that I know I used to know," and struggling to remember things that used to be learned easily. In general, it's harder for new information to get processed, and what does get in seems to be forgotten more quickly.

SLOWNESS AND INEFFICIENCY.   Things take longer to do. And they may have to be done over and over again. In many cases, the basic skills and knowledge necessary to perform a task may be relatively preserved, but the quickness and efficiency of problem-solving, the ease and smoothness with which those abilities are applied to the task at hand—these are what have been affected.

One example of this is often seen on standardized neuropsychological testing. The kinds of cognitive tasks these patients do worst on are those that have time limits or earn bonus points for quick performance. Given sufficient time to work at his own pace, however, the patient may do all right. But he may have to go back and repeat steps many times, or take two or three times as long to decide on the next step of a problem to be solved. When slowness is combined with actual loss of skill on a task, performance suffers still more.

CONCRETENESS.   In the way the term is used here, *concrete* head injury patients generally do better with tasks and in situations that are familiar rather than novel, structured rather than open-ended, and specific rather than ambiguous. They may not appreciate jokes that involve shifting or reversing one's point of view, and they may have difficulty perceiving more than one side (their own) of an argument or putting themselves in another person's shoes, which is often interpreted by others as shallowness or selfishness.

Emotional, Behavioral, and Psychosocial Problems

Many of the problems experienced after head injury are not just in memory and reasoning, but involve feeling, behaving, and interacting with others. Commonly reported changes include excessive tiredness, indifference, impaired attention and concentration, inflexibility, a tendency toward repetitive speech and behavior, impaired ability to anticipate consequences of one's actions, disinhibition and loss of control over behavior, impaired capacity to acquire new skills or apply old ones, irritability, and reduced quality of relationships, especially in the direction of less intimacy and greater superficiality. Obsessive-compulsive symptoms and overconcern for order and stability may also be seen (Lishman, 1973; Miller, 1993c; Slagle, 1990).

Brooks, Campsie, and Symington (1986) polled the relatives of head injury patients and arrived at a list of the ten most frequent patient problems that continued to plague family members at one and five years postinjury: (1) personality change, (2) slowness, (3) poor memory, (4) irritability, (5) bad temper, (6) tiredness, (7) depression, (8) rapid mood swings, (9) tension and anxiety, (10) threats of violence. Families often had particular difficulty dealing with aggression and hypersexuality. Previously subtle personality traits that were, at worst, irksome before the head injury may subsequently become exaggerated to the point of dysfunctional chaos in the postconcussion period.

In fact, the single most significant factor in post-injury job adjustment, quality of family relations, and overall life satisfaction is not how well the patient can think, reason, concentrate, or remember. Rather, the behavioral and psychosocial status of the person, that is, how well he gets along with others, controls his own impulses, does what he is supposed to do, and acts appropriately in social settings, is what makes or breaks back-to-the-real-world adaptation. To a point, families and workmates alike will usually put up with, even empathize with and support, someone who forgets, bungles, and fails, so long as his actions are perceived as basically well-meaning and his demeanor relatively pleasant. But the impulsive, short-tempered, egocentric, and overemotional employee or spouse or neighbor quickly exhausts the good will of those around him, with a resulting vicious cycle of ostracism and bitterness.

A number of emotional and psychosocial problems that are common after head injury include the following.

DEPRESSION AND MOOD SWINGS.   The patient may show a "Jekyll and Hyde" lability of emotional responsiveness over the course of minutes, hours, or days. Irritable outbursts or crying spells may occur with minimal provocation. Manic highs may alternate with depressive lows. Posttraumatic mania may present itself as euphoria, lack of insight into deficits, irritability, impaired judgment, sleeplessness, pressured speech, flight of ideas, grandiose thinking, preoccupation with religious, philosophical, or political themes, distractibility, hyperactivity, hypersexuality, or even assaultive behavior. In some cases, this may progress to frank delusional psychosis. Family members and caretakers may feel yoked to the patient's emotional roller-coaster, the observers never relaxed, always vigilant for the next stormlike mood surge.

Mood disorders can result from direct injury to the emotional processing systems of the brain. Jeste, Lohr, and Goodwin's (1988) review of neuropsychological studies of mood disorders caused by penetrating head injuries, tumor, trauma, epilepsy, and stroke found a tendency for depression to be associated with damage to the left frontal and right posterior parts of the brain, while mania was associated with damage to right frontal and left posterior brain regions. However, this is only a general correlation, and there may be marked individual differences in how the brain controls thought, feeling, and action (Miller, 1990b).

AGITATION, PARANOIA, IRRITABILITY, AND RAGE.   A smoldering chip-on-the-shoulder edginess may be seen, and "little things" may be more aggravating than usual. Constant complaining and hostility may strain family, job, and other interpersonal relationships. At times, this may flare into aggression and rage. Actual physical violence occurs mainly in the early recovery period when the patient may become combative if restrained or if he feels threatened while in a confusional state. Later on, many patients seem to develop a "short fuse" that persists into the postconcussion period. Some of this may be attributable to the increased suspiciousness and paranoia that sometimes develop after head injury. Confused, insecure, and unable to make sense of the world around him, the patient may easily become frustrated and misinterpret the motives and actions of others as hostile or demeaning.

IMPULSIVITY AND INERTIA.   This is a basic problem with motivation. The patient may alternate between mute inactivity and frenetic running about, starting and leaving unfinished all sorts of tasks and projects, going on irresponsible buying sprees, taking dangerous physical and social risks, and generally showing little foresight or judgment. This type of syndrome may be especially associated with damage to the brain's frontal lobes, the "executive control system" for modulating thought, feeling, and action.

"POSITIVE" PERSONALITY CHANGE.   It's difficult to imagine how traumatic brain injury could produce any kind of change for the better, but at least one report (Ranseen, 1990) has described several cases in which the posttraumatic personality changes were perceived by the family as improvements over what had gone before. All of these patients' premorbid personalities were described as being introverted, inhibited, quiet, and perhaps somewhat obsessive and depressed. They were viewed as previously unhappy individuals, and one suffered from clinical depression. Following brain injury, the patients appeared happier, were more talkative, and generally seemed more extroverted. They were also viewed as being more content with their lives.

The downside, however, consisted of a heightened tendency toward impulsivity and irritability. This occasionally translated into inappropriate assertiveness or tactless bids for attention. Yet, by all accounts, this didn't seem to get too out of hand, and interpersonal relationships were not unduly disrupted. Furthermore, this syndrome did not seem to represent some variant of dementia: the patients themselves retained insight and awareness of their change in personality. The changes were regarded as most consistent with those seen after frontal lobe and/or right hemisphere injury (Heilman, Bowers, Valenstein, & Watson, 1986; Stuss & Benson, 1984; Stuss, Gow, & Hetherington, 1992) and appeared to represent a somewhat more benign variant of the overall disinhibition and euphoric lack of concern commonly seen in these syndromes.

Reportedly, the family members had been frustrated in the past by their husbands' or sons' having been overly aloof, withdrawn, and constricted. Consequently, the personality changes of talkativeness, mild disinhibition, and a more affable, if somewhat unstable, demeanor allowed the patients to achieve fuller, more satisfactory relationships with their families than ever before.

Is brain injury good for you? I doubt it. Rather, I suspect that if you start at the overly reserved extreme of the temperamental continuum, the disinhibition produced by brain injury may swing you more toward the center, or perhaps past the center and a little in the other direction, but just far enough that the change is perceived as positive, not pathological, as joie de vivre, not lack of conscience. But if you're already a little brash or impulsive, brain injury will most likely push you temperamentally over the edge into a dangerously disinhibited tailspin (Miller, 1990b, 1993c). At any rate, I wouldn't prescribe brain damage as a way to lighten up.

NEUROPSYCHOLOGY AND PATHOPHYSIOLOGY OF "MILD" BRAIN INJURY AND THE POSTCONCUSSION SYNDROME

Skull and Brain Dynamics

In an *open head injury* the skull has been penetrated and there is contact between brain tissue and the outside environment, as in a gunshot or stab wound, or skull fracture from a fall onto a hard surface or blow with a blunt object. In a *closed head injury* there is no penetration or breach of the skull, and the kinetic energy force of the trauma is retained within the bony skull cavity (Miller, 1993c).

In severe closed head trauma, gross movements of the brain within the skull result in widespread diffuse damage. In contast, movement effects during mild head trauma are usually limited to the anterior frontal and temporal poles and their brainstem connections, affecting mainly the functions of attention, concentration, memory, abstract reasoning, and judgment (Davidoff, Kessler, Laibstain, & Mark, 1988; Kwentus, Hart, Peck, & Kornstein, 1985). *Rotational acceleration*, in which the brain sharply bends and twists on the brainstem axis, is more likely to cause concussion and damage to nerve cell axons. *Linear acceleration*, which tends to damage the observable surface of the cerebral cortex, is more likely to produce focal lesions that affect discrete functions such as language, perception, and movement (Binder, 1986). Centripetally (inwardly) directed forces may be more likely to damage subcortical diencephalic structures related to emotion, motivation, and visceral functions (Parker, 1990).

When the head is accelerated, the brain lags behind the skull because of its inertia. Head accelerations frequently associated with mild head injury almost always involve a combination of *translational* (foward-backward) and *rotational* (bending and twisting) movements. Brain tissue is compressed next to the point of application of force (*coup* injury) and tends to pull away on the opposite side (*contre-coup* injury). Although the brain motion is slight, it causes shear strains to develop in many neuroanatomical areas, including the cerebral cortex, brainstem, cerebellum, and corpus callosum (Elson & Ward, 1994).

Microstructural Damage: Diffuse Axonal Injury

Most neurons transmit information to one another and to other structures in the body (glands, muscles) by way of their slender axons. In 1835, Gama wrote that "fibers as delicate as those of which the organ of mind is composed are liable to break as a result of violence to the head." Nearly a century later, Cajal (1928) described the *retraction balls* that develop at the severed ends of axons in the peripheral nervous system. Strich (1956, 1961) first described what has come to be called *diffuse axonal injury* (DAI) resulting from shear strain damage that had the histological appearance of peripheral retraction balls but occurred in the brain itself after trauma. Evidence for DAI in cases of mild head trauma was presented by Oppenheimer (1968) in five such cases who had died of other causes. Postmortem histology revealed numerous axonal retraction balls, as well as destruction of myelin (Evans, 1992).

Modern research has provided both experimental and clinical evidence that axons are diffusely injured throughout the brain in mild head injury. For example, in patients who die from nonneurological causes (e.g., chest wound) soon after injury, damaged and swollen reactive axons can be identified, while in patients who survive for a more prolonged period, microglial scarring and axonal degeneration are also observed. Further research has suggested that axons are typically stretched, but not severed, in the immediate impact injury. This causes a focal disruption of the axonal cytoskeleton, leading to localized swelling and eventual axonal detachment. In humans, these degenerative changes take about 12 hours and are preceded by axonal stretching and subsequent accordian-like infolding of the axonal membrane (Christman, Grady, Walker, Holloway, & Povlishock, 1994; Gennarelli, 1993; Povlishock, 1992). Intriguingly, the fact that this process requires several hours to evolve suggests the potential for therapeutic intervention within this window of opportunity if the precise pathophysiological mechanisms could be identified and controlled (Hayes, Povlishock, & Singhe, 1992).

Apparently, only a small percentage of the brain's axons in widespread areas of the brain are damaged by mild head injury (hence, "diffuse" axonal injury). The degeneration of the synaptic terminals derived from the damaged axons ultimately translates into diffuse deafferentation of the synaptic target sites of those destroyed terminals. It is this diffuse loss of neuronal input to diverse and multiple target sites in the brain that most likely accounts for the cognitive, emotional, and behavioral symptoms of mild head injury and the postconcussion syndrome (Christman et al., 1994; Erb & Povlishock, 1991; Hayes et al., 1992).

Recent experimental research has shown that diffusely deafferented postsynaptic sites can be reoccupied over time by terminals derived from related intact fiber populations. This model of DAI implies the possibility of subtle dynamic reorganization of the brain in postconcussion syndrome. Thus, DAI and its subsequent diffuse deafferentation most likely contribute to the early clinical impairment syndrome seen in mild head injury, whereas the compensatory neuroplastic reorganizational changes would account for the typical three-to-twelve-month posttraumatic recovery course seen after mild head injury (Elson & Ward, 1994; Erb & Povlishock, 1991; Hayes et al., 1992). In cases of persisting or delayed-onset postconcussion symptoms, what may well be occurring is a less-than-optimal reafferentation of traumatically damaged synaptic pathways—a "defective rewiring" of brain circuits mediating subtle but important aspects of cognition, emotion, personality, and behavior (Miller, 1996, 1997b).

TRAUMATIC BRAIN INJURY AND POSTTRAUMATIC STRESS DISORDER

It seems obvious that any injury that affects so many aspects of a person's cognition, personality, and relationships could have a potentially devastating, psychologically traumatic effect on the brain injury survivor. Brain injury may be viewed as a unique form of stress event because, in a sense, the very organ of coping, the brain itself, has been damaged. This has wide-ranging effects, impinging on virtually every area of life—job, family, school, friends, and recreation. Until recently, however, the role of posttraumatic stress reactions in brain injury syndromes has been little understood.

Characteristics of Postconcussion PTSD

Frequently, the injury occurs in the context of frightening experiences at the time of the event or during the recovery period. In most cases, traumatic brain injury is both totally unexpected and beyond the person's control. Worse, there may be impaired memory for events surrounding the injury, which further contributes to the patient's sense of confusion and fragmentation. Furthermore, there may be a delayed onset of PTSD symptoms until after the physical and cognitive sequelae of the postconcussion syndrome have begun to resolve. In other cases, PTSD symptoms complicate recovery from the postconcussion syndrome from the start, and often must be carefully uncovered and addressed for full recovery to occur. Within three months of injury, 50 to 85 percent of mild head injury patients report some symptoms of PTSD, which are often quite persistent (Evans, 1992; Packard, 1993), and I have found PTSD and other types of posttraumatic stress reactions to be quite common complicators of postconcussion recovery, often accompanied by the additional burden of chronic pain (see Chapter 4).

Several important features of postconcussion stress reactions have been described (Andrasik & Wincze, 1994; Miller, 1993d; Parker, 1990). The brain-injured patient may be preoccupied with the trauma, numbing and denial alternating with intrusive thoughts and images. This may be especially disturbing where impaired memory for the accident impels a frantic yet scattered search for "the facts." The sting of victimization may be all the more intense if the patient is physically scarred, functionally disabled, sexually impaired, or reduced in social status in the eyes of friends, workmates, or family. Impaired ability to comprehend the world around him or to control his own behavior may be particularly frightening and demoralizing.

Brain injury causes the patient's sense of self to become less solid and predictable. A common feeling is that of having become "damaged goods"—deformed, disabled, incompetent, and conspicuously repulsive. The feeling that everybody is staring at his grotesque infirmity arouses feelings of vulnerability and defensiveness. This hair-trigger sensitivity may then alienate the very people from whom the patient most fears rejection, confirming his worst fears and entrenching his standoffishness—yet another vicious cycle. The patient may feel that the injury occurred as a result of an overwhelming or irresistible force, further fueling his sense of powerlessness and vulnerability. He may resent his new dependency on others but fear being left on his own with only his cracked mental compass to guide him. The prospect of having to give up cherished goals and relationships fills the patient with dread and resentment (Parker, 1990).

One of my patients, Frank, suffered an injury right out of those old Saturday-morning cartoons: a piano fell on him. Well, not actually *on* him, but close enough. He was rushing to a business appointment in a busy warehouse district, when the huge instrument suddenly plunged from a faulty scaffold above. The piano grazed the left side of his skull and face with sufficient oblique force to render him unconscious for several hours. Fortunately, the medics responded quickly and "they knew exactly what to do—I have no complaint about those guys, they were great," he later said.

When I saw him, clinical history and neuropsychological testing revealed some typical postconcussion effects on cognitive functioning, but this was not Frank's major problem. The most disturbing aspect of his injury was the effect on his appearance. He had to undergo numerous facial reconstructive surgeries and reparative dental work, and even two years later he felt he didn't look "normal." Objectively, the surgeons had done a fine job; you could hardly tell he'd been disfigured unless you peered close enough to observe some hairline scars and a slight facial asymmetry.

But the emotional toll was devastating. A handsome, single MBA with a previously active dating life, he had gone from zooming in the fast track to stewing in isolation and depression. Even though he had done a lot of business there, he couldn't bring himself to visit the warehouse district where the accident occurred. Formerly invested in his good looks, yuppified entrepreneurship, and bon vivant persona, he now regarded himself as a freak and a failure and stopped socializing entirely. It took several months of psychotherapy to deal with the self-image issues before the actual active rehabilitation of his memory deficits could begin.

"Cryptotrauma"

In many cases of mild TBI, persistent disability may appear to have no explanation because patients are reluctant to report psychological trauma for fear of being thought of as weak or crazy. Pilowsky (1985, 1992) has drawn attention to a syndrome he terms *cryptotrauma* ("hidden trauma") and provides several case studies, two of which are relevant to our present discussion.

A mining engineer was struck on the head by a hopper. He was not unconscious at the time and sustained no lasting physical impairment apart from a headache and a fractured cheekbone. However, the multiton hopper had locked his head against a steel railing, threatening to crush it slowly. He recalled "hearing the bones in his head cracking and wondering how much more he could take before his skull burst." Another case involved a railway worker who fell head first into a hole and suffered only some muscle and ligament damage, yet complained of pain and disability many months later. When queried, he recalled lying head down in the dark hole with an excruciating pain in his neck, "believing his neck was broken and fearing that he would die before he was found" (Pilowsky, 1985).

Two of my own cases closely resemble these reports. A bright, young special education tutor fell down a flight of stairs during a home visit with a physically and mentally disabled student, sustaining a combined traumatic brain injury and cervical fracture. She recalls feeling severe pain in her neck and knowing it was broken but "willing" herself to stay conscious. In fact, during the emergency she was able to keep sufficient presence of mind to instruct the confused student to dial for help. She still experiences vivid, intrusive memories and nightmares about lying in a cramped space at the bottom of the stairs, fearing she would die or be paralyzed for life.

Another patient, a male construction worker nearing retirement, slipped on some loose tiles and fell from a roof, landing on his back and missing by inches being impaled on a vertical 18-inch iron piling. He recalls lying on his back, afraid to move, with the "piling staring me in the face." He suffered a mild concussion, two herniated disks, and some ligament damage. He successfully completed a rehab program, but to this day reports fearful images of how "they could have found me stabbed through the heart."

Brain Injury and Posttraumatic Stress: Short-term and Long-term Interactions

At this point, it should be fairly obvious that brain injury and posttraumatic stress can exacerbate one another, yet until recently few controlled studies existed to back up the wealth of anecdotal clinical evidence. From a short-term perspective, one group of researchers (Bryant & Harvey, 1995) asked brain-injured and control subjects to monitor their degree of stress and postconcussion symptoms across a six-week period. Results showed that the higher the level of stress experienced by the subjects, the worse their postconcussion symptoms were felt to be.

It may be that, in the early convalescent phase of recovery from traumatic brain injury, disturbing symptoms are minimal because the patient hasn't yet had to confront the daily tasks and responsibilities that he used to take for granted. Upon returning home or to the jobsite, however, his cognitive impairment now interferes with smooth, adaptive functioning, causing tension and frustration to mount, and precipitating the development of disturbing posttraumatic stress symptoms. The situation is probably even worse for patients with "mild" head injuries because, looking so normal on the outside, they're expected to get back on the beam right away.

This issue of "You look fine, what are you complaining about?" continues to plague many postconcussion patients who nevertheless experience profound disturbances in their abilities and self-concept months or years following their injury (Lewis & Rosenberg, 1990; Miller, 1993c; Parker, 1990; Tyerman & Humphrey, 1984). Fifty patients with mild head injury were interviewed six months and three years postinjury (Wright & Telford, 1996). As a group, they showed PTSD and other signs of psychological distress. A prominent theme that emerged was the discontinuity in the patients' sense of self following the head injury, and these changes were significantly related to their symptoms of psychological distress. They also showed marked impairment in social functioning and interpersonal relationships.

Another prominent theme that emerged from Wright and Telford's study—which is consistent with the experience of all clinicians who work with these groups—was the widespread attitude among family, friends, coworkers, and health care providers that "There's nothing really wrong with you" or "Okay, you have some problems, but they're not so bad, and besides, there's nothing we can do about them, so learn to live with it and get on with your life." This imputed wimpishness only adds another thick layer of humiliation to the patient's already crushing burden of wrecked self-esteem.

Wright and Telford (1996) agree with others in the brain injury field (Lewis & Rosenberg, 1990; Parker, 1990; Small, 1980; Tyerman & Humphrey, 1984) that, while mollycoddling patients into enforced invalidism is of course counterproductive, any real move toward "getting over it" is predicated on the reshaping of a coherent postinjury identity— reclaiming the shattered self (Miller, 1993c). There has to be a "me" that wants to go back to work, be a loving spouse, a responsible parent, and so on. This reintegration can occur with the help of the therapist's carefully crafting bridges between the patient's current and former personalities, as well as developing new areas of competency to spackle in the more gaping cracks of the self-structure, which will hopefully then harden into the permanent edifice of a new identity.

Can PTSD Occur with Loss of Consciousness and Amnesia for the Trauma?

Controversy—much of it fueled by legal and compensation issues (Taylor, 1996)—continues to swirl around the question of whether an event that is not consciously processed or recalled can in fact be "traumatic." Some authorities (Sbordone, 1992; Zasler, 1995) argue that posttraumatic amnesia and PTSD categorically exclude one another, while others (Brooks, 1995; Layton & Ward-Zonna, 1995) insist that the two syndromes are not incompatible and present case studies to support this conclusion.

Several recent studies have systematically attempted to address this question. Bryant and Harvey (1995) investigated acute stress responses in 38 head-injured and 38 nonhead-injured motor vehicle accident survivors between one and fifteen days following the accident. Results showed that, while both groups reported comparably high levels of general anxiety, amnesia for the traumatic event was associated with fewer acute intrusive symptoms in subjects with head injury than in noninjured subjects.

In a follow-up study, Bryant (1996) assessed posttraumatic stress in a sample of 114 motor vehicle accident survivors, including 38 patients who had sustained a mild head injury. Subjects were evaluated within two weeks of hospital admission. Again, patients who were amnesic for the accident tended not to show posttraumatic intrusive symptoms related to the accident itself, leading the authors to conclude that conscious recall of the traumatic event is a prerequisite for the development of posttraumatic symptoms.

With the presence of such major theoretical and practical controversy (and associated legal and financial axes to grind), it is doubtful that the amnesia/PTSD issue will be definitively answered soon. I think that part of the problem lies in a perhaps too-narrow definition of "trauma" and the traumatic event. Discrete, brief, one-hit-and-it's-over traumatic events, such as car accidents, represent only one type of traumatic event. What about head injury that occurs during a natural disaster or in the course of a frightening crime? Even in traffic accidents, the traumatic aspect may involve pain during extrication from the vehicle, the confusion and fear of emergency medical procedures, or witnessing passengers hurt or killed (Shalev, 1992; see also Chapter 6).

My own clinical experience with brain-injured patients is that full-blown PTSD is a fairly common accompaniment to the head injury in motor vehicle crashes, criminal assaults, and worksite accidents. Even Bryant and Harvey (1995) point out that case studies exist indicating a tendency for some brain-injured patients to suffer intrusive symptoms (MacMillan, 1991). Obviously, one cannot recall events that took place during a period of unconsciousness. But I have had several patients report complete amnesia for apparently lucid intervals—backed up by police and emergency medical reports—where they got out of their cars and even conversed with rescuers, only to lose consciousness seconds or minutes later and subsequently have no recall of the episode. These patients typically experience a visceral type of intrusion—recapitulating the fear and distress of the accident—rather than an imagistic one of reexperiencing the "scene." This seems to support the idea of multiple neuropsychological pathways in processing trauma (see Chapter 1).

PSYCHOTHERAPY OF THE POSTCONCUSSION/ POSTTRAUMATIC PATIENT

I have covered the broad field of brain injury psychotherapy in previous publications (Miller, 1990a, 1991a, 1991b, 1991c, 1992a, 1992b, 1992c, 1992d, 1993a, 1993b, 1993c, 1994a, 1998). This section will present an overview of the main principles of therapy for those patients whose postconcussion syndromes are especially entangled in, and complicated by, a coexisting posttraumatic stress disorder, producing a cumulatively severe traumatic disability syndrome.

General Considerations

Brain injury levels the cognitive and emotional playing field, and, as noted above, there is a range of "typical" postconcussive syndromes. But each patient still brings his individual personality, coping style, and unique history to the recovery process. Therefore, to repeat one of this book's guiding themes, each patient needs to be treated as an individual. As always, you as the clinician must understand the syndrome *and* know your patient.

In addition, working with traumatized patients in general, and brain-injured patients in particular, necessitates a stretching of the psychotherapeutic role to include multiple modalities, such as concrete guidance, remedial instruction, special training, environmental restructuring, referral and monitoring of medication, educational and vocational counseling, behavior modification, psychotherapy, and working with the family, educators, and employers (Miller, 1993c; Small, 1980).

An effective program of psychotherapy must address three major areas of functioning: (1) *cognition*, with emphasis on rehabilitation; (2) *emotion*, with attention to long-term personality traits, adjustment reactions to trauma, and temperamental and personality changes caused by the injury; and (3) *behavior*, including management of physical disabilities, pain, and postconcussive symptoms, as well as realistic goal-setting and the careful structuring of successful experiences for the patient (O'Hara, 1988).

In fact, cognitive and emotional issues are rarely separable in the real clinical world of brain injury, and brain injury psychotherapy—indeed, all psychotherapy—necessarily includes some element of practical cognitive rehabilitation (Ben-Yishay & Diller, 1983; Carberry & Burd, 1986; Miller, 1992a, 1992b, 1993c; Novack, Roth & Boll, 1988; Parente & Herrmann, 1996; Prigatano, Fordyce, Zeiner, Roueche, Pepping, & Wood, 1986; Smith & Godfrey, 1995).

For example, patients who are cognitively impaired are typically also confused about their own emotional states. When the disorientation begins to subside, feelings of anger, depression, and remorse may emerge. Many of the interpersonal problems experienced by brain-injured patients are related to inaccurate perceptions and assumptions about themselves and others in social situations, and to cover-up of deficits by alternating rigidity and lability of thought, speech, and action. Interpersonal dialogue and social interactions are thus often characterized by concreteness, loose associations, missing the main point, cognitive "tunnel vision," and egocentricity.

Many of the so-called "postconcussive personality changes" may be secondary to cognitive deficits such as decreased speed and efficiency of information-processing, increased distractibility, and decreased ability to focus and sustain attention (Bennett, 1987, 1989). This can result in the brain-injured person's missing part of what he is told or what he observes in the actions of others. This in turn may lead to the belief that others are being hypercritical, "taking over," and/or talking about or plotting against the patient as he tries to make sense of the incomplete messages he is straining to comprehend. The end result may range from hypersensitivity, to wary suspiciousness, to outright delusional paranoia. Such a situation is best resolved through careful explanation to, and continued positive regard for, the brain-injured patient and significant others.

Cognition and Psychodynamics in Brain
Injury Psychotherapy

Traditional psychotherapy places substantial cognitive demands on patients, which few brain-injured individuals can adequately meet (Bennett, 1989; Cicerone, 1989; Small, 1980). Typically, the successful psychotherapy patient must possess good receptive and expressive language skills and must be able to understand and communicate inflection, innuendo, metaphor, and other subtle and abstract language cues. Attention must be adequate to track the conversation for relatively extended periods of time. Within- and between-session memory must be reasonably intact if continuity and cumulative gains are to be maintained. Reasoning ability and self-insight must be adequate, and the patient should be able to autonomously apply general principles discussed in therapy to specific instances in his or her everyday life.

In contrast, the cognitively impaired brain-injured patient may be quite concrete in his language skills, may interpret everything literally, and may totally miss subtleties of language. The ability to remember what transpired during the session or in the patient's daily life may be fragmented. Difficulties with reasoning ability and insight can not only prevent the patient from successfully participating in psychotherapy but also increase psychological distress when his inability to handle these higher-level cognitive processes becomes apparent. Thus, experiential/insight-oriented psychotherapy, which depends in part upon fairly intact cognitive functioning, may upset and demoralize the brain-injured patient, rather than help.

Brain damage often results in behavioral regression, due in large part to the dissolution of higher integrative cognitive skills necessary for complex adaptational tasks. Even as recovery and improvement in cognitive functioning occur, the patient may cling to the more regressed mode because it has become predictable and manageable. Careful encouragement, support, and step-by-step retraining may be necessary to enable such a patient to utilize his or her recovering capacities. Forcing a too-early renunciation of "immature" defenses and coping patterns may precipitate a catastrophic reaction and instill massive resistance to further therapeutic progress (Small, 1980).

Denial, especially when severe and pervasive, is probably the most difficult of the defenses to deal with, and organic denial is often refractory to virtually any kind of psychotherapeutic approach. In other cases, denial serves a more psychodynamically-based, ego-protective function, which, however, may maladaptively prevent the development of a realistic self-concept and divert the therapeutic focus from areas where true progress could be made. The treatment approach, then, should consist not so much of a confrontation or challenge as a gradual focus on reality that continually monitors the patient's ego tolerance as it proceeds. Partial insights and provisional interpretations should take precedence over grand therapeutic "breakthroughs," so that sufficient time is allowed for thorough digestion of each small bite of self-awareness (Small, 1980).

Brain-injured patients who freely acknowledge or even flaunt their physical symptoms may staunchly deny any cognitive, behavioral, or emotional disability. Within the psychological realm itself, patients may acknowledge problems with memory much more readily than problems with reasoning or personality. It seems that impairment of physical functioning and, to a lesser degree, memory are more objectifiable, more easily separated from the person's core sense of self, and therefore less psychologically threatening than "mental problems" that connote loss of emotional control or personality dissolution (Cicerone, 1989).

However, it is also possible that the comprehension of our own styles of thinking and character requires a greater capacity for self-reflection, and therefore represents knowledge that is less accessible to the patient with impaired conceptual ability and organic unawareness. In still other cases, denial may represent an emotional reaction and protective response in the face of distress caused by increasing recognition of disability.

One major goal of psychotherapy, then, is to increase the brain-injured patient's capacity for self-observation. Patients who are frankly unaware of their deficits may benefit from informative and educational aspects of therapy. Successful patients themselves report that concrete feedback is often the most effective means of dealing with resistance to treatment. Helpful strategies include the use of formal checklists, self-monitoring inventories, and videotapes. Such feedback can be repeated as required to allow patients to objectify the evaluation of their own performance and to practice self-monitoring and self-assessment skills in a relatively nonthreatening environment. This can be extended to group therapeutic modalities. Such overt self-observation and mutual group correction may thereby help compensate for the organic loss of internalized self-monitoring (Cicerone, 1989; Prigatano et al., 1986).

Any discussion of psychodynamically-oriented psychotherapy with brain-injured patients must consider the effects of patients' premorbid personalities in determining whether the therapy process itself is seen as a benefit or as a threat and a burden (Lewis & Rosenberg, 1990). Patients whose preexisting level of ego organization was already only in the borderline range probably never fully developed the capacity to use ideation and self-reflection in the service of adaptation. When they are encouraged to reflect on their experiences, therapy quickly becomes an onerous chore, as their ability to use thinking in the service of self-understanding, problem-solving, and adaptive planning—vestigial at best, even before the brain injury—is now further taxed (Miller, 1992a, 1992b). Many such patients, therefore, show marked "resistance," and the therapist must then continually tread the fine line between stimulating the patient's latent capacities for adaptive thought and action and pushing the patient beyond his limits, thereby creating the set-up for a catastrophic reaction.

To varying degrees, many brain-injured patients see psychotherapy as a threat to the safety of their dependency wishes (Lewis & Rosenberg, 1990). In fact, they may not necessarily experience their neurological dysfunction entirely negatively—a phenomenon clinicians working with chronic pain and somatization patients will recognize (Miller, 1993e). By virtue of their physical and neuropsychological deficits, brain-injured patients may be exempted from many of the demands and responsibilities of normal adult life, and they have often found an acceptable way of having their dependency needs met by others. Psychotherapy, with its thrust toward growth and autonomy, may be viewed by such patients with some degree of ambivalence, if not outright protest.

Also, patients may be reluctant to make changes that are genuinely within their capacity for fear that others will perceive them as more competent, or less impaired, than they actually are, and then abandon them. Further, patients are sometimes plagued by guilt, with the injury perceived as cosmic punishment. Psychotherapy, with its implicit promise of a fuller and more productive life, may therefore be viewed as "too good" for the patient. As in all trauma therapy, these postconcussion feelings of guilt and "badness" must be addressed directly in psychotherapy (Lewis & Rosenberg, 1990).

Existential Issues

In a sense, all effective psychotherapy with wounded, shattered persons is by definition "existential," as it necessarily deals with the ultimate questions of life's purpose (Baumeister, 1991). Perhaps nowhere else do issues of selfhood, identity, and the meaning of life emerge so starkly as at the interface between brain injury and traumatization (Miller, 1993d; Parker, 1990). Yalom (1980) has identified four central concerns of a psychoexistential approach to psychotherapy: death, isolation, meaninglessness, and freedom. This has been applied directly to brain-injured patients by Nadell (1991) and can be extended here to the treatment of combined postconcussion syndrome and PTSD.

DEATH. As much as any threat to physical survival, traumatic brain injury and the exposure to traumatic stress underscore our fragile and finite nature, forcing the injured individual to come to grips with his mortality in a sudden and radical fashion. Brain-injured and traumatized patients frequently comment that they can never look at life the same way again. They envy "normal" people with their petty everyday concerns; these others are seen as living in a now-irretrievable Edenic garden of ignorant bliss that the patients have been cast out of. Therapists are advised to initially validate the patient's sense of alienation, while not reinforcing it. Later in treatment, one focus will be on repairing the salvageable past links, and forging new ones, between the patient's reshaped sense of self and the world of other people.

FREEDOM. Beyond the boundaries of autonomy and freedom we all struggle with, brain injury in the context of trauma can impose crippling limitations on virtually every aspect of life, from basic activities of daily living to more complex academic, vocational, social, family, recreational, and communicative functions. These limitations may, especially at first, be so dramatic as to crush any motivation for positive self-change, even under the guidance of the most dedicated therapist. In such cases, the best course is not to "push it"; the clinician must bide his or her time and wait for the right existential opening to begin the process of dealing with limitations.

MEANINGLESSNESS. The alterations in the interpersonal, vocational, and recreational spheres of existence that follow brain injury and traumatization can strike insurmountable blows to the patient's sense of the meaning of life. Clinicians and well-intentioned friends and family members often tell the patient to "just relax" and "enjoy life," without realizing that even the seemingly safe and simplistically pleasureable pastimes we all take for granted may present demoralizing cognitive obstacles for the brain-injured patient (Forrest, 1987). Reading novels, taking a drive, playing checkers or shooting pool, following the plot of a movie or TV show, taking a crocheting or computer course—all may challenge the brain-injured patient's diminished capacities and further erode his self-esteem.

Add to this the unpleasant effect of many TV shows or aversive neighborhood locales on the postconcussion patient with comorbid PTSD and it is easy to see why many such patients eventually find it easier to seclude themselves into near-total hermitage. Here again, finding some "hook" into the outside world where the patient can feel any kind of human connection and sense of competence is often the necessary first step to productive therapy.

ISOLATION.   Indeed, isolation often becomes the dominant coping strategy of the brain-injured patient with PTSD, with "Leave me alone!" the prevailing response to any attempt at contact. It is not unusual to find such patients literally spending all their time in a darkened room, often in bed, day in and day out, immune to the most earnest remonstrations by family or clinicians to come out into the light. The brain-injured patient experiences an alienation and estrangement from the self, a wrenching separation of the individual from qualities that had been vital extensions of himself, including skills, talents, abilities, and the familiar reality that all of us create in our lives.

Self-alienation may further distance the patient from others, as the individual is typically reluctant to reach out and socially engage others, defending against the pain of anticipated rejection, and thereby producing yet another vicious cycle. In such cases, it is often useful to encourage the patient to secure a link to one outside person, a "safe" person, as one plank in the bridge to social relatedness. Since many close friends and family members may be burned out from their intense interactions with the patient, the therapist often has to assume this transitional interpersonal role. The therapist should allow time, as the relationship may take a while to develop, and in the meantime do all he can to make this relationship as constructive as possible.

Existential Psychotherapy of the Brain-injured, Traumatized Patient

In addition to the above recommendations, some general principles of existentially oriented psychotherapy with brain-injured, traumatized patients can be offered. In the ordinary course of life, people are able to gradually confront and integrate the existential realities of mortality and vulnerability in a developmentally timely manner, through the deaths of elderly loved ones, expectable life changes and illnesses encountered in the normal aging process, and with the comfort of spiritual, philosophical, and religious belief systems (Nadell, 1991). Brain injury and trauma contract and contort this developmental pathway, and therapy must therefore help the patient deal with his now all-too-glaring perception of the precarious grasp we all have on life but that most of us keep dimmed and proportioned by the filtering lenses of normal health, work, and relationships.

Prigatano et al. (1986) point out that the concept of God has extraordinary psychological significance for many brain-injured patients. God can represent a coming to grips with reality, a connecting of one's core self to something beyond a limited biological existence. When this takes place, the patient has a sense of integration and individuation that is necessary for acceptance of the tragedy of his life. For many patients, this may be the only thing that allows them to move ahead psychologically. The same is obviously true for traumatized patients generally.

Swinton (1997) makes the compelling argument that faith and spirituality are not really intellectual concepts at all, but rather *relational* realities. In this view, only through the transcendent power of human relationships can mortals learn anything about the divine. A relational orientation to faith avoids evaluating the traumatized, brain-injured person's spiritual life according to abstract or doctrinal criteria, but rather allows the patient to search for new ways of sharing faith, even in the presence of impaired communication or cognitive understanding.

As a result of this elevated awareness, the patient's sense of the urgency of the moment may help him seize satisfaction in "little things" that might have previously gone unnoticed. The taste of food, the sights and sounds of nature, the companionship of friends and family, a favorite song, the reading of a good book, and so on may all be experienced with a greater intensity, enhancing the quality of life. This enhanced quality of life may in turn allow the patient to cope more effectively, softening the blows of his ever-present limitations and deficits, easing his depression, and enabling him to channel more of his energies into rehabilitation (Prigatano et al., 1986; Swinton, 1997).

The centrality of meaning to life makes it incumbent on the psychotherapist working with the traumatized brain-injured patient to act as a vehicle for helping him reconstruct a viable sense of terrestrial meaning. While important, the issue of cosmic meaning, says Nadell (1991), should not be something the therapist "takes sides" on, but only validates in terms of its importance to the patient as a source of strength, motivation, support, and meaning.

Again, therapists should help the patient develop interpretive options, but avoid pushing them. As with my caveat about existential psychotherapy cited in Chapter 2, here, too—perhaps here especially—therapists must be cautious about promoting a particular religious or philosphical orientation, or any religious view at all. Once again, take your cue from the patient and develop it accordingly. Don't feel you have to play priest, rabbi, minister, or guru if you're uncomfortable with this role, and refer the patient to the appropriate clergy for more extensive religious work, if this is indicated.

As noted above, a central theme of psychotherapy with wounded patients is personality continuity and reintegration. While recognition of losses is a painful process for the patient, one can emphasize the qualities that are still, in part or in whole, defining features of who the person was and still is. Among these essential characteristics may be various aspects of his personality, interests, knowledge, skill areas, religious beliefs, and so on. Through this exploration process, the gap between the patient's premorbid and postinjury self can be partially closed, reducing the sense of self-alienation and isolation with its accompanying ego-dystonic states.

At some point in the therapy process, I find it useful for the patient to begin to develop a few short- and long-term projects that can serve as concrete sources of accomplishment and satisfaction. Here, the therapist treads another thin line, this time between empowering the patient by potential success and risking psychic disembowelment by potential failure at even "baby tasks." Needless to say, good clinical judgment and empathic skill are required to reduce the chances of such unintendedly pernicious set-ups.

Bennett (1987) notes that brain injury, at least mild brain injury, may be an opportunity for personal growth (see also Chapter 12). After several years have elapsed and the recovery period and residual deficits have been put in perspective, a number of successfully treated brain-injured patients may come to believe that some good things have resulted from the ordeal. Some have told Bennett (1987) that the injury "knocked some sense" into them, which may represent the adaptive coping strategy of making lemonade out of lemons; alternatively, it may reflect an internalization of the encouraging sentiments of others. In any case, while significant personal growth is possible during the recovery period, this should not be "expected" and additional undue existential pressure should not be placed on the patient.

According to Bennett (1987), having had a brain injury may leave one with a greater appreciation of life and a greater respect for its fragile nature. This kind of trauma is a sobering experience that may render the patient more serious overall. Indeed, the new seriousness is one reason why some adolescent and young adult brain injury patients lose friends; they seem too mature, "not fun anymore." (Caveat: Don't mistake organic emotional flattening and loss of abstract humor appreciation for existential seriousness.) The greater appreciation of life and the experiences of abandonment and isolation can leave the brain-injured person exquisitely sensitive to the needs and feelings of others. (Caveat: Sometimes the opposite occurs, i.e., egocentricity and cynicism.) Finally, for the patient who makes a good recovery, the brain injury may signal a time to settle down and to be more goal-directed, in a sense forcing that quotidian but oft-evaded existential question, "What do I want to do with my life?"

Again, the posttraumatic brain injury mural of religious, existential, interpersonal, and intellectual meaning and identity needs to be crafted with a fine brush, not splattered with a paint gun. For persons who have sustained traumatic brain injury—indeed, as this book shows, for all recovering traumatic disability patients—ultimately it's the patient's responsibility and privilege to effect the recreation of self. The therapist must initially serve as a guide and mentor, and then gradually step back and let other, normal support systems—family, job, church, community—move in to help the patient continue the work, a work of evolving identity that in the best cases shades seamlessly into the larger canvas of ongoing life.

Chapter 4

NO RELIEF

Traumatic Pain and the Chronic Pain Syndrome

Suffering is the sole origin of consciousness.

—Fyodor Dostoyevsky

There was never yet philosopher,
That could endure the toothache patiently.

—William Shakespeare

Many of the traumas discussed in this book involve physical injuries that require some sort of emergency medical treatment. All too frequently, the trauma of physical and emotional injury doesn't end when the patient has been whisked to safety. In many cases, the greatest trauma occurs—or at least continues—long after the acute medical treatment has been concluded. In some cases, the trauma stems from the treatment procedures themselves; in other cases, the problem originates in the patient and her response to the injury and recovery.

TRAUMATIC PAIN

Pain and Trauma

Aside from actual threat to life, perhaps the most traumatically stressful aspect of many accidents or acts of violence is the unavoidable pain that is sometimes involved in the injury or its treatment. In both military and civilian traumas, research has shown that posttraumatic stress reactions occur more frequently among painfully injured survivors than in those emerging physically intact (Helzer, Robins, & McEnvoi, 1987; Pitman, Orr, Forgue, de Jong, & Claiborn, 1989). Paradoxically, however, sometimes the opposite occurs. That is, bodily injury may actually defuse and delimit the stress response by giving the patient something "real" and "physical" on which to focus her anxiety and distress.

Even in the case of clear-cut military trauma, it may be necessary to tease out what aspects of the posttraumatic stress reaction come from the field of battle itself and what ones emerge later as the wounded warriors deal with their pain and injury. One soldier on riot control duty in the Middle East lost an eye to a rock thrown by a member of an angry mob (Schreiber & Galai-Gat, 1993). He developed a typical posttraumatic stress response which the army doctors assumed was related to being attacked and blinded, his eyeball literally spilling into his hand. No, he later pointed out, the eye loss, although terrible, was something he could deal with. Far worse was the traumatic experience of sitting for hours in what seemed like interminable agony, waiting for medical help to arrive.

Similar cases from civilian life are common, and more enlightened authorities in pain management are now starting to advocate adequate pain control as an essential component of injury treatment and recovery (Coderre, Katz, Vaccarino, & Melzack, 1993; Flor, Birbaumer, & Turk, 1990). Since persistent postinjury pain can prolong and intensify the posttraumatic stress response, as well as measurably delay medical recovery, it must be recognized and treated as soon and as effectively as possible.

Medical Emergency Procedures

We take for granted the lifesaving achievements of modern emergency medicine and surgery, and indeed, medics and emergency rescue teams should be justly praised for their routinely heroic activities (see Chapter 10). Only a few generations ago, wounded soldiers and injured workers feared for good reason the company "sawbones" who was sent to patch them up. Today, injuries that used to routinely kill or maim now produce only temporary or mild disability because of rapid treatment with state-of-the-art technology.

However, many lifesaving procedures employ complex, invasive techniques for which the patient has little or no preparation. The emotional impact of the injury itself may thus be compounded by painful and frightening medical procedures. In fact, these procedures may constitute bona fide traumatic events, as they are often associated with sudden onset, lack of control, and perceived or actual threat to life.

Shalev, Schreiber, Galai, and Melmed (1993) have reported a number of cases in which posttraumatic stress reactions followed lifesaving medical procedures. One 45-year-old, skilled blue-collar worker suffered a heart attack during a cardiac catheterization. He showed a flat EKG and required electric shock to restart his heart. Physically, he recovered and went home, but during the next few weeks he began to experience heightened arousal, insomnia, difficulty concentrating, restlessness, and repeated flashbacks to the episode. He tried to avoid any reminders of his hospital stay, but he had frequent nightmares of being back in the operating room with the entire resuscitation scene going on around him. While watching TV, he experienced dissociative states in which the screen suddenly became an EKG monitor with a flat line.

More gravely, he began to flout his doctor's advice and to purposely try to "challenge" his heart, as he put it, by engaging in intense physical effort. Two years of psychotherapy and psychotropic medication helped him partially recover from this stress syndrome, but his symptoms were occasionally reactivated by doctors' visits or on the anniversary of his heart attack.

Another case in this series was a 32-year-old wife and mother who had experienced years of vague physical and mental symptoms without a definitive diagnosis, until eventually one comprehensive exam turned up a meningioma. The neurosurgeon was able to remove this benign brain tumor without leaving any permanent neurological deficit, and the case was considered successfully closed as the woman began getting back into her daily routine.

Then, abruptly, she "collapsed." For the next year, she struggled with crippling depression, accompanied by recurring intrusive recollections of her operation and the surrounding events. This alternated with periods of emotional numbing when she would stubbornly avoid anything that reminded her of doctors or hospitals, including, unfortunately, necessary medical checkups. Psychotherapy helped her work through the effects of her traumatic experience, and she returned to her normal life without any further difficulties.

One of my own patients was a lifelong Christian Scientist in her late fifties who had literally never seen the inside of a hospital or doctor's office in her entire life. Her first contact with modern medicine came jarringly one evening when she began to experience numbness, weakness, blurred vision, and trouble speaking. In fear, she did the unthinkable and dialed 911. The ambulance wailed to her door and the medical team burst in, probing and poking her face and body with all manner of alien devices, then trundling her off to the emergency room where she was further assailed by glaring lights, blaring sounds, and loud voices, before finally slipping into oblivion.

She awoke in a hospital bed hours later and was told she had suffered a mild stroke. Several weeks later, she had more or less recovered neurologically, left with only a mild residual weakness of the right arm and hand. But she was now subject to almost constant jumpiness and irritability, punctuated by bouts of panic-level anxiety, and she described recurring nightmares of her medical ordeal. Most disturbingly, she suffered excruciating guilt over having violated her religious convictions by seeking medical help. Even seeing me, a psychologist, was stretching things, but was rationalized as acceptable because I wasn't really providing medical treatment per se—"It's like seeking counsel," she reasoned, "and I guess that's permitted." Unfortunately, she only attended two sessions and disappeared from follow-up, no doubt turning her psychological and spiritual recovery over to God.

Another of my patients, a businessman in his thirties, seemed at first to be a fairly straightforward closed head injury case (see Chapter 3). His car was rear-ended in a rainstorm and he suffered a combination skull impact plus whiplash injury, causing a few moments of unconsciousness and a residual postconcussion syndrome and neck pain, all of which mostly abated over the next six months. The truly "traumatic" aspect of this event, however, occurred during his treatment by the ambulance team and emergency room staff. "They scared the hell out of me," he related, by telling him "not to move or I might be paralyzed." In addition, the ER physicians' discussions of possible brain damage or paralysis during his first few hours of treatment frightened him sufficiently to produce a full-blown PTSD syndrome, with hypervigilance, numbing, intrusive daytime recollections, and nightmares. Once I was able to explain to him what was going on, brief psychotherapy was quite effective in helping this otherwise normal man work through his traumatic experience and get on with his life.

Medical professionals and rescue personnel need to be sensitive to the fact that their well-meaning and often crucially lifesaving ministrations may sometimes produce as much or more distress in their patients than the injuries themselves. This argues strongly for preparing patients as much as possible for what they will undergo and explaining to them, in as simple and realistically reassuring terms as possible, the nature of their injury and what will be done to treat it. Certainly, any questions that patients ask should be answered to the best of the clinician's knowledge and patient's level of understanding, and any expressed concerns should be sensitively addressed.

Burns

Sometimes, however, all the reassurance and preparation in the world can't mitigate the effects of a particularly painful injury, its treatment, and the recovery process. Burn patients are confronted by at least two stressors: first, the traumatic event that caused the burn and, second, the pain, disability, and cosmetic injury associated with recovery (Davis & Breslau, 1994). Severe burns are catastrophic, life-threatening events that alter body-image and can produce lifelong medical difficulties. Exposure to a severe burn is commonly followed by painful months in a hospital burn unit, multiple painful debridements and other procedures, mind-numbing doses of powerful narcotics, repeated reconstructive surgeries, and the prospect of lifelong disfigurement and disability.

One particularly devilish aspect of a burn stressor is that the patient is frequently and persistently reexposed to the pain of the injury. The constant reminder of the injury may impair recovery and contribute to the persistence of posttraumatic stress symptoms. This feature of burns is also common in other stressors where physical injury, impaired relationships, or material loss serves to remind the victim of the traumatic event. This kind of "flashback" is not of the mind only; it has a very real, here-and-now substantive basis. In these cases, a certain degree of pain relief, "damage control," physical recovery, and provision of basic resources is almost always necessary before moving on to the more psychological reparative aspects of trauma therapy (see also Chapter 7).

Health Care Workers

Not just patients, but clinicians, too—the helpers—may suffer trauma connected with their activities. Hospitals, clinics, and emergency rooms can sometimes be dangerous places to work. In addition to the stresses of making life-and-death decisions and dealing with innumerable daily hassles, nurses, aides, physicians, and other health care providers are sometimes exposed to violence or threats from patients (Davis & Breslau, 1994; Miller, 1997a; see also Chapters 9, 10, and 11).

One of the special challenges that injured, traumatized clinicians face is the conflict between the roles of victim and caregiver, a dilemma also experienced by injured teachers. Although health care personnel who are victims of violence may later associate their symptoms with the specific traumatic event, chronic exposure to cumulative daily stresses may be important as well. It's the straw and the camel again: when a clinician develops PTSD following a specific experience associated with injury and pain, the intrusive thoughts and flashbacks often recall prior stressors that have heretofore been kept under psychological wraps. The most recent, physically painful, trauma is the trigger that evokes reactions to traumas past.

One of my patients, an experienced nursing home nurse, was assisting in the ambulation of an elderly resident with dementia, when the deceptively frail-looking man abruptly hauled off and hit her, literally knocking her across the room. To add irony to injury, this occurred during National Nurses Week. She sustained a broken jaw and a sprained neck, both of which healed fairly quickly, but she has never felt truly relaxed or safe at her job again. Each time she gets a twinge in her neck or jaw, she experiences a mental wince as well. "I feel for these old people, I really do," she says, "but I watch myself now—and I watch them."

CHRONIC PAIN

"At first it didn't seem so bad," Joe told me. "I was lifting this pile of boards on the construction site, and I heard a snap and it felt like a tearing sensation in my lower back, but it also felt kind of numb and I was able to straighten up right away and finish out the day. I really figured I'd rest up over the weekend and go back to work on Monday."

But in the days that followed, the back pain worsened to the point where Joe could barely move. Walking caused pain. Standing caused pain. Sitting caused pain. Eventually, just breathing caused pain. "Okay, so I go to the doctor, figuring he'll give me something and I'll be okay in a week or two. After all, how bad could this be?" That was three years ago, and Joe hasn't been back to work since.

The Chronic Pain Syndrome

Chronic pain is a problem that affects tens of millions of Americans, disrupts job, family, and social functioning, and is responsible for four billion lost work days every year (Hanson & Gerber, 1990; Osterweis, Kleinman, & Mechanic, 1987). Continuing research supports the view of chronic pain as a complex, multidimensional clinical entity that involves not only sensory elements but motivational, cognitive, and emotional components as well (Keefe & Williams, 1989; Miller, 1990, 1991b, 1992a, 1993a). Despite this, most doctors, including many "pain specialists," persist in regarding the physical and psychological aspects of chronic pain in a narrow, either-or way. This leads to much needless suffering.

Based on cumulative clinical observations and empirical studies of pain patients, it is possible to describe a fairly characteristic course of events for the chronic pain syndrome (Hanson & Gerber, 1990; Hendler, 1982; Miller, 1991b, 1992a, 1993a; Miller & Kraus, 1990). While the following scenario is certainly not preordained for all chronic pain patients, it occurs often enough to frustrate many a practitioner in the pain rehab field who just can't understand why, if so many patients get better without a fuss, a significant proportion of others, with seemingly similar physical injuries, remain disabled, often for life.

The problem typically begins with some accident or injury that causes a degree of acute pain requiring treatment. For example, the patient hurts her back in an auto accident or job injury but doesn't feel too bad right away. Nevertheless, she goes to the emergency room or company doctor, gets a brief exam and a few X-rays, and is told "there's nothing really wrong with you, take the rest of the day off, go home and rest up for a couple of days, and get back to work." But over the next few days, the pain gets worse and the patient visits her doctor again, or sees another doctor who does another exam, takes more X-rays or perhaps an MRI, and prescribes muscle relaxants and anti-inflammatories, reassuring the patient that she'll be all right in a week or two.

However, here it is several weeks later, and the pain is no better; in fact, if anything, it's gotten worse. At this point, the patient is referred to a "specialist," typically an orthopedist or physiatrist, who performs yet another exam, takes yet another MRI, and places the patient in physical therapy, often located right there in the doctor's office or outpatient pain clinic or rehab center.

Several months go by with little or no improvement. Now begins what Hendler (1982) calls the "chronic pain odyssey." The patient travels from doctor to doctor, clinic to clinic, pain center to pain center. Various medical treatments are applied, but none of these seems to work, and the pain just won't go away. Each new treatment or physician briefly raises hope, which is then quickly dashed when the new procedure fails to cure the pain. The patient now discovers that the "experts" in the pain field won't even see her because they don't take accident or Workers Compensation cases. Or she may wait months for an appointment with one of these medical bigshots, who then barely glances at the voluminous records the patient has so painstakingly compiled, performs whatever perfunctory exam the doctor's packed schedule permits, takes still another set of MRIs and pronounces that "it's just soft tissue injury" (typically without taking the time to explain what that means), and "there's nothing really wrong with you."

The patient is now left with no choice but to cycle through the original set of doctors once again, who continue to find "nothing wrong" based on their brief exams and the limited tests they conduct. The patient's growing disappointment, resentment, and bitterness toward the medical profession is matched by commensurate hostility from the other direction, as doctors come to dread another visit from the "crock."

Meanwhile, the insurance company is threatening to cut off benefits, bills are mounting because of the patient's unemployment, the family is bickering, and the pain is getting worse, so at some point a lawyer is called in to "straighten things out." One of the first things the attorney does is send the patient to yet another pain specialist or orthopedic surgeon who—surprise!—does another exam, takes more MRIs, and sends a lukewarm report to the attorney, but one that holds out a glimmer of hope that "something can be done," either through surgery (but making no promises, of course), more physical therapy, or classifying the patient as disabled with entitlement to a cash payout.

Naturally, the insurance company is entitled to its own independent medical examination (IME)—another exam, more MRIs—typically carried out by an insurance company physician with a reputation for being "tough on pain cases." Predictably, the IME finds no significant pathology and makes a determination of maximum medical improvement, or MMI, which essentially means that the patient is as better as she's going to get and therefore requires no further treatment. Patient's translation: we've wasted enough money on this crock—dump her. At this point, with the case dragging on, the patient's attorney recommends "settling out," mainly so the lawyer can get paid and move on to other cases.

The ongoing struggle with persistent pain, ineffective treatment, and life stresses caused by debt and disability continually grinds the patient down. There develops a growing tendency to conceptualize all areas of life in terms of greater or lesser degrees of pain. Depression, hypochondriacal preoccupation, and death anxiety increasingly dominate the clinical picture. Disturbed sleep and appetite compound the fatigue and disability, and excessive or inappropriate medication makes the patient even more groggy and irritable.

By now, pain has become the overwhelming central focus of the patient's life. External attachments and interests are abandoned as she devotes more and more time to the crusade of finding a miracle cure, obtaining sufficient medication, or seeking compensation. As family and friends tire of their conscripted service to this lost cause, they begin to withdraw and avoid the patient: "We've had it. We've done everything for you, put ourselves in debt, waited on you hand and foot, taken you to every doctor in the world, and you still won't get better." The patient's reaction is typically one of wounded outrage at this perceived abandonment and betrayal, fueling resentment still more, and further contributing to her near-total isolation.

Pain now becomes the sole coping mechanism for all of life's stresses, continuing the downward spiral to total invalidism. Abuse of medication, illicit drugs, or alcohol may further compound the situation. In too many cases, the patient just crashes, sinking into depressed oblivion. Or she may achieve an unstable, unhealthy psychic equilibrium, continuing to struggle year after year, exhausting the good will of doctors, lawyers, family, and all those around her, and remaining a lone voice crying in her agonized wilderness.

THE PSYCHOLOGY OF CHRONIC PAIN

Psychosocial variables are among the most important factors affecting recovery from disabling pain syndromes. Research shows that individuals suffering from daily stress are more likely to report a variety of types of pain and to suffer from more frequent pain episodes. Those with a more external locus of control, who typically see events in their lives as being determined by forces beyond their control, report a higher incidence and severity of pain than those with a more internal locus of control, who view their experiences and actions as largely self-determined (Sternbach, 1986). For example, individuals who report lower levels of general psychological well-being have significantly higher scores on indices of back pain (Mechanic & Angel, 1987).

Although rehab clinicians have traditionally dichotomized chronic pain patients into those with "physical" vs. "psychological" disorders, this is hardly ever a clear-cut distinction (Benjamin, 1989). Pain is the commonest symptom in most medical settings and the second most common complaint of psychiatric patients. It is present in up to 40 percent of new psychiatric admissions, and less than half these patients have an identifiable physical cause for their pain (Delapaine, Ifabamuyi, Merskey, & Zarfas, 1978; Merskey, 1980). In patients referred to pain clinics, about 60 percent have a diagnosable physical disorder, and at least half have some kind of psychological disorder, with a considerable overlap between these groups (Benjamin, Barnes, Berger, Clarke, & Jeacock, 1988). Physiological studies show that sustained nerve root compression or pinching typically leads to numbness rather than pain, further arguing for at least some psychogenic contribution to the symptom complex in most cases of chronic low back pain (Coen & Sarno, 1989; Rosomoff, 1985).

Personality and Psychopathology

Minnesota Multiphasic Personality Inventory (MMPI) profiles of chronic pain patients reflect a tendency to manifest marked somatic concern, to use denial and repression as major psychological defenses, and to interpret problems of living in rationalized and socially acceptable terms. This is associated with poor prognosis for remotivation and a contrasting appearance of being externally extroverted and sociable, while internally self-centered, demanding, and dependent (Naliboff, Cohen, & Yellen, 1983).

In a university medical center pain clinic, Reich, Tupin, and Abramow-itz (1983) found a relatively high frequency of somatoform disorders, substance abuse disorders, affective disorders, and a diagnostic category called "psychologic factors affecting physical condition." Somewhat more histrionic and dependent personality disorder diagnoses were found, although the presence of any type of personality disorder may be a more salient characteristic of the chronic pain syndrome than any specific type—a finding also true of traumatic brain injury and substance abuse populations (Miller, 1991a, 1992b).

Pain and Depression

The commonest diagnostic association of chronic pain is with depression (Benjamin et al., 1988; Fishbain, Goldberg, Meagher, Steele, & Roso-moff, 1986; Kramlinger, Swanson, & Maruta, 1983; Krishnan, France, Pelton, McCann, Davidson, & Urban, 1985). Depending on the subject series, between 10 and 100 percent of chronic pain patients report depression at some point (Blumer & Heilbronn, 1981; Pilowsky, Chapman, & Bonica, 1977). Pain-related depression seems for the most part to improve with adequate rehabilitation, although antidepressant medication is also sometimes effective (Ward, Bloom, & Friedel, 1979).

Many clinicians and researchers have accepted the pain-depression link as axiomatic and have attempted to provide a neurobiological rationale. According to the now-classic biogenic amine theory of affective disorders, depression reflects underactivity in the catecholamine and serotonin neurotransmitter systems of the brain (Schildkraut, 1965; Shaw, Camps, & Eccleston, 1967). More recently, dysregulation of other transmitter systems, including brain enkephalins, have been added to the list (Butler, 1984; von Knorring, 1988). A key argument for the biogenic amine theory of pain and depression is that many antidepressants which are known to increase brain levels of catecholamines and serotonin are effective in alleviating both depression and pain. However, antidepressants do not relieve all pain states—or, for that matter, all depressions—and so the pain-depression link is unlikely to rest entirely on any such one-to-one biochemical association (Tunks, 1990).

Nevertheless, many of the pain patients we see in clinical practice appear depressed, although not necessarily all for the same reasons. I have found it useful to distinguish between depression, in the clinical-syndromic sense, and *demoralization*, which frequently accompanies chronic pain. This demoralization need not be associated with severe personality disorder or other significant psychopathology, and may often be quite quickly responsive to supportive psychotherapeutic intervention. In other cases, it represents the decompensation of a premorbidly superachieving individual who has characteristically coped with repressed dependency needs by extreme hard work and independence, and who has now crashed because the pain and disability no longer allow this overcompensated striving (Ford, 1977–78). Finally, many personality-disordered patients with chronic pain syndromes may have been coping with bouts of depression long before the pain syndrome began. In such cases, the depression is just another stable part of the clinical picture and should be treated accordingly.

Pain and Anger

Less well recognized is the association of pain with anger. Anger may be underestimated because of patient denial, but the triad of anger, fear, and depression may be the commonest emotional constellation in the chronic pain syndrome (Fernandez & Turk, 1995). Unexpressed anger may directly contribute to increases in pain mediated by elevated muscle tension and autonomic nervous system arousal (Kerns, Rosenberg, & Jacob, 1994), or the anger may leach out in the form of resistance to treatment, medicolegal power struggles, family manipulation, or other acts of overt or covert retaliation designed to "get back at" the patient's sense of being wronged and victimized (Braha & Catchlove, 1986; Fernandez & Turk, 1995; Miller, 1993a; Turk & Rudy, 1990). Many pain patients I encounter look angry, sound angry, and make no bones about their fierce resentment of the medical, legal, and insurance systems.

One study (Kerns et al., 1994) found that subjects who tended to internalize angry feelings and avoid interpersonal conflicts reported higher levels of pain and pain behavior, leading the authors to hypothesize a bidirectional relationship between anger and pain disability. Pervasive feelings of anger and associated hostile thoughts and aggressive behavior may interfere with effective interpersonal functioning and more generally disrupt efforts at adaptation. Conversely, failed efforts to maintain or resume a patient's premorbid level of functioning may be understandably frustrating and even irritating. Perception of a loss of control and impaired self-efficacy related to changes in functioning may further mediate the experience of anger and resentment. Untreated anger may lead to another kind of vicious cycle in which treatment fails, thus aggravating the levels of frustration and anger (Turk & Rudy, 1990, 1991).

Pain and Somatization

An often-cited major diagnostic association of chronic pain is with so-called somatoform disorder in *DSM-III* and *DSM-III-R*, (APA, 1980, 1987), this diagnosis being applied to about 10 to 15 percent of pain patients (Benjamin et al., 1988; Reich et al., 1983). These patients typically present with severe pain at single or multiple body sites. Because, in theory, these patients are using somatic complaints as a defense against disturbing emotional issues, they tend to be quite reluctant to pursue a psychological course of evaluation and treatment (Miller, 1984).

DSM-IV (APA, 1994) has included a new diagnostic subcategory, "Pain Disorder Associated With Both Psychological Factors and a General Medical Condition," recognizing that psychological disturbances can often be a consequence of persistent pain, disability, psychosocial disruption, and medicolegal aggravation following an injury, as well as other times being caused by symptom amplification due to premorbid personality or dysfunctional psychological adjustment.

Some patients complain of pain in order to establish and maintain their invalid status, with its ensuing benefits and relief from responsibility. They consult doctors repeatedly, not to obtain effective treatment, but to seek medical endorsement of their invalidism. Their covert communications usually invite the doctor to accept responsibility for treating and "curing" the patient; in fact, the patient, all the while appearing to be highly compliant, has in reality taken control of the treatment course. The doctor who fails to recognize this is likely to end up fruitlessly trying treatment after treatment, all providing only temporary benefit, thereby fulfilling the patient's need to be a permanent patient (Benjamin, 1989; Matheson, 1988; Sternbach, 1974).

Pain as a true *conversion* phenomenon—i.e., the psychodynamically symbolic transformation of an unconscious fear, wish, or conflict into a physical symptom—is generally thought to be rare in modern clinical practice (Coen & Sarno, 1989; Merskey & Buhrich, 1975; Ziegler, Imboden, & Meyer, 1960). However, I have seen a number of cases where the pain syndrome has been accompanied by other "classically hysterical" symptoms. One case involved conversion paralysis of a single leg in a male trucker with back pain who was experiencing conflicts about going back to work, anger at his job, and unrecognized dependency needs. Another case involved glove-and-stocking anesthesia in a female bookkeeper and computer operator with temporomandibular joint pain who had a history of sexual abuse and severe control/dependency/individuation issues related to feeling trapped in her family business.

Pain and PTSD

As noted above, the higher association of PTSD with traumas involving physical injury than those without (Helzer et al., 1987; Kuch, Evans, Watson, & Bubela, 1991; Pitman et al., 1989) virtually guarantees an association between pain and PTSD in at least some cases. The addition of depression to the PTSD picture often presents a particularly refractory clinical problem (Geisser, Gaskin, Robinson, & Greene, 1993).

Patients involved in motor vehicle accidents who were diagnosed with PTSD reported higher pain levels than accident patients without PTSD; they also had increased emotional distress and greater functional disability (Geisser, Roth, Bachman, & Eckert, 1996; see also Chapter 6). Pain and PTSD may feed off each other in a vicious cycle. Particularly important to consider is the diagnostic possibility that poor functional recovery in pain patients may be due in some part to undiagnosed and/or undertreated PTSD, as is the case with many cases of PTSD and traumatic brain injury (Miller, 1993b; see Chapter 3).

Chronic Pain, Personality, and Cognitive Style

How patients think about and conceptualize their pain and its implications for their future may be an important factor influencing response to treatment and long-term outcome. Cognitive distortion is a factor that can have important emotional and behavioral effects (Keefe & Williams, 1989). Chronic low back pain patients are prone to catastrophizing, overgeneralization, personalization, and selective abstraction, and patients who engage in high levels of cognitive distortion tend to be much more depressed than patients who don't (Lefebvre, 1981).

Catastrophizing and overgeneralizing are especially related to excessive disability in back pain patients, particularly with regard to sleep disturbance and impaired social relationships. Similarly, in rheumatoid arthritis patients, cognitive distortion has been found to be associated with increased depression and physical disability, even when controlling for disease severity (Smith, Follick, & Ahern, 1986; Smith, Peck, Milano, & Ward, 1986). The overwhelming majority of chronic pain patients may overestimate their baseline pain when asked to recall it following treatment (Linton & Gotestam, 1983), and subjects' recall of the reactive and emotional quality of their pain appears to be particularly subject to distortion (Roche & Gijbers, 1986).

Patients' beliefs about chronic pain strongly influence the nature of the syndrome. Patients who regard their pain as an unexplained mystery are less apt to comply with treatment and typically show an overall poorer outcome. Interestingly, patients who blame themselves for their pain tend to have lower pain levels (Keefe & Williams, 1989). Perhaps pain caused by one's own misjudgment or foolish excess is easier to bear than that which is attributed to the neglectful or malign actions of others. Indeed, a commonplace angry complaint from pain patients regarding those believed responsible (surgeon, auto driver, industrial foreman, etc.) is "How could they do that to me and get away with it?"

A strong relationship is found between *self-efficacy*—the belief in one's own effective coping abilities—and better treatment outcome in chronic pain patients, both in terms of patient self-ratings and lower medication use (Kores, Murphy, Rosenthal, Elias, & Rosenthal, 1985). Active coping strategies are generally more effective for resisting stress than passive ones (Tan, 1982; Turk, Meichenbaum, & Genest, 1983), and certain patterns of thinking may be intrinsically pathogenic, for example, resentfulness, avoidance, or catastrophizing (Crook, Tunks, Kalaher, & Roberts, 1988; Lefebvre, 1981). Cognitive impairment, which may arise from the distraction of the pain itself or from coexisting head injury and/or PTSD, appears to be related to the psychological distress and emotional disruption that are frequently associated with chronic pain (Dufton, 1989).

Family and Social Systems

Chronic pain affects others beyond the patient and the clinician, especially family, coworkers, and other familiar social systems (Miller & Kraus, 1990), and a formerly energetic, productive individual may become a social and economic liability (Gallagher, 1976; Hendler, 1982). Family and workmates may have to compensate for the patient's loss of working capacity, which tends to weaken support for the pain patient and lead to mutual resentment.

On the other hand, many relatives of chronic pain patients appear to derive "tertiary gain" (Benjamin, 1989), that is, the patient's pain and disability help other family members deny or deflect their own conflicts, and in some families, the presence of a disabled member serves to maintain intrafamilial homeostasis (Hughes, Medley, Turner, & Bond, 1987; Roy, 1985). In this context, reports of marital disharmony may actually have positive therapeutic implications, since this may mean that the spouse is failing to endorse the patient's invalidism (Benjamin, 1989). By contrast, an overly solicitous spouse has been found to be the single most important predictor of a patient's failure to comply with a behavioral pain rehabilitation program (Funch & Gale, 1986).

Indeed, there is a strong overall relationship between pain behavior and perceived quality of social support. Patients who report high satisfaction with social support show significantly higher levels of pain behavior than those reporting low satisfaction—presumably because those in the high-satisfaction group receive more positive reinforcement for their pain behavior (Gil, Keefe, Crisson, & Van Dalfsen, 1987). Patients who perceive their spouses as solicitous have higher levels of pain and lower levels of activity (Flor, Kerns, & Turk, 1987). Similar relationships between family and social support and level of disability have been described for traumatic brain injury patients (Miller, 1993c, 1993d; see Chapter 3).

Litigation Issues

Issues of litigation and compensation related to chronic pain may lead to increased suffering for the patient, which adversely affects prognosis. Pursuing claims, no matter how legitimate, may serve to focus the patient's attention on having been wronged and on restoring wounded pride, rather than on trying to adjust to a difficult situation while leading as normal a life as possible (Miller & Kraus, 1990).

However, according to some authorities (Benjamin, 1989; Tunks, 1990; Woodward, 1982), there is little to support the widely held view that dramatic improvement occurs swiftly and spontaneously after litigation has been completed. H. Miller (1961a, 1961b) originally argued that litigation was responsible for prolonging disability after injury. Since then, many studies and reviews have failed to confirm this opinion: Thus, pain symptoms and disability do not automatically evaporate after claims are settled and sufferers do not as a general rule have automatic resolution of their symptoms after settlement of their claims (Gotten, 1956; Hohl, 1974; McNab, 1964). Patients who are actively engaged in litigation tend to have about the same prevalence of symptoms as those who have had their cases settled or who were never involved in lawsuits (Hohl, 1974; Schutt & Dohan, 1968).

Several studies have found that, after case settlement, many patients do not return to work, and many of those who do end up with lighter, lower-paying jobs (Balla & Moraitis, 1970; Encel & Johnson, 1978; Mendelson, 1982; Tarsh & Royston, 1985). Here again, there is a parallel with closed head injury: Despite the widespread belief in litigation-related malingering of cognitive symptoms in this group, there is little actual evidence that this occurs on a wide scale (Miller, 1998; Oddy, 1984).

My own experience with both chronic pain and brain injury patients (Miller, 1991b, 1992a, 1993a,b,c,d, 1996a, 1996b, 1998) is that when the syndrome derives most of its motivating force from the desire to evade work and other responsibilities and/or to "cash in" on the disability, litigation issues by themselves may be sufficient to entrench the syndrome. On the other hand, where the problem is more a part of overall personality dysfunction, litigation issues are often less important from an actual monetary standpoint and more related to efforts at legitimizing the patient's outrage by suing and punishing the "guilty" party.

The Psychodynamics of Chronic Pain

Psychodynamic approaches have been advocated for a variety of somatization phenomena since the time of Breur and Freud (1895). Modern authorities seem to agree on the potential value of understanding the personality dynamics of individual pain patients, but there is far less consensus on how these insights might translate into more effective treatment.

Pain commonly signals a threat to the person, and therefore the integrity of the ego requires an adjustment, a sense of protective closure (Swanson, 1984). Whether the threat is an observable injury, loss, guilt, or existential anxiety, for most people it is more psychologically acceptable to cope with an assumed tangible bodily event than a "mental problem." It has been observed that many pain patients seem to have led "painful lives," including childhood trauma, family disruption, personal loss and failure, death of loved ones, and so on. They seem to be unable to release emotional pain through appropriate verbal communicative channels. Thus, when a physical injury or illness fortuitously occurs, the physical pain is latched onto and prolonged as a substitute for the emotional expression (Dorsel, 1989).

It has been observed that many pain patients tend to be unassertive, passive, and martyrlike. They are overly dependent on others and constantly fearful of both specific situations and life in general, which leads to withdrawal and further inaction. Helplessness is the hallmark of many chronic pain patients, and they induce others to take care of them through a variety of tactics, including threatening, demanding, acting hurt, projecting guilt, feigning compliance, and blaming others. Since these patients tend to be deficient in basic social, family, academic, job and/or leisure skills—any means, that is, for expressing themselves or dealing with their psychologically painful lives other than by somatic complaints and invalidism—what would seem to be a relatively nonserious injury is blown way out of proportion due to the concentration of intense psychological pain "escaping" through the site of the physical injury (Dorsel, 1989).

Coen and Sarno (1989) have provided similar insights from their experiences in treating chronic low back pain patients. In this view, intolerance of emotion and conflict is the main psychodynamic factor, and this increases the patient's state of anxiety, tension, guardedness, and defensiveness, which expresses itself through the musculoskeletal system. Conflict is sidestepped, rather than adaptively coped with, and a secondary absorption in, and preoccupation with, the somatic symptoms further avoids, and at the same time is infiltrated by, the underlying conflicts. Hypervigilant attentiveness to symptoms is abetted by the patient's fear of what will become of her, and by some physicians' misguided, if well-intentioned, admonitions about the need for "rest" and the dangers of "overexertion."

Although many patients respond adequately to expressive and supportive psychotherapeutic approaches, Coen and Sarno (1989) report that about five to ten percent of their low back pain patients require more intensive treatment because of the persistence and/or debilitating effects of the chronic pain syndrome. This subgroup of patients tend to have especially rigid character defenses against experiencing feelings and wishes that they fear might lead others to make unfavorable judgments and withdraw their support. For example, awareness and expression of intense angry criticism make such patients anxious, penitent, and placating. Fears of being gotten rid of or of being unloved are heightened by awareness of their feelings of overriding "badness." They become more anxious, try to protect themselves from awareness of such angry/destructive feelings, and seek proof of acceptance through self-torture and demonstration of their martyred "goodness."

Coen and Sarno (1989) note that once back pain occurs, "these patients make use of it as expression of dependent longings (to be cared for as ill), defense against affects and wishes that cannot be tolerated and integrated (by preoccupation with the somatic symptoms, emphasis on passivity and helplessness), punishment through pain and suffering, and (unacknowledged) angry and sadistic attacks on caretakers (internal and external objects) through one's suffering" (p. 368). Because of their difficulty tolerating and integrating their perceived negative qualities, these rigid characters are relatively unable to rely on themselves to provide ongoing self-assessment, self-guidance, and self-direction. As a consequence, everyone suffers.

PSYCHOPHYSIOLOGY OF
CHRONIC PAIN

As in many of the other traumatic disability syndromes considered in this book, the interaction of neurobiology and psychodynamics in the genesis and persistence of chronic pain typically involves a vicious mind-body cycle.

The psychophysiology of the pain response has been reviewed by Flor et al. (1990). Pain episodes, as well as other stressors, may trigger increased sympathetic nervous system activation and elevated muscle tension. If stress- or pain-related muscular contractions occur in a sustained or repeated pattern, this information is transmitted to the spinal cord via specialized mechanoreceptors. This then sets off a neuromuscular and sympathetic reflex that leads to further increases in muscle tension and constriction of blood vessels, aggravating the pain still more.

As muscle tension is sustained for prolonged periods of time, impaired blood supply and oxygenation may develop in the affected muscle, leading to the release of pain-producing substances, such as bradykinin, that activate chemosensitive pain receptors. The ensuing pain experience increases muscle tension and sympathetic activity still more, thus exacerbating the vicious cycle of chronic pain. Moreover, pain receptor input may be enhanced through sympathetic "overflow" due to increased stress, anxiety, or anger. This results in the release of even greater amounts of adrenalin and noradrenalin, further heightening pain receptor sensitivity. Combined with the effects of catastrophizing cognitions ("This is horrible! I'll never get better!"), overall pain perception may climb to subjectively unbearable levels under states of anger, fear, or stress.

Extending the above conceptualization, Coderre et al. (1993) have proposed a *central neuroplasticity model* of chronic pain in which peripheral injury produces CNS changes that persist even after input from the injury ceases or is removed. In this model, prolonged sensory disturbances associated with tissue injury result from either a reduction in the threshold of pain receptors or an increase in the excitability of CNS neurons involved in pain transmission. With repeated pain stimulation, sensitization of pain-responsive neurons within the spinal cord, brainstem, and other CNS sites contributes to the worsening levels of chronic pain over time. The pain, originally caused by noxious peripheral stimulation, has now "moved into" the nervous system, where it takes on a life of its own.

In the brain, neurons in the somatosensory thalamus of chronic pain patients display high spontaneous firing rates, abnormal bursts of electrical activity, and evoked responses to stimulation of body areas that do not normally activate these neurons. According to this model, a closed neural circuit within the limbic system progressively induces a sensitized state in such limbic structures as the hippocampus, mamillary bodies, anterior thalamic nuclei, and cingulate cortex—the same limbic loop that is responsible for mediating the heightened stress response in PTSD (see Chapter 1). This may partially explain the frequent association of chronic pain with PTSD—recall the "somatomorphic type" of PTSD from Chapter 1 (Alarcon, Deering, Glover, Ready, & Eddleman, 1997)—and why treatment of one syndrome may not be effective without addressing the other.

With regard to treatment (see also below), Coderre et al. (1993) review the clinical evidence suggesting that the central pain-sensitizing effects of surgical procedures may in fact be prevented by the appropriate administration of analgesic agents. When given sufficient medication up front, so that the pathological pain loop is not allowed to develop in the first place, the patient may actually require lower doses of pain medication postoperatively, with the duration of postoperative analgesia in many cases outlasting the direct pharmacological effect of the drug. In these cases, the CNS seems to have, in effect, been "taught" to "keep the pain out" of the nervous system by blocking the physiological component of the chronic pain syndrome. Other evidence suggests that in cases of sudden traumatic injury, where analgesic pretreatment is of course impossible, diligent pain relief efforts in the acute stages and in the first few weeks of recovery may help forestall a debilitating chronic pain syndrome.

But medications are not the only treatment of choice for dealing with acute and chronic pain. As Coderre et al. (1993) point out, and as will be discussed further below, the effectiveness of behavioral, suggestive, coping-skills, and other psychotherapeutic techniques may involve a similar kind of psychophysiological preemption of persistent refractory pathological pain memory traces.

PSYCHOLOGICAL TREATMENT OF CHRONIC PAIN

Given the complex, intertwining psychophysiological nature of the chronic pain syndrome, it follows that any kind of successful treatment program will have to address the patient at both physical and psychological levels of dysfunction.

Pain Management and Pain Clinics

In the past 20 years, a veritable industry of "pain rehab" centers has sprung up across the U.S. and around the world. Although there are individual variations, treatment approaches at these facilities generally follow one or a combination of two main models. First, there are treatments based on the concept of *operant pain behaviors* (Fordyce, Fowler, Lehman, Delateur, Sand, & Trieschmann, 1973; Fordyce, Roberts, & Sternbach, 1985). Following the operant model, behaviors related to pain may be positively reinforced by their desirable consequences, such as increased care, sympathy, and nurturance, and at the same time negatively reinforced by avoidance of aversive consequences, such as an unrewarding job or having to face unpleasant family and social responsibilities. Treatment therefore consists of changing environmental contingencies to stop reinforcing learned pain behaviors, while systematically rewarding "well" behaviors (Benjamin, 1989).

Second, *cognitive-behavioral* approaches generally involve training the patient to identify inappropriate negative beliefs and expectations about pain and to use specific cognitive strategies and skills—often along with biofeedback, hypnosis, relaxation, stress management, and attention-diversion techniques—to replace these with more appropriate positive ideation and coping responses (Hanson & Gerber, 1990; Phillips, 1988; Turk et al., 1983; Turner & Chapman, 1982).

Linton (1982) reviewed 15 reports of operant behavioral treatment and found that all showed improvement on some measures for some patients. Similarly, of 21 studies of biofeedback-assisted and nonassisted relaxation, all except one reported some improvement in pain, although the successful cases involved mainly electromyograph (EMG) biofeedback for headache pain. There is far less evidence for the value of other biofeedback modalities, and it has also been suggested that while relaxation may be a useful coping strategy, biofeedback may encourage somatization and chronicity (Benjamin, 1989; Turner & Chapman, 1982). Moreover, in some cases relaxation itself may not be without its adverse side effects (Lazarus & Mayne, 1990; Miller, 1994). Six studies of various cognitive strategies all claimed some improvement (Linton, 1982; Tan, 1982), as did 16 studies of hypnosis (Turner & Chapman, 1982). However, methodological limitations of these studies may limit their clinical generalizability (Benjamin, 1989).

The overall impression is that the majority of pain patients who are willing to accept and comply with these kinds of treatments improve to a considerable extent and maintain improvement at follow-up (Benjamin, 1989; Shealy & Cady, 1998). There is some evidence that more strictly operant treatments are more effective in increasing physical activity, reducing medication, and preventing unnecessary disability, but tend to ignore beliefs and feelings about pain (Doleys, Crocker, & Patton, 1982; Draspa, 1959; Fordyce et al., 1973; Fordyce et al., 1985; Fordyce, Brockway, Bergman, & Spengler, 1986; Linton, Melin, & Stjernlof, 1985; Tunks, 1988, 1990). On the other hand, cognitive-behavioral methods result in a greater reduction in pain complaints but fail to alter environmental contingencies, including inappropriate medical treatments and family attitudes and behaviors, that help reinforce pain behavior and ongoing disability (Benjamin, 1989; Turner & Chapman, 1982).

Most inpatient or outpatient coordinated programs for chronic pain involve a treatment "package." Usually the underlying approach is based on physical therapy and rehabilitation to improve physical function, despite the acceptable continuation of at least some pain. The quest for a specific physical cause leading to a specific "cure" that can be administered to the passively recipient patient is discouraged, and the patient is urged to take increasing responsibility for her progress toward recovery. Most pain treatment packages rely on some combination of operant and cognitive-behavioral approaches (Benjamin, 1989; Hanson & Gerber, 1990; Phillips, 1988; Shealy & Cady, 1998).

Components of most pain treatment packages include the following: (1) the identification of specific behavioral goals, such as return to family, employment, or recreational activities; (2) a contract, treatment plan, or other agreement specifying treatment offered and accepted, and mutual commitments; (3) operant-based activity programs to increase appropriate behaviors and reduce such inappropriate pain behaviors as verbal complaints, inactivity, and inappropriate use of physical treatments; (4) exercise and increased activity level; (5) liaison with other involved agencies—medical, social, vocational, and others—to establish a consistent and coordinated approach; (6) marital or family therapy to ensure consistency in reinforcement schedules and to resolve associated problems in relationships; (7) cognitive-behavioral strategies to identify and replace inappropriate thoughts about pain; (8) relaxation training, sometimes with biofeedback and/or hypnosis, to provide a sense of self-control and mastery over pain; (9) problem-solving, communication skills, assertiveness training, and social skills training; (10) medication monitoring, with the goal typically being the reduction and eventual elimination of unnecessary pain medication, especially narcotics; (11) individual psychotherapy for specific personal issues, where indicated (Benjamin, 1989; Hanson & Gerber, 1990; Phillips, 1988; Shealy & Cady, 1998; Turk et al., 1983). With regard to outcome, the overriding impression seems to be that these "packages" lead to worthwhile improvements for the majority of patients who comply with them (Benjamin, 1989; Hanson & Gerber, 1990; Shealy & Cady, 1998).

One application of the cognitive-behavioral approach to the outpatient treatment of chronic pain (Skinner, Erskine, Pearce, Rubenstein, Taylor, & Foster, 1990) has particular relevance for the development of effective, yet low-cost pain management programs. The authors point out that outpatient programs are less expensive to run and may be more effective in the long term, as patients remain in contact with their normal environment while learning and practicing new behaviors in the clinic. Their program, which takes place one afternoon per week for seven weeks and is conducted by a multidisciplinary team, aims to increase patients' skills for coping with chronic pain and its social, emotional, and physical consequences. In this model, ideas of helpless passivity and constant cure-seeking are challenged and the notion of active control over pain management is encouraged (Turk et al., 1983).

In Skinner et al.'s (1990) program, each afternoon's schedule is highly structured. In the *group discussion* period (one hour), patients are first encouraged to shift from a purely sensory view of pain to a multicomponent view modeled after the gate control theory of pain (Melzack & Wall, 1965). The influence of psychological factors on pain of all kinds is emphasized, and patients are taught cognitive skills to deal with stress and pain. Next follows one hour of *physical exercise* designed to improve general fitness and confidence in performance of physical activity. After a break, a one-hour *lifestyle planning group* session develops individual goals in the areas of paid work, self-care, analgesic medication reduction, and social life. Wherever possible, these involve close friends or relatives. Thirty minutes each afternoon are spent practicing a *progressive relaxation exercise*, and patients are given a tape recording for home use between sessions.

Skinner et al.'s (1990) study demonstrated the clear feasibility and efficacy of an outpatient pain program, all patients showing a significant improvement from baseline functioning on admission. As a result of this program, patients were less depressed, less anxious, more active, and more likely to report that they could cope with life and with their pain. The generally successful outcome in terms of overall life functioning occurred despite the fact that measures of pain intensity, per se, were largely unchanged. In sum, this study suggests that results comparable to those reported from expensive inpatient residential pain treatment programs can be achieved in less time and at lower cost when done on an outpatient basis.

Another study (Heynemann, Fremouw, Gano, Kirkland, & Heiden, 1990) emphasizes the necessity of taking into account individual differences in personality and cognitive style in the application of cognitive-behavioral therapies. Cognitive coping strategies may be divided into two broad subtypes: *self-instructional training* that attempts to alter subjects' self-statements and cognitive appraisal of the pain; and *attentional diversion training* that attempts to divert attention away from the pain (Turk & Genest, 1979).

Heynemann et al. (1990) found that, for subjects classified as catas-trophizers, self-instruction works better in terms of improving pain toler-ance scores, while attention diversion is the more effective strategy for noncatastrophizers. These findings highlight the importance of individual differences in mediating the effectiveness of cognitive-behavioral thera-pies for pain (Kendall & Watson, 1981). Failure to take such personality and cognitive style variables into account may be one reason for lack of optimum effectiveness of "generic" pain management programs applied indiscriminantly to diverse patient populations.

Psychotherapy of Chronic Pain

But you can't just treat people like machines. Especially in cases of posttraumatic pain syndromes, appropriate psychotherapy that is able to deal with "messy" psychodynamic variables is essential for lasting recovery. Given the seemingly wide interest in personality variables contributing to the chronic pain syndrome, there are surprisingly few published studies dealing with the psychodynamic treatment of chronic pain. The general consensus from recent reviews is that, while a psycho-dynamic perspective may be helpful in understanding the process of psychogenic pain development, patients with these disorders are gener-ally regarded as unsuitable for "true" psychotherapy; instead, treatment techniques are typically limited to information, explanation, and support (Benjamin, 1989; Kellner, 1986). Indeed, one gets the impression from reading clinical accounts of such cases that many therapists find these patients irritating, frustrating, and distasteful to work with.

In line with the psychodynamic conception of physical pain as an expression of psychological pain, Dorsel (1989) sees the first step in therapy as bringing this psychological pain into awareness, affirming its significance, and encouraging the patient to accept personal issues that have been the source of considerable stress in her life. This lays the groundwork for teaching the patient new outlets and techniques for handling future psychological pain. The patient must learn through guided and monitored practice how to express emotions appropriately, how to be more assertive, how to relax and cope with daily stresses, how to communicate effectively with family members and others, and how to develop her academic, occupational, and recreational potential as nec-essary for overall well-being.

In my practice, I find that chronic pain is often an expression of longing for other types of somatic stimulation, particularly that related to affection. Patients who feel rejected or neglected by their mates, who long for close physical contact, or who experience a dearth of physical, sexual, or emotional intimacy may channel this deprived feeling into heightened pain sensations. Accordingly, encouraging physical and emotional intimacy—hugging, holding hands, giving each other a massage, playing contact games such as "Twister," cooking a meal together, or watching a funny movie and sharing the viscerally intimate communication of a good laugh—often goes a long way in ameliorating the feeling of somatic deprivation.

Coen and Sarno (1989) maintain that the majority of their chronic back pain patients show some degree of recovery simply as the result of plain-spoken, empathic explanation of the role of anxiety and defensive states in causing back pain, together with reassurance that this is a reversible, self-limited syndrome. For patients with more refractory pain syndromes, the therapist must project a sense of resolute confidence that the pain is not due to undiscovered physical injury, but is psychologically derived and self-limited. The patient must be gently but firmly confronted with her intolerance and fear of her own wishes and feelings. The more severe the case, the more imperative it is that the patient's hypervigilance and character rigidity be interpreted early on. She must be made aware of how strongly she believes that anything negative in her makes her unacceptable, and assured that her pain will not disappear until she is able to stop scrutinizing her physical symptoms and believing that she can be worthwhile only if she is "all good."

In effect, the capacity to tolerate one's own affective life seems to portend a break in the vicious cycle of dysfunctionally disabling back pain. When patients are able to accept themselves, the residual, organic chronic pain that continues to persist typically recedes into the background of life, instead of cannibalizing the patient's whole consciousness. The patient may still get a nasty twinge from time to time, but she says her "ouch," rubs the tender spot with perhaps a momentary moue of self-sympathy, shrugs, and gets on with what she's doing.

In summary, dealing with anger, dependency/control issues, and inability to verbally and directly express emotions are crucial elements of virtually all effective courses of psychotherapy for chronic pain. This is particularly true when the pain has its origin in a traumatically frightening and disorganizing experience. As with all traumatic disability syndromes, the more a patient's chronic pain entwines and expresses her characterologically dysfunctional style of coping with distress, the more intensive must be the therapeutic effort to unknot the stranglehold of the mind on the body.

Just as important, taking the time and care to make an accurate diagnosis and provide appropriate treatment for the legitimate physical aspects of a patient's pain, instead of dismissively labeling refractory cases as "crocks," demonstrates respect for the patient that is fundamental to any therapeutic relationship, and which, when absent, virtually guarantees an adversarial maelstrom designed to sink the treatment process.

The various therapeutic approaches discussed in this chapter, and the models from which they stem, should not be seen as competing; on the contrary, there is some evidence to suggest that, within reason, the more such treatments are used together, the greater their therapeutic effect (Benjamin, 1989; Hanson & Gerber, 1990). The effectiveness of this multimodal approach to treatment seems to apply not just for pain and other traumatic disability syndromes, but also for the personality disorders and other psychological syndromes that frequently underlie them (Sperry, 1995). Probably, the most important question will turn out to be not which treatment is most effective but which treatments work best with which pain patients (and their families) with which kinds of pain disorders (Benjamin, 1989; Shealy & Cady, 1998; Turk & Rudy, 1991).

Finally, as with traumatic disability syndromes generally (see Chapter 12), we should study the vast majority of pain sufferers who are coping well and who therefore manage to stay *out* of the pain treatment centers. Lessons from such success stories may yield valuable clues to improving our treatment of those patients who persistently remain tormented in body, mind, and spirit.

Chapter 5

POISONED MINDS

Toxic Trauma, Chemical Sensitivity, and Electrical Injury

The diseases which destroy a man are no less
natural than the instincts which preserve him.

—George Santayana

The call came in just as they were going off shift. Warehouse fire, unknown extent, possible occupants, possible arson, police already called to the scene. The three paramedic firefighters, Freddy, Jean, and Carlos, grumbled about the late call, but called for a backup fire unit and raced to the incident location. When they arrived, a two-man police cruiser was already on the scene, one officer on the car radio, the other already in the building, searching for the reported occupants.

There didn't seem to be much smoke, so Carlos and Jean began to make their way inside the warehouse, while Freddy ran back to the truck to get breathing gear. The backup fire engine then arrived, and three more firefighters jumped off the rig and began to make their way toward the warehouse, gear on, hoses ready. Meanwhile, the police officer by the car apparently couldn't wait and went inside the building to search for his missing partner.

Just then, Carlos staggered from the building, practically dragging Jean along with him with one hand and pushing the protesting police officer outside with the other. Their faces and clothes were covered with a brownish, greasy, acrid-smelling substance, and their voices were a rasp. Freddy turned his attention to giving medical aid to his coworkers, who had now collapsed in a heap next to the ambulance.

Meanwhile, two of the later-arriving firefighters were carrying the unconscious police officer out of the building and making for the ambulance, expecting help. Then one of the firefighters brought out another man, an unknown civilian, who had been inside the warehouse before the police car arrived. By this time, Jean was feeling well enough to attempt rescusitation on this unidentified victim. The standing officer had radioed for more help, and another fire truck and a civilian ambulance pulled up. All of the injured were taken to a nearby hospital, while the remaining firefighters handled the blaze.

This is the story I was able to reconstruct more than twelve months after the incident. Several years ago this case came to my attention in the course of a complex insurance and litigation dispute. Carlos and Jean were referred for a neuropsychological evaluation to see if the strange assortment of symptoms and complaints they were reporting were "just psychosomatic," as one insurance company attorney had put it. Both had been off work status and on full disability since the incident.

I interviewed each of these patients individually, and they both reported the same basic cluster of symptoms. Both had shown marked, persistent increases in blood pressure, and Carlos was now on antihypertensive medication. They experienced bouts of headache, nausea, and dizziness. Their arms and legs became weak, tremulous, and numb whenever they attempted any kind of strenuous work. They were prone to drenching sweats, especially at night or in hot weather. They had trouble concentrating and remembering. They slept poorly, often jarred awake by nightmares. They had become more irritable and emotionally labile. The taste of many foods seemed to have gotten either too bland or too sharp; both had lost weight. And they were plagued with an ever-present, acrid, "turpentiney" smell and taste that no amount of toothbrushing, mouthwash, breathmints, nasal sprays, or, in Jean's case, even dental work could eradicate.

Reportedly, one of the later-arriving firefighters had developed similar symptoms, and the unconscious police officer and the civilian—a warehouse employee, it turned out—were supposedly "messed up pretty bad," but reliable information was hard to pin down because of the legal issues.

Neuropsychological assessment of these firefighters showed mild deficits in concentration, memory, and complex problem-solving, as well as impaired spatial reasoning, motor speed, and manual dexterity. Their current overall IQs were in the low average to borderline retarded range, probably at least somewhat lower than what one would expect in trained emergency medical technicians and firefighters. Worse than the cognitive effects, however, was the emotional impact. Both of these workers had excellent prior service records and had enjoyed good health. After the incident—probably at least partly in response to the insurance claims and litigation issues—they had been treated like fakers, slackers, nut jobs, and pariahs by doctors, lawyers, claims adjusters, and many of their own supervisors and coworkers. Nobody seemed to have any definitive answers as to what was wrong with them. "How could this happen?" Jean exclaimed at one point. "I feel like my mind's been poisoned, my whole life's been poisoned. Doesn't anybody know about these things?"

I wish I knew then what I know now. Less than a decade ago, there was virtually no readily available published information on the neuropsychological and emotional effects of toxic exposure. In fact, I became interested in this area largely because of a few referred cases such as the above one that traditional clinical explanations couldn't account for. In the last few years, some research findings and clinical insights have started to appear from the emerging field of *neurotoxicology* (Hartman, 1995; Valciukas, 1991). This chapter will describe the main types of toxic substances known to affect thought, mood, and behavior. Then, the kinds of posttraumatic toxic stress syndromes that may develop following such exposures will be described. Finally, the chapter will describe the effective psychotherapeutic strategies that are beginning to be developed for this patient group.

TOXIC INJURY: A SPECIAL KIND OF TRAUMA?

Approximately 60 thousand chemicals and two million mixtures are currently used in manufacturing and industry, and more than a thousand new chemicals are developed every year. Only a fraction of these substances have been adequately studied to determine their effect on human health and behavior. In the United States alone, as many as 20 million workers a year are exposed to chemicals that can potentially injure the nervous system. Uncounted millions more come into daily contact with commercial products or other substances that can affect the brain and behavior (Koestner & Norton, 1991).

In addition, exposure to hazardous substances is often a traumatic event. Being "poisoned" has a frightening connotation that goes deep into the collective psychological and cultural unconscious of humankind. It conjures up fears of diabolical possession, the casting of evil spells, moral and spiritual uncleanness, ostracism and banishment from the community, and—especially in more modern times—insidious contami-

nation and conspiracy. In fairness, these industrial and commercial chemical products are obviously useful in our daily lives, or we wouldn't be
producing and using them in such quantities. But let's hope that as a
result of the accumulating knowledge from toxic injury cases, increased
attention will be paid to these substances' potentially harmful effects,
and more responsibility exercised in their manufacture and use.

EFFECTS OF TOXIC INJURY ON THE
BRAIN AND BEHAVIOR

The nervous system is a sensitive target for toxic agents in several ways
(Koestner & Norton, 1991). First, the adult neuron does not replicate
and, therefore, replacement of lost brain cells is not possible. Second,
while the blood-brain barrier prevents the passage of many substances
into the brain, it permits many others to enter. Third, since the normal
functioning of the nervous system requires complex, integrated networks
of activity, damage to even a small portion of the brain can result in
marked effects on behavior. Fourth, neurons are dependent on glucose
and oxygen as constant sources of energy, and cell bodies and fiber
processes in some brain areas exist at borderline levels of vascularization.
If high energy demands are placed on the system or if delivery of oxygen
or glucose to the neurons is reduced by any pathophysiological mechanism, selective neuronal death can occur.

The reaction of the nervous system to toxic substances is varied for
several reasons. Exposures to toxic agents may result in microscopic
lesions restricted to specific neuronal sites, e.g., cell body, axon, dendrites,
myelin, or vascular tissue, and often to selectively vulnerable groups of
neurons. Acute and long-term exposures may have markedly different
consequences for the central nervous system. The neuronal injury caused
by toxicity may further depend on the species, age, or sex of the exposed organism.

There are marked regional differences in the structural and biochemical composition of different parts of the nervous system, and the propensity for many toxic agents to cause localized damage reflects this.
Generally, low doses of toxic substances produce more selective effects,
whereas large doses or prolonged exposures increase the number of areas
and types of cells that are affected. After injury, functional recovery may
not be complete for months or years after a single exposure to a toxic
agent. Once the immediate damage from cell death is resolved, regrowth
of brain tissue, which includes capillaries as well as glial and neuronal
structures, may be a prolonged and incomplete process, if it occurs at all.

Toxic Substances that Produce
Neurobehavioral Impairment

Given the enormous number of chemicals in common use, it's not surprising that neurotoxicologists have so far systematically studied only a few of the more widely used varieties. Nevertheless, we are beginning to learn a great deal about the effects of these substances on the brain and behavior (Eskenazi & Maizlish, 1988; Hartman, 1995; Miller, 1993b, 1995; Valciukas, 1991). To date, the classes of toxic substances on which there exists a reasonable neuropsychological data base include the following.

ORGANIC SOLVENTS.   Organic solvents have a special affinity for fatty tissues such as brain. The intoxication states resulting from acute, high exposure to many organic solvents is widely recognized; indeed, the short-term euphoric effects of many such substances have led to their abuse by habitual sniffers of glue and paint thinner. More common, however, are the effects of chronic, lower-level exposure to such substances in the workplace. A number of different organic solvents have been studied.

- *Styrene* is used as an industrial solvent.
- *Toluene* is commonly used as a solvent, in dyes, and in the manufacture of some kinds of explosives (e.g., "TNT" = trinitrotoluene). Toluene's main notoriety comes from being the active intoxicating ingredient that glue-sniffers enjoy.
- *Carbon disulfide* is used primarily in the rayon industry and as a grain fumigant.
- *Methyl chloride* is currently used in the production of silicones, butyl rubber, and organic lead compounds, and as a blowing agent for polystyrene packing foams.
- *Trichloroethylene (TCE)*, once used in the dry cleaning industry (now replaced by perchloroethylene, see below), is currently used for degreasing metal parts, as an adhesive in the shoe industry, and as an ingredient in inks, lacquers, and varnishes.
- *Perchloroethylene (PCE, or "Perc")* is currently the most widely used solvent in the dry cleaning industry. Garments are immersed in this degreasing agent, then as much of the chemical as possible is removed for reuse by heating and spin-drying. Perc is regulated as an air pollutant under the Clean Air Act and constitutes an environmental contaminant when found in soil and water. Measurable exposure to Perc occurs by wearing recently dry-cleaned clothes or storing them indoors, and such clothes can raise Perc levels in the house for several days. Clinically significant toxic exposure can occur in persons who

work in, or live near, dry-cleaning establishments. Perc levels hundreds of times higher than acceptable have been found in the air of apartments located over dry-cleaning stores. Recently, nontoxic alternatives to Perc and other polluting compounds have begun to be tested by the dry cleaning industry (Consumers Union, 1992; Wu, 1997).

• *Trichloroethane*, or *methyl chloroform*, is used primarily in cold cleaning and metal degreasing.

ORGANOPHOSPHATE PESTICIDES.   The organophosphate pesticides are fat-soluble compounds that are rapidly absorbed through the skin, eyes, and respiratory tract. These substances are ubiquitous in the agricultural and pest control industries. The toxic effects on neurobehavioral functioning are caused by an inhibition of cholinesterase, resulting in the excessive accumulation of the neurotransmitter acetylcholine at neuronal synapses in the central and peripheral nervous system—the same mechanism of action as in many military "nerve gasses." Pesticide poisoning is especially common in agricultural workers (Reidy, Bowler, Rauch, & Pedroza, 1992).

LEAD.   The toxic effects of lead exposure have been recognized for over 2000 years; indeed, one historical theory links the fall of the Roman Empire with the widespread use of lead plumbing and utensils. Lead is common in the modern industrialized environment and most of us growing up and living in these societies have a measurable body burden of lead. *Lead encephalopathy* can result from a single severe exposure or from lower-level chronic exposure. Chronic low levels of lead, insufficient to produce a classic syndrome of lead encephalopathy, can still subtly affect nervous system functioning, especially in exposed children (Boivin & Giordani, 1995).

OTHER SUBSTANCES.   Information on the neuropsychological effects of other toxic substances is more limited; the following reports have been culled from the recent literature (see Miller, 1993b, 1998 for reviews).

• *Formaldehyde* is a popular industrial chemical used in the manufacture of many furniture and paper products, and present in many home and office environments as an airborne gas at various concentrations. Sufficiently high concentrations are detectable by a pungent odor and will irritate the eyes and respiratory tract (Eskenazi & Maizlish, 1988).
• *Manganese* is often used as a component of metal alloys, as an antiknock agent in lead-free gasoline, in the coloring of glass and soaps,

and in the manufacture of chlorine gas, electrical batteries, paints, varnish, enamel, and linoleum. Manganese ore can enter the body through inhalation or swallowing of dust particles containing manganese dioxide, and can produce cognitive impairment, emotional dyscontrol, and a movement disorder resembling Parkinson's disease (Hua & Huang, 1991).

- *Hydrogen sulfide* is a gas emitted from decaying organic matter and can produce hypoxic damage to the brain. Tvedt, Skyberg, Aaserud, Hobbesland, and Mathiesen (1991) report severe dementing brain injury in several patients exposed for varying lengths of time to hydrogen sulfide gas from the following: decaying shrimp offal at a sewage treatment plant; swine manure in an agricultural pump; a ship's hold filled with rotting fish; a tannery waste tank; and a pool of fetid water on an oil rig.

Types of Impairment Due to Toxic Exposure

Not all substances will produce all of the reported effects, and not all persons exposed to the same chemicals will show the same symptoms. However, the following classes of persistent postexposure effects seem to be reported consistently with a wide variety of toxic substances (Miller, 1993b, 1998).

- *Neurobehavioral signs and symptoms*: headache, nausea, dizziness, giddiness, fatigue, lethargy, tremor, disturbed walking, impaired coordination, muscle weakness, visual disturbances, changes in smell and taste, excessive perspiration, heart palpitations, increased blood pressure, chest tightness, intolerance of alcohol, anxiety, depression, social withdrawal, irritability, disturbed sleep, poor appetite, impaired sexual functioning, posttraumatic stress disorder.
- *Neuropsychological test findings*: impaired reaction time, impaired motor speed and dexterity, impaired vigilance, impaired learning and memory, impaired visuospatial perception and reasoning, impaired speed and efficiency of thinking, impaired problem-solving, deficits in mental arithmetic, deficits in attention and concentration, lowering of overall intellectual ability.
- *Diagnostic neurological findings*: abnormal EEGs, abnormal processing in sensory pathways, peripheral nerve damage, impaired nerve conduction.

Clearly, appropriate evaluation will yield a wide range of pathological findings in toxic exposure subjects. Where the exposure has been severe and the effects dramatic, little doubt will exist as to the presence of impairment and its relationship to the toxic injury. In milder cases, cursory medical examination may be unrevealing or ambiguous, and subjective symptoms dismissed as anxiety, hypochondriasis, or malingering. This may be a special problem for emergency services personnel who must deal with the double task of attending to civilians in toxic emergencies while maintaining their own safety and peak functional performance levels (Hermann, 1992; Howes, 1994; Kilburn, Warsaw, & Shields, 1989). It is in such cases that a careful and informed neuropsychological workup may be most useful.

CHEMICAL SENSITIVITY AND THE TOXIC STRESS SYNDROME

During the mid-1980s, when real estate values and mortgage rates were skyrocketing, Dave and Lynn, a thirty-something married couple, worked hard and saved their money for a downpayment on a beautiful home in a pleasant suburban neighborhood. It was only after they moved in that they discovered that their dream house had a few bugs in it—literally. To deal with the newly uncovered termite infestation they called a local exterminating company who tented and fumigated the house for a few days, assuring the couple that the process was "perfectly harmless to humans."

A few days after the fumigation, after what they were told was a safe interval of ventilation, the couple moved back into their home. But the house still had a chemical smell. Over the next several days, their eyes became grainy and watery, and they had trouble breathing. They developed a dry cough. At night, they sank into a dead, dreamless sleep and awoke feeling drained instead of rested. In fact, they seemed to be tired all the time. They had trouble concentrating at work. Finally, after about two weeks, they moved out of the house and in with relatives. The coughing, breathing, and eye problems abated, but the fatigue, impaired thinking, and disturbed sleep persisted.

When I first met the couple, both their faces registered extreme anger and they could barely spit out their story. "Our lives are ruined," Lynn pronounced. They were both currently unemployed and suffered from chronic fatigue, headaches, high blood pressure, dizziness, impaired memory and concentration, and anxiety about possible genetic damage and the risk to future children. Moreover, they couldn't seem to "get that bug spray smell out of our nostrils."

The couple could find no doctor who would give them a definitive diagnosis of their condition or prognosis about their recovery. If anything, their desperate search for medical validation seemed to have led to more than one cool dismissal and—adding insult to injury—a psychiatric referral. So lawyers were called in, more medical and psychological evaluations were made, and eventually this couple had gotten to me.

The Nose (Sometimes) Knows: Normal and Pathological Olfaction

Smell has a long history. The first primitive sensors possessed by the earliest primordial simple-celled creatures were chemosensory receptors that would later develop into the organs of olfaction. A couple of billion years later, most land-dwelling mammals make far greater use of smell than man, but the human olfactory sense is far from rudimentary. Moreover, the brain mechanisms that process smell and taste coevolved with the structures subserving emotion and motivation, hunting and evasion, sex and survival, learning and recall.

Smell has a long memory. Ordinarily, olfaction is a very adaptable sense, and workers in malodorous occupations, such as coroners, sanitation workers, and chemical plant operators, soon become inured to smells that would gag the novice. It seems that high exposures to even the most foul environments eventually cease to bother those who regularly live and work in them, as long as these exposures are regarded as safe and as part of business as usual.

But when exposure to strong odors occurs in the context of frightening circumstances, an opposite sort of adaptation occurs. War prisoners forced to tend decaying bodies, neighborhood residents chased out of their homes by a toxic spill, workers spattered with chemicals from a ruptured storage tank—these individuals often develop an intensified, not diminished, replication of the traumatic smell. The smell-memory connection seems to have been hyperactivated and the emotional distress manifests itself as a cloying visceral revulsion. Smell becomes a curse.

Cacosmia

A frequent complaint of individuals exposed to toxic substances, especially organic solvents, is that their sense of smell has changed. Odors seem sharper, duller, or altered in quality—food smelling like paint or smoke, for example. Odors that most people would regard as neutral or mildly annoying at most, e.g., hair spray, perfumes, gasoline, or household products, may now be perceived as noxiously pungent. This hypersensitivity to odors is often accompanied by headaches, dizziness, nausea, and other symptoms.

This postexposure syndrome has been termed *cacosmia* (Morrow, Ryan, Goldstein, & Hodgson, 1989), and it can persist for weeks or longer following a toxic exposure. It may affect as much as 15 percent of the elderly and young adult populations, 30 percent of office workers, and up to 60 percent of solvent-exposed workers (Bell, Schwartz, Amend, Peterson, & Stini, 1994; Bell, Schwartz, Peterson, & Amend, 1993). It is more common in women than men, and many sufferers are found to have a preexisting history of allergies and food sensitivities. Cacosmia is frequently misdiagnosed as a manifestation of depression, malingering, hysteria, hypochondriasis, or olfactory seizure disorder. Patients with the syndrome typically encounter a succession of examining experts who doubt the validity of their symptoms, and many such patients eventually end up as mental health referrals.

Workers with cacosmia and a documented history of solvent exposure have been found to show impairment across a wide variety of cognitive domains, such as verbal learning, visual memory, and spatial reasoning. Brief periods of sudden, intense toxic exposure seem to have a more severe impact than steady, longer-lasting, but lower-level exposures. Also, neuropsychological functioning is worse in subjects who report feeling nauseous after the exposure, which is probably a correlate of dose level. Based on these results, Ryan, Morrow, and Hodgson (1988) have hypothesized that chronic solvent exposure may affect phylogenetically ancient limbic system structures deep within the brain that subserve both smell and memory.

Multiple Chemical Sensitivity

Sometimes, however, there is no identifiable dramatic toxic event. A number of individuals seem, for all or most of their lives, to have been unusually sensitive to many different kinds of odors and substances that other people easily ignore. Those who suffer from this syndrome often resort to complicated restrictions on their activities and lifestyles in an attempt to forestall or ameliorate their symptoms. This "sensitive-to-everything," or "environmental illness," or "environmental somatization" syndrome, has been caricatured in both the scientific literature and popular press and is frequently a target of skepticism, if not downright derision and contempt, by clinicians of every specialty (Brodsky, 1983; Cone, Harrison, & Reiter, 1987; Cullen, 1987; Gothe, Odont, & Nilsson, 1995; Less-Haley & Williams, 1997; Schottenfeld, 1987; Terr, 1986,

1987); one study goes so far as to compare it to the experience of UFO abduction (Wilson, 1990).

Bell, Miller, and Schwartz (1992) and Haller (1993) have described a syndrome called *multiple chemical sensitivity*, or MCS. The symptoms may include chronic fatigue, daytime drowsiness, nightime insomnia, impaired concentration and memory, irritability, anxiety, depression, food cravings, headaches, nausea, dizziness, nasal congestion, irritation of mucous membranes, muscle and joint pain, ringing in the ears, stomach upset, heart palpitations, and inflammation of the blood vessels.

Some sufferers do trace the onset of MCS to an intial high-dose chemical exposure, for example, from moving to a new home or office, or to having their residence or workplace fumigated for pests. Or it may involve a type of substance or level of exposure that most people would not find "toxic" in the usual sense, such as furniture wax, bug spray, scented soap, or a particular kind of food. The initial exposure seems to sensitize the patient to the substance in question, so that a future encounter with even minute amounts of the chemical or foodstuff produces an even more unpleasant reaction. If the patient is forced into repeated encounters with the substance, some degree of adaptation occurs, so that the aversive response becomes blunted over time. But reexposure after a period away from the substance causes a rebound effect, so that now even smaller amounts than before produce an exaggerated sensitivity response.

Once the MCS syndrome has developed, the sensitivity generalizes from the original substance to lower and lower doses of more and more kinds of chemicals, such as perfumes, tobacco smoke, auto exhaust, newsprint, common foods, beverages (especially alcohol), and even previously tolerated medications; many of these may be entirely unrelated to the original sensitizing chemical. Total avoidance of the growing list of offending substances necessitates increasing restrictions on everyday activities, impairing overall adaptive functioning and quality of life.

The Toxic Stress Syndrome

Living with a disturbing and in some cases disabling syndrome that causes multiple symptoms, disrupts job, family, and social functioning, yet resists diagnosis and incurs clinical skepticism, cannot help but be overwhelmingly stressful. In many cases of toxic exposure, the emotional and behavioral disturbances—anxiety, depression, irritability, and general withdrawal—are more distressing and disabling than the physical symptoms themselves, and it is these emotional disturbances that may finally impel the patient toward clinical treatment, including psychotherapy (Morrow et al., 1989; Morrow, Ryan, Hodgson, & Robin, 1990, 1991).

In fact, there are striking parallels between the symptoms experienced by chemically exposed workers and reports of soldiers who have experienced wartime PTSD.

Indeed, war and toxic exposure often go together. Accounts from the First World War describe how the psychological disturbance of soldiers gassed in combat often outweighed the physical effects. Levy (1988) found a particularly high incidence of PTSD symptoms in Vietnam veterans who had been exposed to the neurotoxic defoliant Agent Orange. Interestingly, veterans who believed they had been exposed to Agent Orange were assessed as more emotionally disturbed than those who were closer to the actual spraying but had no actual knowledge of their exposure (Korgeski & Leon, 1983).

A generation later, hundreds of military service personnel developed a variety of mysterious symptoms, including chronic fevers, joint pain, fatigue, shortness of breath, sleep disturbance, impaired coordination, memory deficits, gastrointestinal disturbances, and skin rashes, upon returning home from the Iraqi war in 1991. This was named the *Gulf War Syndrome* (Adler, 1994; Milner, Axelrod, Pasquantonio, & Sillanpaa, 1994; Persian Gulf Veterans Coordinating Board, 1995), and it has been blamed on a number of suspiciously plausible, but unproved causes, such as parasitic infection, uranium poisoning from artillery shell coatings, oil and diesel fuel contamination of water supplies, or secret enemy use of nerve gas.

Of particular interest is that many of the affected soldiers spent up to six months spraying military vehicles with potentially toxic paints or solvents, such as *chemical agent-resistant coating*, or CARC. Reportedly, soldiers often worked 12-hour shifts in poorly ventilated maintenance tents. Respiratory equipment, when it was available, was largely ineffective. Over the course of a day, some soldiers reportedly breathed in so much CARC that by quitting time they were literally coughing the stuff up. When doctors at the American Academy of Environmental Medicine exposed 25 CARC-affected soldiers to normally harmless concentrations of alcohol, formaldehyde, and phenol, the soldiers all developed extreme adverse reactions characteristic of MCS.

In civilian life, Schottenfeld and Cullen (1985) found that approximately 20 percent of industrial workers referred to their clinic experienced persistent or recurrent symptoms following toxic exposure that could not be explained solely by the known effects of the chemicals themselves. Many of these patients were severely disabled by their symptoms, which included heightened physical arousal, intrusive recollections, and dreams about their exposure experiences. Some patients reported the typical PTSD symptoms of intrusive recollections or dreams of the traumatic chemical exposure event, while others experienced recurrent symptoms outside the workplace that were identical to their exposure-related symptoms. For this latter group, reliving the trauma seemed to occur in the form of reexperiencing the bodily state and somatic symptoms associated with the event, rather than in the form of intrusive words, images, or dreams. These traumatic reexperiencing episodes were frequently triggered by the odor of perfumes, newsprint, auto fumes, or other normally innocuous substances. All of these patients took great pains to avoid exposure to these offending odors, often limiting work, hobbies, socializing, or other activities. One patient wore a gas mask whenever she left the house.

ETIOLOGY OF CHEMICAL SENSITIVITY SYNDROMES

Not surprisingly, such incompletely understood syndromes as toxic trauma and multiple chemical sensitivity have spawned a variety of explanatory theories to account for their development and persistence. This section will review the main theoretical formulations most relevant to treatment.

Neurobiological Theories

To explain MCS, Bell et al. (1992) appeal to a neural sensitization model, known as *kindling,* in which repeated subconvulsive doses of stimulation to neural tissue, especially in the brain's sensitive limbic system, produce a cumulative and longlasting change in the neurophysiological response characteristics to triggering stimuli. Applied to MCS, many environmental chemicals gain access to the central nervous system via olfactory and limbic pathways, induce lasting changes in limbic neuronal activity and overall arousal levels, and thereby alter a broad spectrum of behavioral and physiological functions to produce MCS symptoms.

The lack of a blood-brain barrier in the olfactory system permits direct access via the nasal mucosa to the olfactory bulb for a wide range of environmental chemicals, including aromatic hydrocarbon solvents, aluminum, and cadmium. Macromolecular substances can move transneuronally from the primary sensory neurons in the nose to the olfactory bulb, and from there to multiple sites within the limbic system. In the present model, subconvulsive chemical kindling in the olfactory bulb, amygdala, piriform cortex, and hippocampus would act to amplify reactivity to low-level chemical exposures and to provide an initial common pathway for a variety of clinical phenomena, including cognitive and affective dysfunctions.

Bell et al. (1992) hypothesize that a range of environmental chemicals can kindle and perpetuate emotional and cognitive disorders, as well as related somatic disabilities, in vulnerable individuals via kindling mechanisms. Fat-soluble chemicals with convulsant properties, such as certain pesticides, could initiate olfactory-limbic kindling, while other agents could perpetuate the illness in a variety of target neural, endocrine, and immune systems. In this model, the individuals who would be most vulnerable to kindling and related phenomena from low levels of environmental chemicals would be those genetically predisposed to certain affective spectrum disorders such as bipolar disorder, major depression, and panic disorder, as well as those high on the variables of trait shyness and avoidant temperament.

The most important psychological factors involved in kindled MCS and toxic stress syndromes may be (1) the perception of inescapable stress either from life circumstances or from the chronic illness itself; and (2) the novelty or unfamiliarity of the setting in which chemical exposures occur. Numerous animal and human studies have shown that inescapable stress and unfamiliar environments interact with drugs and other chemical exposures to accentuate adverse effects beyond those induced by the chemical agents alone. Depressed patients who perceive themselves as helpless or extremely shy persons who react with fear to novel stimuli would be prime candidates for such biopsychosocial interactions (Bell et al., 1992).

Again, the neurophysiological similarities of MCS to chronic pain, postconcussion syndrome, and PTSD are intriguing. All of these traumatic disability syndromes involve the pathological reorganization of central nervous system mechanisms that are ordinarily adaptive for the person's healthy functioning. In response to some extraordinary environmental stressor—whether a blow to the head, exposure to a toxic chemical, ruptured lumbar disk, or frightening experience—the entire neurophysiological apparatus of the person is placed on permanent emergency standby, like a faulty computer program that won't shut down or, to use an older metaphor, a "broken record" that continues to play the same shrill, scratchy, irritating note, until it all but drives the listener crazy.

Psychological Theories

Psychotherapists understand that emotional, social, familial, and economic factors may cause symptoms to persist following almost any kind of medical illness or injury. However, some specific and distinct psychological conflicts and social disturbances seem to arise regularly following toxic exposure in the workplace. Workers often experience occupational exposure or any kind of potentially avoidable work injury as a violation of their security expectations, i.e., that employers or supervisors will provide a safe environment and financial security. When this implied understanding is breached, anger, resentment, and feelings of betrayal may interfere with recovery. In this context, physical symptoms—"real" illnesses—may represent attempts to validate injustice and legitimize dependency wishes (Horowitz, 1986; Nemiah, 1963; Weinstein, 1978).

In addition, fears about exposure to chemicals, often intensified because of lack of information or misinformation about their long-term effects, may contribute to persisting psychological impairment. Secondary gain, including reduction in marital, occupational, or social responsibilities, as well as disability payments or litigation, may further entrench persistent symptoms in the context of work-related illness or injury (Balla & Moraitis, 1970).

Morrow et al. (1989) found that over 90 percent of a sample of solvent-exposed workers showed clinically significant MMPI profile elevations on scales reflecting anxiety, depression, difficulty concentrating, heightened somatic concern, feelings of unreality, and disturbances of thinking. In a subsequent study (Morrow et al., 1991), lack of improvement or even deterioration in cognitive functioning, as measured by follow-up neuropsychological testing, occurred in solvent-exposed subjects with the highest initial MMPI scale elevations.

Some authorities have suggested that toxic trauma or chemical sensitivity may be a variant of somatoform disorder or somatization syndrome (Gothe et al., 1995; Simon, Katon, & Sparks, 1990). Brodsky (1983) characterized eight chemical sensitivity patients as longtime somatizers with histories of unexplained illnesses and high utilization of health care services. Stewart and Raskin (1985) found current, active psychiatric illness in 18 chemical sensitivity patients referred for consultation. Eight of these patients appeared to have long histories of somatization that predated the exposures.

Other authorities (Bolla-Wilson, Wilson, & Bleeker, 1988; Haller, 1993; Shusterman, Balmes, & Cone, 1988) suggest a classical conditioning model for the development of chemical sensitivity syndromes. In this conceptualization, the unconditioned stimulus of a strongly odorous chemical irritant evokes an unconditioned response of various physical and anxiety symptoms. Subsequently, the same odor, even at physiologically nontoxic or nonirritant levels, becomes a conditioned stimulus for the same (conditioned response) symptoms. Through stimulus general-ization, completely different odors can also become conditioned stimuli leading to the same conditioned response symptoms.

Guglielmi, Cox, and Spyker (1994) posit a two-factor model, i.e., classical plus operant conditioning, to explain the chemical sensitivity syndrome, which they conceptualize as similar to a phobia. According to the original two-factor model of conditioned avoidance (Mowrer, 1947), classical conditioning is responsible for the development of conditioned aversive physiological reactions to the feared stimulus, while operant conditioning provides reinforcement of avoidance and escape behaviors by a reduction of fear and distress. In the case of chemical sensitivity, escape and avoidance behaviors (e.g., staying away from "contaminated" locales or activities) are reinforced by a reduction in classically conditioned psychological and somatic distress.

Other contributory factors include observational learning and cognitive mediation. The frequently observed "contagious" nature of chemical sensitivity, the tendency of these patients to read avidly in the clinical ecology literature, to form support groups and websites, and to become environmental activists suggests that social modeling may have an important role in the development and maintenance of this syndrome. In addition, catastrophic cognitions ("I'm poisoned!" "My life's ruined!") are likely to fuel the patients' avoidance behaviors (Guglielmi et al., 1994).

Using structured diagnostic interviews and standardized self-report measures, Simon et al. (1990) studied the psychological factors associated with an outbreak of chemical-induced illness in an aerospace equipment manufacturing plant. Their findings did not support Schottenfeld and Cullen's (1985) view that chemical sensitivity syndrome, or environmental illness, is a variant of PTSD. None of these subjects met the formal diagnostic criteria for PTSD or attributed their symptoms to a single, discrete trauma. Many case histories, however, suggested that a conditioning mechanism similar to that proposed to operate in some PTSD cases may also explain the development of environmental illness. In fact, the affected subjects typically described anxiety and symptoms of autonomic arousal in response to odors of plastics or petroleum products. However, the researchers note that a prior tendency toward symptom amplification may enhance this conditioning process; for some subjects, exposure to chemicals did not appear to precipitate new symptoms as much as provide a new and convenient explanation for longstanding, chronic physical symptoms and psychological distress.

Of course, brain models and conditioning models are hardly incompatible—indeed, one implies the other, in that kindling and sensitization could provide the neurophysiological substrate for conditioned toxic stress and chemical sensitivity responses, which would then be cognitively, emotionally, and psychodynamically elaborated into one or more kinds of somatization syndrome. The main point of controversy in all these conceptualizations seems to surround the precise role of the triggering chemical agents themselves. Theory notwithstanding, however, a number of psychotherapeutic approaches have been developed for treating and managing these syndromes.

PSYCHOTHERAPY OF TOXIC TRAUMA AND CHEMICAL SENSITIVITY

Clinical Ecology

For many chemical exposure patients, the field of *clinical ecology* has heretofore been the only refuge where their complaints have been taken seriously (i.e., not "all in your head") and hopeful treatments offered (Golos, O'Shea, Waickman, & Golbitz, 1987). Support and validation can, after all, be powerful therapeutic factors in their own right—as long as they contribute to, and not detract from, other appropriate treatment.

A number of clinical ecology clinics have sprung up in recent years, most run by osteopaths, chiropractors, nutritionists, and other members of disciplines that tend to pride themselves as being relatively unfettered by conventional medical authority. Often subscribing to an allergic etiology conceptualization, clinical ecologists typically prescribe strict avoidance of provocative agents, special diets, and sometimes the use of antifungal agents (Levin & Byers, 1987; McLellan, 1987; Terr, 1987). Some forbid the wearing of cosmetics and perfumes, or the use of certain foods or products, in their presence.

While the contribution of this field must be acknowledged in terms of raising consciousness about chemical exposure effects, progress in this area has been hampered by an often far less enthusiastic adherence to basic principles of empirical science and rational clinical practice, and thus the bona fide gains of this discipline risk being overshadowed and discredited by unsubstantiated hype (Spyker, 1995). Indeed, I have worked with about half a dozen specialists in clinical ecology, and in terms of their scientific sophistication and clinical ethics, I have found them to run the gamut from well-intentioned, knowledgeable practitioners to frank crackpots and charlatans. Of course, they might say the same about many psychotherapists. In general, though, it is only quite recently that psychotherapists have begun to address toxic trauma syndromes at all.

Individual Psychotherapeutic Approaches

Recently, a number of treatment approaches for individuals with MCS have been described; most parallel the models posited for its etiology (Haller, 1993).

BEHAVIORAL AND COGNITIVE-BEHAVIORAL THERAPIES.   Classical and operant conditioning proponents favor behavioral modification treatment approaches, built around graded exposure to noxious stimuli accompanied by response prevention. That is, the patient is gradually exposed to the offending substance but helped to remain in its presence and to maintain as normal a level of functioning as possible. Relaxation exercises and/or distraction with a pleasant odor may be used to achieve response prevention and eventual extinction of the conditioned response (Bolla-Wilson et al., 1988; Shusterman et al., 1988).

A modified behavioral approach was used by Guglielmi et al. (1994) to treat three patients with MCS. The authors point out that every effort was made to take their patients "seriously" and not treat them as malingerers. The patients underwent an intensive desensitization program consisting of two-hour sessions over five consecutive days, employing biofeedback-assisted relaxation training, in-vivo exposure to the offending chemicals, and cognitive restructuring techniques. The in-vivo exposure was based on a hierarchy of noxious stimuli developed for each patient. Between sessions, the patients were asked to perform self-exposure homework assignments in their natural environments.

All three patients reportedly completed the course of therapy with success. They had acquired significant relaxation skills and were able to sustain prolonged exposure to a wide variety of noxious chemicals without demonstrating physiological or symptomatic activation. However, two patients were lost to follow-up, as they had come under treatment of clinical ecologists, and one was in therapy with a psychologist who was a fellow MCS sufferer.

SUPPORTIVE-EXPRESSIVE AND EDUCATIVE APPROACHES.   Other authorities have emphasized a more supportive form of therapy with a focus on acquiring knowledge and developing healthy coping behaviors (Haller, 1993; McLellan, 1987). In this approach, the clinician acknowledges that the patient's symptoms are real and frightening to the individual, regardless of etiology. However, focusing treatment solely on determining the etiology of patients' difficulties may only add to their feelings of frustration and anger, and therefore should be avoided. Rather than advocating strict avoidance as prescribed by clinical ecologists, the therapist encourages patients to remain social and active and to limit their avoidant behavior (Brodsky, 1987; Cone et al., 1987; Goethe et al., 1995). Inasmuch as many of these patients have led lonely, isolated lives, I recommend that the therapist instruct and model concretely the kinds of socialization skills the patient may need to function adequately in the social world.

Haller (1993) reports the application of this supportive therapy model with three female patients suffering from MCS. The treatment staff took the nonjudgmental, validating approach that each patient truly experienced the symptoms she reported, regardless of the presence or absence of observable organic pathology. Success was not measured by whether specific organic diagnoses were made, but rather by each patient's improved understanding of the impact of stress on her illness and acquisition of newfound skills for coping with effects of the illness on her life.

Techniques used to achieve these goals included supportive group and individual psychotherapy, hypnosis, and guided imagery with music. Medication regimens were simplified to reduce the risk of drug effects. At the patients' request, staff were asked to avoid personal use of perfumes and hair conditioners. However, a goal of treatment was being able to live in the real world, and patients were therefore told that a totally irritant-free environment on the unit was neither guaranteed nor desirable. Thus, air filters and special diets were not used. Instead of focusing on avoiding noxious stimuli, the main treatment focus was to help the patients lessen the illness' impact on their lives.

This approach appeared to work, since at discharge each patient had greater tolerance for noxious odors, fewer MCS "attacks," improved insight, and new awareness of a variety of coping strategies. Haller (1993) points out that approaching the evaluation and treatment from a purely psychological point of view may alienate many patients, thus sabotaging any potential for improvement. Conversely, using a purely biological model may reinforce continued isolation and functional impairment, as patients seek safe refuge from the increasing numbers of substances to which they become sensitized. In this middle-path model, individuals with MCS will benefit most from clinicians who evaluate and manage their multiple somatic complaints using a serious and nonjudgmental approach without unduly focusing on the necessity of elucidating an underlying etiology.

My main concern here is that these kinds of "open" approaches may be perceived as—and in many cases represent—a kind of diagnostic fence-sitting on the clinician's part. Remember that most of these patients have long histories of being bounced from doctor to doctor, test to test, exam to exam. They've been clucked over, dismissed, ridiculed, accused of malingering or worse, impugned by lawyers and insurance companies, and re-re-re-referred by the time they get to the psychotherapist. To the extent that trust is a basic ingredient in all forms of effective psychotherapy, the clinician at some point must usually take a stand, one way or the other, as to whether he accepts a primary chemical etiology or not.

I have found that the identification, at least provisionally, of a legitimate etiological precipitant or predisposing factor often provides a much-needed dose of diagnostic validation that can have a powerful therapeutic anti-ambiguity effect—a "reality check"—for many patients (Miller, 1997b, 1998). Similarly, Spyker (1995) notes that one of the most helpful aspects of treatment for many patients is simply having a doctor who really understands their syndrome. Yet, where no definitive precipitant can be identified, the therapist should avoid fishing for remote explanations and help the patient deal with the diagnostic uncertainty. Certainly, putative causes should not be "made up."

To this end, I find the kindling-neurosensitization model described above to provide a reasonable scientific rationale for understanding toxic trauma and chemical sensitivity syndromes, as well as a number of other traumatic disability syndromes addressed in this book (see Chapters 1, 3, and 4). There is a powerful positive therapeutic effect when a patient realizes that his disorder is understood, that there is a name and a scientifically-informed conceptual etiological mechanism for it, and that, even if treatment efficacy still lags behind diagnostic accuracy, a knowledgeable and concerned clinician is prepared to roll up his sleeves and do whatever it reasonably takes to help.

PSYCHODYNAMIC AND EXISTENTIAL THERAPIES.   Schottenfeld and Cullen (1985) suggest that some patients with toxic posttraumatic stress disorder may be amenable to exploring the relationship of their symptoms to actual or perceived exposure and to their psychological response to exposure. To the extent that preexisting personality traits influence the momentum for repetitive resensitization (Bell et al., 1992), dealing with psychodynamic issues may be a necessary component of the treatment of toxic stress in general. In this regard, toxic trauma is treated as a subspecies of posttraumatic stress disorder (PTSD), and many of the treatment recommendations discussed in Chapter 2 apply here as well.

Schottenfield and Cullen (1985) present the case of a 34-year-old married man who was exposed to a chemical solvent at work. Following the exposure, he did not recall having "typical" PTSD symptoms such as nightmares, dreams, or recurring thoughts about the exposure. However, even though medical tests were normal, he experienced recurring bouts of severe chest pain and difficulty breathing, often accompanied by nausea, dizziness, and just "feeling out of it." These symptoms could last for days and were virtually incapacitating. Since they were provoked by exposure to paints, diesel exhaust, or the fumes from a wood stove, the patient tried at all costs to avoid these substances.

The patient described the original exposure event as a terrifying experience: first being blinded by the solvent, then gasping for air, and finally passing out. He stated that he had been "too busy trying to breathe to feel scared." Currently, after a typical bout of breathlessness and chest pain, he would retire to bed, isolate himself from his family, and go over and over the details of his activities immediately prior to the accident "to see if I made any mistake." In psychotherapy, the therapist helped him to begin to think of his recurring symptoms as an "early warning system" designed to alert him to dangerous situations, but sounding many false alarms. He was gradually able to expose himself to potentially aversive situations to desensitize himself or, as he put it, "turn off the false alarm."

One of my own patients, an athletic college freshman, was referred initially for biofeedback treatment of irritable bowel syndrome. It turned out that these had begun about a year earlier, following an accident during a post-high school summer job at a local chemical plant. The patient was walking along a catwalk, which was later reportedly found to be covered with grease spots. The hapless young man slipped and plunged into a vat of viscous, bubbling chemicals, submerging completely for several seconds, and even swallowing some of the goo before being pulled out. The substance itself turned out not to be a seriously dangerous one for everyday use—indeed, as I recall, it was used as a fire-retardent component in children's clothing—but certainly was not intended for that kind of close human contact or ingestion.

In treatment, it quickly became apparent that symptom control would depend on more than biofeedback. A comprehensive medical and toxicological workup was unable to establish any direct connection between the effects of the chemical and the patient's bouts of severe cramping and diarrhea. However, the toxic traumatization had apparently reevoked a host of parental dependency issues that worked themselves out in the form of surrogate parental medical treatment-shopping and doctor-hopping. In psychotherapy, the patient was able to get in contact with the conflicts surrounding his striving for autonomy vs. his wish for someone—parent, physician, psychotherapist—to "take care of" him. Having a seemingly legitimate medical illness seemed to serve the purpose of keeping him tied in with the support-dependency systems that surrounded him. Yet, both taking the chemical plant job in the first place and actively pursuing his medical and legal claims on his own behalf represented a drive for independence.

Partway through the course of psychotherapy, the patient left town to start a business with a friend. At first I suspected this to be a "flight from treatment." However, via several follow-up calls with the patient and his family, I was satisfied that, at least for the time being, he had become more autonomous and independent in pursuing his own life's goals and doing what he truly wanted to do. Almost as a "side effect," the gastrointestinal symptoms were much improved as well.

In general, I find that individual psychotherapy with toxic trauma and chemical sensitivity patients almost inevitably moves between traditional psychodynamic and more current practical and existential issues involving trust and betrayal, autonomy and dependency, potency and helplessness, justice and victimization. While traumatization of any type reaches back into an individual's history and calls forth all manner of past psychic wounds, the psychotherapist should be careful not to overinterpret present symptomatology in terms of regressive reactions and wishes. Enough traumatization has probably occurred in the here and now, and many patients may resent the clinician's "dredging up" past experiences that seem to have no bearing on the present problem. Of course, in some cases, real therapeutic progress cannot occur unless past traumatization or other experiences are dealt with (see Chapter 2).

Probably a combination of coping skills training, real-world practical guidance, empathic support, delicate psychodynamic exploration where appropriate, and sensitivity to economic, legal, and cultural factors represents the best general approach. For many industrial employees, who are typically young, male, blue-collar workers, a straightforward, rehabilitation-like, behavioral deconditioning approach as described above and in Chapter 4 is most effective. For persistent somatizers or patients with longstanding personality disorders, a more extensive, supportive-expressive/psychodynamic approach may be necessary.

Group and Family Modalities

Many patients with MCS experience severe interpersonal and relationship problems in the course of their illness and may benefit from couples or family therapy modalities (Haller, 1993). Here, as with other types of traumatic disability syndromes, the focus is on helping the family to revise role relationships, deal with feelings of denial, isolation, hostility, and guilt, and come to grips with sexual and work role issues (Miller, 1993a, 1993c, 1994).

The recommendation for support group participation in toxic trauma and MCS cases is mixed, based on my experience with other kinds of traumatic disability support groups (Miller, 1992). To the extent that such groups foster a sense of cohesion, support, and empowerment directed at assuming some measure of responsibility for recovery and taking control of the controllable aspects of life, they are a valuable adjunct and follow-up to formal clinical intervention. But if they entrench dependency and fuel feelings of victimhood and impotent entitlement, they will have a destructive effect on the patients, their loved ones, and the community at large. Here, as in all good clinical work, the effective psychotherapist must serve as guide, teacher, and advocate to help patients negotiate between the Scylla of wasteful confrontation and the Charybdis of help-less capitulation.

SHOCKING DEVELOPMENTS: ELECTRICAL TRAUMA

We chuckle uncomfortably when Wiley Coyote or Curly the Stooge sticks his finger in a light socket or unintentionally picks up a high voltage wire, and—Zzzzap!! Our humor reflects the culture we live in, not to mention the things we fear. Electricity is so new in human consciousness that it still retains an air of dangerous spiritlikeness, an as-yet unreliable taming of Zeus's bolts for our own petty purposes. Mortals that we are, such a force of nature may strike back and zap us when we least expect it. So we do what mortals do to assuage our fears: we laugh it off.

Demographics of Electrical Injury

But it's no joke. Each year, electrical injuries result in approximately 1,200 deaths in the United States, with similar statistics reported for such other industrialized countries as Canada, France, Switzerland, and Germany. Men suffer more electrical injuries on the job than women, primarily because men's work more commonly exposes them to high-voltage electrical equipment. However, in the home, electrical injuries are equal-opportunity zingers, in these cases usually due to malfunctioning or misused appliances. Bathtub electrocutions account for approximately 25 deaths per year in the United States as of last decade, but as more "shower radios" and other waterproof appliances become available, it is likely that at least this particular hazard will be reduced (Patten, 1992).

Electric Shock Effects on the Brain and Behavior

Accumulated research and clinical study (Hooshmand, Radfar, & Beckner, 1989; Patten, 1992; Primeau, Engelstatter, & Bares, 1995) have shown that there are a number of ways that electrical current can harm the nervous system and affect behavioral, cognitive, and emotional functioning. Sensory and motor nerves in the limbs can suffer burn injuries. Swelling of the brain may occur due to fluid accumulation. Electric shock may disturb the heart's rhythm enough to interfere with proper blood supply to the brain; this may be aggravated by shock-induced disturbances of breathing. The result is essentially a shock-induced stroke.

The force of the shock may cause the victim to lurch forward or backward, which produces the equivalent of a whiplash concussion, the brain impacting on the inner skull surface. The victim may also fall to the ground or against some other hard surface, adding a true impact concussion to the injury pattern (see also Chapter 3). In a rather grim line of research, postmortem pathology reports from state electric chair executions indicate that capillary hemorrhages are frequent in the brain and spinal cord, along with destruction of neurons.

In the majority of patients revived from electrical shock, there are no lasting disturbances, or at least none documented by examining physicians. In others, symptoms abound. Headaches are common, but it is often difficult to attribute these to the shock itself. Urinary inhibition and constipation may continue for weeks. In severe cases, cerebral edema (brain swelling) may require treatment. All types and degrees of paralysis may be seen. If these are present acutely, they typically clear completely, but if they develop after apparent full recovery, they may progress and even prove fatal.

Neuropsychological deficits associated with electric shock tend to be nonspecific and to resemble those seen after traumatic brain injury (see also Chapter 3). Disturbances of language, visuospatial skills, and fundamental orientation and awareness are rare, but impairment of attention, concentration, learning, and memory are common, affecting occupational and social functioning. Unlike the case of typical postconcussion syndrome, however, electric shock cognitive impairment may be delayed and/or progressive, in some cases resulting in a dementia-like clinical picture.

The experience of electric shock is, in a sense, the prototype of one-trial aversive conditioning, and thus may naturally be a potent inducer of PTSD. When the shock affects many people simultaneously, as in a lightning strike on a busy golf course or an electrical accident on a crowded shop floor, a comparison may be made to the effects of any natural or man-made disaster, complete with survivor guilt and secondary trauma (see Chapter 7). Even without full-blown PTSD, electric shock may be followed by persistent anxiety, depression, and phobic responses. The consensus of studies suggests that up to 20 percent of electrical injury survivors will experience lasting psychological disability, many presenting with atypical or diffuse complaints, thus risking clinical mis-judgments of somatization or malingering.

Follow-up studies and clinical experience suggest that the first twelve months following electrical injury are crucial in the recovery process, the most substantial gains being observed during that time, with recovery continuing up to three years postinjury. Then recovery plateaus, and the remaining symptoms reflect chronic dysfunction. As in other traumatic disability syndromes, premorbid psychological adjustment and physical health play an important role in the individual response to injury and the recovery process, as well as in the ultimate extent of the disability.

Hooshmand et al. (1989) extensively studied 13 men and three women with early and late complications of alternating current (AC) electrical injuries. Their ages at the time of injury ranged from 21 to 47. Twelve of the patients were shocked while at work, either by accidentally coming in contact with high voltage overhead wires or by touching poorly insu-lated electrical connections in a wet environment. The four subjects who were shocked at home came in contact with poor wiring on appliances, such as washers and dryers, or household electrical outlet connections.

All of these electrically shocked patients needed to be hospitalized due to loss of consciousness, pain in the extremities, seizures, abnormal reflexes, impaired memory and concentration, clouded judgment, and severe anxiety and depression. Later complications included seizures, dizziness, ringing in the ears, balance problems, trouble with hearing, facial weakness, cataracts and other visual disturbances, and deterioration in spinal cord functioning. In addition, impairment was seen in memory, attention, concentration, judgment, and overall intellectual ability.

All of the patients reported disturbances in their daily lives, and most suffered from depression, irritability, and increased sensitivity. The pa-tients lost their normal motivation and initiative and had trouble activat-ing their thought processes and making long-term plans. The deteriora-tion in interpersonal functioning strained their marriages and caused problems with family relationships. After five years, most of the patients had lost their jobs and the majority of married patients had been divorced.

Electrical injury cases do not commonly come to the attention of psychotherapists, and certainly less frequently than head injury or even toxic trauma cases. As awareness of the electrical trauma syndrome grows, no doubt so will the number of clinical referrals. However, I'll present a few of my own cases and a few related to me by colleagues that illustrate some common features of this electrical trauma syndrome.

One of my patients was a 22-year-old waiter who was asked by a coworker to help remove a stuck AC wire plug from a wall socket in the restaurant kitchen where they both worked. To get a better grip on the wire, he braced himself with his free hand on a metal sink which, unbeknownst to him, was filled with dishwater and wet utensils. The shock threw him back against the wall and onto the floor. Although momentarily dazed, he did not think he lost consciousness. Immediately following the accident he started shaking, and he kept shaking for several days. In addition, his speech was slurred and he had difficulty walking, which also lasted for several days.

In the weeks and months that followed, he developed chronic back and shoulder pain. He described numbness over the right side of his body. His sleep was disturbed, and he became irritable, anxious, and depressed. Family and friends who observed him said he seemed "spacy." About nine months following the original accident, he tried to return to work but collapsed on the first day back. This young man had completed high school and one year of college, and was on the management career fast track of the restaurant chain he worked for. Two years following the accident, he had not gone back to work.

Another case involved a female electric pole line splicer for a local power company who was also an amateur bodybuilder—"no weak chickie," as she described herself. While on a repair climb, she accidentally touched the wrong wire and was knocked unconscious by the resulting shock. Fortunately, her work harness kept her from falling from the top of the 30-foot pole, and she was retrieved by coworkers minutes later. One rescuer recalled that when she was first brought down, her hair was literally standing on end, "like a fright wig."

For the next few days, she experienced shaking "on and off, especially when I get tired." Her whole body seemed "numb." She also felt fatigued much of the time and was unable to work out in the gym, mainly because her "sense of heaviness and strength" seemed to be impaired. She had become increasingly irritable, which caused problems with her roommate and other friends. She claimed that her memory was as "sharp as ever," but acquaintances had pointed out that she often didn't seem "with it." "I want to get better," she told me. "Don't they have a cure for this?"

Another patient, a successful shipbuilder, Navy veteran, and accomplished seaman, sustained a combination electrical injury and closed head trauma when the shock from a poorly insulated wire slammed his head into a low crossbeam at a ship construction site. His biggest issue was the effect of the injury on his previously productive work life, as well as the purported negligence that allegedly led to the accident. Through psychotherapy and by dint of his own dogged perseverence in trying to overcome the posttraumatic and postconcussive effects of his injury, he was able to resolve the major personal identity issues tied in with his disability and ultimately to return to work.

A colleague has related to me the case of a middle-aged contracting foreman who got too close to a live wire on a construction site. The shock knocked him off his feet, but he did not black out. Immediately, however, he started experiencing "shakiness" in his arms, hands, and upper body, and this persisted over the course of the day. Gamely, he wanted to stay on the job, but his crew insisted he go home and see a doctor. He decided to rest up and, if he didn't feel better in the morning, he'd get himself checked out. That night he began having palpitations, which soon turned into dangerous heart arrhythmias, and the next day he suffered a stroke which left him with numbness, weakness, tremors, partial blindness, gait and balance problems, mood swings and depression, as well as impaired concentration, memory, reading, arithmetic, and spatial reasoning.

Another colleague relates the case of a woman who sustained an AC current electrical shock. Although she could recall the shock and the events preceding it, there was about a 15-minute gap of time following the shock that she had no recollection of. Subsequently, she experienced headaches, irritability, impaired memory, decreased performance on the job, and occasional feelings of numbness, tingling, and weakness in her hands. Neuropsychological assessment showed impaired verbal and spatial memory, concentration, and sensorimotor functioning, as well as anxiety and depression.

Psychotherapy of Electric Shock Trauma

In contrast to traumatic brain injury or toxic trauma, virtually nothing concerning the psychotherapeutic treatment of electrical injury exists in the literature. All I could find were some basic recommendations by Primeau et al. (1995), who point out that even for cases likely to have a substantial or complete recovery, supportive psychotherapy may prevent reactive disorders and facilitate return to previous roles. Anxiety disorders and depression may be amenable to behavioral and cognitive-behavioral psychotherapy. For cases with significant loss of function, the treatment goal would be to assist in adaptation and adjustment to disability. These authors' clinical impression is that most patients do improve and that the clinician has the opportunity to influence the outcome through his reassurance, patience, and attitude of acceptance.

My experience with electrical trauma patients is more limited than with other traumatic disability patients—even toxic cases are more common—but, in general, many of the recommendations made in this chapter and in Chapter 2 apply. More specifically, I have found that a key issue for electric shock trauma patients that must be addressed in therapy is their almost universal feeling of being "singled out," which is even more pronounced than for PTSD patients generally. The literal, metaphoric, and even cosmic significance of being "zapped" by fate may have particular trenchancy for electric shock victims.

As uncommon as industrial electric shock patients are in most therapists' caseloads, rarer still must be the "mother of all zappings": getting hit by lightning and living to tell about it. In the single lightning strike case I've consulted on, a middle-aged man survived a strike on a boat that killed two of his companions. In this case, the main issue was clearly survivor guilt—even more than his own physical and cognitive impairment, which was considerable.

We live in a rapidly evolving technological world, where physical and psychological traumatization by chemicals, electricity, radiation, and who knows what next will become more common facts of life into the next century. Our human psyches—and the therapeutic approaches we devise and adapt to treat them—must be able to keep up. There's no going back to a Luddite state of nature: instead, let's enjoy the comforts of our gadgets and conveniences, but let's all be responsible for ensuring that the products of our cleverness don't become the instruments of our needless suffering.

Chapter 6

ROADS TO RUIN

Traffic and Transportation Accidents

The machine does not isolate man from the
great problems of nature, but plunges him more
deeply into them.

—Saint-Exupery

Many of the traumatic experiences described in this book are, if
admittedly awful, nevertheless reassuringly rare or unusual. After
all, how likely is it that any of us will be swept away in a flood, kidnapped
by terrorists, find ourselves downwind from a toxic spill, or be called to
pitch in for disaster relief? But almost all of us work and travel on a
regular basis, and a traumatic road or rail accident can be as psychologically shattering as an earthquake if it violates our sense of a safe and
secure world.

AUTOMOBILE TRAFFIC ACCIDENTS

It's almost impossible to imagine modern life without our high-speed
motorized modes of individual transportation—American culture is indeed a car culture. Yet there's a downside to all this zipping around.
Traffic accidents bring about injury, pain, and loss, and are the major
cause of death in young adults in Western society (Baum, Fleming, &
Singer, 1983; Blanchard, Hickling, Taylor, & Loos, 1995a; Blanchard,
Hickling, Vollmer, Loos, Buckley, & Jaccard, 1995b). Unfortunately, the

121

psychological aftermath of auto accidents usually receives little attention, unless famous personalities or spectacular court cases are involved.

The survivor of a serious motor vehicle accident may be afraid to ride in cars or may be such a jittery passenger that she becomes a pest to drive around with. She may develop a paralyzing preoccupation with physical symptoms or injuries resulting from the accident. She may suffer headaches and other aches and pains, even when no physical injury has occurred. Anxiety, irritability, and depression are common. She may be unable to read or watch news stories of traffic accidents, hear traffic reports on the radio, or even tolerate automobile commercials on TV. Phobias to particular models of cars involved in the accident may develop, even to colors that remind her of the vehicles. Some patients develop a curious perceptual distortion in which cars or street corners appear closer than they actually are. The usual posttraumatic stress reactions of intrusive recollection and emotional numbing are typically seen (Hodge, 1971; Kuch, 1987; Kuch, Cox, Evans, & Shulman, 1994; Munjack, 1984; Parker, 1977).

In addition to such anecdodal reports, systematic research (Foeckler, Garrard, Williams, Thomas, & Jones, 1978) supports a link between auto accidents and posttraumatic stress syndromes. About a third of car drivers who have been in an accident involving a fatality suffer from persistent psychological aftereffects. Fear, depression, shame, and work disruption may be seen in a large proportion of traffic accident victims, as long as five years later. A particularly high incidence of headache has been noted in patients with posttraumatic stress reactions, even where there has been no head injury. These headaches often require more than twice as much treatment as nonstress-related headaches. Psychophysiological studies show marked increases in heart rate and blood pressure in individuals with PTSD secondary to car accidents while the subjects imagine scenes related to their accident.

One of my patients, Ivan, was driving home from a pleasant evening of vacation fun with his out-of-town relatives, who had been visiting for the holidays. Some of these relatives had recently been reunited after a long separation in various locations in North America and Eastern Europe. Suddenly, seemingly out of nowhere, a huge off-duty charter bus careened into their lane, forcing the car against a right concrete retaining wall. From the friction and gas spill caused by the collision, the car caught fire. The panicked occupants poured from the burning vehicle and ran for their lives.

But relief at their narrow escape abruptly turned to horror when a head count revealed that one of their number was missing. Several male members of the group ran back to the car to find Ivan's teenaged nephew pinned in the back seat, surrounded by flames. The fire was too hot for the men to get at the trapped youth, and a few of them suffered burns on their hands and faces while struggling to reach through the flames. Ivan's last clear image is of his nephew crying to him for help. In the next hellish moments, Ivan could hear the boy screaming until smoke and flame engulfed him and the anguished voice was stilled.

For several months afterward, Ivan was "a human vegetable." The burn injuries on his hands and a wrenched hip joint required a short period of hospitalization and a few months of rehab, but otherwise his physical injuries were mostly minor cuts and bruises. Because of his general lack of responsiveness in the hospital, the doctors at first feared that Ivan had suffered brain damage in the accident or perhaps an allergic sensitivity reaction from the morphine used for his burn pain. But all the medical tests checked out normal. A psychiatric consult was called in, a tentative diagnosis of depression was made, and medication was prescribed. Physically healed, he was discharged a few days later.

When I first met Ivan, he was curled up in a chair in my office when I arrived for my first appointment of the day. His wife had driven him over, and the reception staff had let him into the office because he could not tolerate being with the other people in the crowded waiting room of a busy group practice on the first day back after a long holiday weekend. A clinical interview with Ivan made it clear that he was suffering the classic PTSD symptoms of intrusive recollections, frightening dreams, emotional numbing alternating with panic and depression, phobic avoidance of car-related activities and materials, and, above all, a crippling depression that no amount of medication could touch.

Because of his withdrawn clinical presentation and because he reported having banged his head while trying to get his nephew out of the car, I administered a standard neuropsychological test battery. Ivan's intellectual and cognitive functioning were surprisingly intact—above average, in fact, on most of the measures. This was all the more surprising, since depression itself can depress neuropsychological test scores. No, Ivan's mortal wound was not in his intellect but in his feelings, in his soul.

Over the course of our sessions, it became clear how the effects of this traumatic event were inextricably tied in with the complex interpersonal dynamics of Ivan's extended family. Virtually all the common themes of psychotherapy were played out in this case: love, hate, loyalty, jealousy, rivalry, religion, politics, money, and the legal aspects of the case. Most important was coming to terms with the death of his nephew and its reverberation with Ivan's sense of family responsibility. Happily, after more than two years of intensive psychotherapy, Ivan was able to work through the trauma and the meaning it had for his personal and family life. He understands that "I'll never be completely over it," but he has learned to live again.

Traumatic Effects of Traffic Accidents

Motor vehicle accidents are a widespread American experience, with over 3.5 million traffic-related personal injuries occurring annually in the United States. Interestingly, however, there has been much more systematic study of traffic accident victims in Europe and Canada than in the United States. Car accidents are a major cause of PTSD (Blanchard, et al., 1995a, 1995b), and accident survivors account for a large share of referrals to both chronic pain treatment centers and anxiety clinics (Kuch, Evans, & Mueller-Busch, 1993).

Fifty victims of recent motor vehicle accidents who sought medical attention, and 40 matched controls, were assessed for psychological morbidity by Blanchard, Hickling, Taylor, Loos, and Gerardi (1994). Almost half of the accident victims met the criteria for PTSD, while an additional 20 percent showed a subsyndromal version consisting of reexperiencing plus either avoidance/numbing or overarousal. The accident victims who displayed PTSD symptoms were significantly more likely to have experienced previous trauma other than traffic accidents and were more likely to have previously met the criteria for PTSD as the result of that trauma. Almost half of the accident victims who met criteria for PTSD also suffered significant depression, and many of these had experienced depressive episodes in the past.

Subsequent studies (Blanchard et al., 1995a, 1995b) have found that for some accident victims, avoidance and numbing symptoms tend to decline within six months following an accident, but hyperarousal symptoms persist. Accident victims with PTSD tend to be more subjectively distressed and to have more impairment in work, school, home functioning, and relationships with family and friends than non-PTSD accident victims. PTSD after car accidents is significantly associated with depression, which in turn is linked with a history of prior depressive episodes and prior PTSD-related events. The lives of auto accident victims are curtailed by the avoidance of travel as driver or passenger. Even if compelled by circumstance or necessity to travel, many victims endure substantial subjective discomfort as they carry out their essential trips to work, school, doctors' visits, or family outings. This is a largely ignored population in need of assistance.

Traffic Accidents and Head Injury

Parker (1996) provides an insightful description of the neuropsychological and emotional reactions following car crashes that may be accompanied by head injury and the postconcussion syndrome (see also Chapter 3). Neuropsychologically, areas vulnerable to concussive head trauma include the anterior frontal and temporal structures that are important for emotional and behavioral self-regulation and adaptive personality functioning. Emotionally, physical injury to the head represents a unique threat to self-image and meaningfulness of life. The stress of a frightening accident, associated with the continuing trauma of recovery, such as waking up in a hospital or coping with slow-healing physical injuries, can have its own traumatic effects. These stress effects can interact with the neuropsychological impairment caused by the brain injury itself to exacerbate deficits in adaptive cognitive functioning, leading to a vicious cycle of depression and demoralization.

Traffic Accidents, Physical Injury, and Chronic Pain

Physical injury with pain is a known predictor of PTSD after accidents (Kilpatrick, Saunders, Amick-McMullan, Best, Veronen, & Resnick, 1989; Parker, 1996), and several factors appear to account for this increase in the likelihood of developing PTSD after accident with injury. First, physical injuries serve as constant visual and proprioceptive cues for intrusive reexperiencing phenomena; it's hard to forget a traumatic event when facial scars or a noticeable limp serve as daily reminders. In addition, physical injury is usually accompanied by significant levels of pain, which typically lowers the patient's overall ability to handle stress.

Accident survivors account for a large share of referrals to chronic pain treatment centers. Conversely, chronic pain populations probably contain a substantial percentage of patients with PTSD and posttraumatic phobias (Kuch, 1989). A variety of interactions have been found between anxiety and chronic pain, which may sometimes be due to the presence of somatization (Kuch, Evans, & Watson, 1991a; Kuch, Evans, Watson, Bubela, & Cox, 1991b; Kuch et al., 1993). Accident-related chronic pain tends to be exacerbated by stress, anxiety, and poor coping, and such pain often remits when PTSD and accident phobias are adequately treated (Kuch, 1989; Kuch & Swinson, 1985; also see Chapter 4).

Traffic Accidents, Anxiety Disorders, Phobias, and Anger

Right after a traffic accident, a posttraumatic stress reaction may not be apparent (Kuch et al., 1994), and minor traffic accidents are often shrugged off as commonplace. Accident-related driving fears are rationalized as "understandable," and impairment of normal daily living from phobias and PTSD is then ignored, often concealed by the victim to avoid ridicule. Accident phobias appear to be particularly prevalent among patients with flexion-extension (whiplash) injuries, sometimes producing a syndrome with the pejorative label, *"whiplash neurosis."*

There also seems to be a difference between specific traffic accident phobia and agoraphobia (fear of open spaces) in general. While agoraphobics typically avoid operating a car out of fear of losing control in the event of a panic attack, many accident phobics actually appear to prefer the control that goes with being in the driver's seat. Given a choice, they'll stay out of the car entirely, but if the family has to go on a trip, the torture of being a passive passenger impels them to commandeer the vehicle, the family typically acquiescing rather than endure the patient's incessant back-seat gasps and flinches.

In fact, car accidents are far more associated with phobias than industrial accidents (Kuch, 1989; Parker, 1977), perhaps due to the more startling nature and unfamiliar surroundings in car accidents. Phobias may be quite specific; for example, a patient who crashed during a rainstorm may be unable to drive when he hears raindrops drumming on the roof of the car but may be able to drive in sunshine or snow (Kuch, 1989).

Worries about illness, whiplash injury, postconcussion syndrome, chronic pain, and other physical injuries may obscure specific phobias in motor vehicle accident survivors and become the presenting complaint. Anxiety disorder impairs the prognosis of medical illnesses in general by adding or magnifying symptoms and evoking illness behaviors. Anxiety disorder patients suffer from dizziness, faintness, palpitations, difficulty breathing, and other signs of excessive somatic arousal, and often attribute these sensations to the effects of physical injury (Kuch, 1989). Of course, such cases require careful differential diagnostic evaluation so that orthopedic, neurological, and psychological etiologies can be teased out and treated appropriately.

Kuch et al. (1993) present a case example of phobic anxiety: a woman was driving her car alongside a parking lot when, without warning, another car went out of control and jumped the snowbank bordering the parking lot, then struck the hood of the patient's car. No demonstrable injuries resulted, but the patient developed intense driving fears that turned commuting to work into an ordeal. She sold her house to be closer to work and gave up pleasure driving. She also developed frequent nightmares about the accident and became very sensitive to news and media reports of other accidents and mishaps.

One of my own patients sustained a postconcussion syndrome, cervical whiplash pain, cervicogenic and oculomotor vertigo, and PTSD in a car accident that left him totally car-phobic for several months, affecting his job and family functioning. In a case that "reads the textbooks," in six months, through a combination of cognitive rehabilitation, psychotherapy, and judicious, graded practice, he was able to go from not even being able to stand next to a parked car to driving to work relatively normally, although some residual symptoms remain. In a "positive cycle," as his abilities continued to recover under his own (albeit clinically guided) efforts, the clear rays of self-confidence began to burn off the depressive fog that had been hampering his social and family functioning, leading to greater confidence, better mood, and better relationships.

Anger problems are also very common in accident survivors, many of whom feel victimized by the "system." In this regard, Kuch (1989) identifies two subgroups of accident victims. One is more highly educated, more likely to self-diagnose phobias, has good coping skills, and is generally less distressed. The other subgroup typically has poor social and problem-solving skills and is less well-informed. Patients in the second group are more inclined to feel helpless, mistreated, and unduly distressed by the adversarial process often involved in the settlement of claims, and are also less likely to actively seek treatment for phobias.

Psychotherapy of Traffic Accident PTSD

GENERAL AND SPECIFIC CONSIDERATIONS.   Length of therapy may vary from just a few sessions to a course of treatment lasting months or longer. Best and Ribbe (1995) recommend that therapeutic interventions first address physical symptoms, followed by cognitive symptoms, and then behavioral symptoms. The entire process should begin with an educational phase that includes goal-setting and explanation of the therapy process, and it should conclude with an evaluation of therapeutic progress.

Best and Ribbe (1995) have attempted to identify the factors associated with positive therapeutic outcomes in treating accident-related PTSD. These include early intervention, few or no prior traumas, a noncomplicated premorbid mental and physical health history, less severe accident-related injury, good premorbid adjustment, and adequate social support. Factors associated with poorer outcomes are late referral, complicated trauma history, complicated mental and physical health history, severe accident-related injury, perceived threat to life, substance abuse currently or by history, poor premorbid adjustment, and poor social support systems.

According to Best and Ribbe (1995), the victim's individual perception of danger is important in determining posttrauma response. Clinically, the most efficacious way of determining perceived life threat is to straightforwardly and empathically ask the victim if she thought that she might be killed or seriously injured during the accident. The victim may not recognize the relationship between life threat and intensity of symptoms in light of the apparent "minor" nature of some traumas and accidents. Therefore, other people, or the victim herself, may impute her high level of distress to "weak character" or malingering, or think that she is "overreacting" to the trauma. Consequently, others may be less willing to offer vital emotional, social, or financial support to the victim.

Best and Ribbe (1995) also emphasize the role of the psychotherapist as patient advocate. For example, in cases of work-related driving trauma (trucks, taxis, delivery vans, service vehicles), the patient may benefit greatly from the clinician's educating employers about PTSD symptomatology and the need to follow a gradual exposure model in order for the worker to ultimately return to his regular route. Or the clinician may need to speak on behalf of the patient to insurance carriers or employers. Also, clinicians may become advocates and guides for victims who become involved in civil or criminal proceedings (see Chapter 8).

TELLING THE STORY.   If the forgoing implies that practitioners must often take an active role in the treatment process, this is certainly not to underemphasize the therapeutic utility of sometimes just letting the patient talk. A great deal of clinically useful information can be obtained by having the patient describe what happened just prior to, during, and immediately after the accident, how things are different for her since the trauma, and how she has been affected by it (Best & Ribbe, 1995). A greater amount of detail and affective information becomes available when the patient first tells her story in an unstructured manner. This also provides the clinician with insight into the patient's particular style of coping with trauma. For example, very detailed and precise accounts may indicate obsessive or intrusive symptomatology. Scattered and disorganized stories, or those containing a paucity of details, may reflect impaired concentration or avoidance caused by anxiety.

In addition to its role in assessment and diagnosis, having the patient tell her story can have tremendous therapeutic benefits. First, the process of telling the story may be cathartic in itself for the patient. Second, it lets the patient know that therapist views her as an individual and wants to understand her unique experience. Third, in contrast to the frequent shocked and defensively minimizing reaction of other people, the narrative process communicates to the patient that it is really "okay" to talk about what may have been a terrifying and embarrassing event, as well as the intense emotional response that has resulted from the experience.

Best and Ribbe (1995) suggest that having the patient tell her story is best accomplished during the first session, prior to completing the rest of the assessment process, but I have found that the full story often emerges in a gradual and piecemeal fashion over time, in the form of islands of recall that slowly emerge from beneath the murky waters of denial, gradually coalescing to form larger and larger narrative land masses, finally interconnected by isthmuses of awareness into past and present, ultimately to create a variably textured continent of personal history. This is why, unlike the standard medical questionnaire, taking a psychological history—especially in trauma cases—often requires its own time. The patient often cannot just pop out the story on demand; rather it surfaces over time as trust and security take root in the therapeutic relationship.

REDUCING AROUSAL. Traumatized auto accident survivors typically show heightened arousal, especially to phobic objects and circumstances associated with their accidents. Since driving is important to virtually all outside activities that most Americans engage in, some form of desensitization is usually the first step to getting the patient safely and comfortably back behind the wheel or in the passenger seat.

Deep *muscle relaxation* techniques, used alone or in a *systematic desensitization* paradigm, can produce a sense of calm and control that the patient can employ when she begins to feel fearful or anxious. Another technique is *cue-controlled breathing*, in which the subject takes a deep breath, then exhales while saying silently such calming words as "calm," "relax," or "peace." Particular benefits of cue-controlled breathing are that it is easily mastered by patients, is an abbreviated method of achieving relaxation compared to other more lengthy methods, and can be done discreetly virtually anywhere and at any time the patient needs to reduce anxiety (Best & Ribbe, 1995).

Other patients, I've found, find relaxation threatening to their sense of control, so that standard low-arousal techniques may actually exacerbate physical and emotional symptoms (Lazarus & Mayne, 1990; Miller, 1994). For these patients, more active coping techniques may be useful in gradually overcoming the fear of driving (see Chapter 2). Remember, "desensitization" need not connote limp and stuporous patients floating on a cloud. Some people cope by "hardening" rather than "softening," as long as the former represents productive coping, not just defensive armoring. Get to know your patient, then choose whatever therapeutic approach will most effectively let her develop a sense of security and mastery that can dissipate, block, or suspend driving anxiety.

COGNITIVE-BEHAVIORAL THERAPY.   Cognitive-behavioral therapies have become a mainstay in treating phobic and posttraumatic stress disorders. Accident victims often develop distorted perceptions of the accident and its consequences. They may elaborate complex belief systems about the conditions, real or imagined, that led to the accident, complicated it, or contributed to a dire outcome. Such cognitions may compound the distress that the accident victim experiences (Best & Ribbe, 1995). In fact, when accident victims begin to act on misinterpretations and distorted beliefs, they may inadvertently create more difficulties in their medical, legal, and social environments, which further impair functioning. The goal of cognitive treatment techniques, then, is to limit and correct faulty thinking about the accident behaviors and consequences of the accident.

Best and Ribbe (1995) identify several modalities of cognitive-behavioral therapy that may prove useful with accident victims. In *rational-emotive therapy*, the goal is to help the patient ease feelings by learning to modify or adapt many of her fundamental belief systems about fairness, causality, and controllability. Similarly, in *cognitive restructuring* the goal is to discover the source of faulty beliefs or misinterpretations and to substitute other beliefs or ideas. Obviously, the terrible circumstances of many traumatic events limit the degree to which complete cognitive restructuring can occur.

Thought-stopping is a cognitive-behavioral technique used to interrupt ruminative thinking (see also Chapter 2). When using this technique with accident victims, the therapist instructs the patient to think about the accident for a brief period. When the patient signals with a raised finger that she has a clear image, the therapist literally shouts, "Stop!" The patient should then be queried to see if the thoughts are continuing. If so, the procedure is repeated until the thoughts cease. The patient can then be trained to stop her own intrusive, distressing, or ruminative thoughts in this way, first overtly (aloud), then covertly (silently). Although not all patients find thought-stopping to be beneficial, for some this technique provides great relief from intrusive PTSD symptomatology.

Following an accident, victims may have some difficulties interacting with other people. Previously acquired interpersonal skills may have temporarily fallen out of their repertoire of behavior as a result of the stress of the accident. *Role playing* can be used to help victims deal with stressful interpersonal situations and engage in behaviors that are more adaptive. In some cases, this will involve learning brand new interpersonal skills that patients can add to their personal repertoire, and the therapist may have to be quite explicit and directive in modelling these skills, especially at the beginning of treatment.

EXPOSURE THERAPY.   In a sense, *exposure therapy* (sometimes called "implosion" therapy) is the antithesis of low-arousal relaxation, and it may actually work best for some patients who want to take an active, "let's-get-it-the-hell-over-with" approach to dealing with posttraumatic anxiety and phobia. Adapted from use with traumatized war veterans, exposure techniques have now been used with a variety of PTSD syndromes. More than with almost any other PTSD therapeutic modality, it is vital that therapists who use these techniques know what they're doing in order to avoid retraumatization and exacerbation of disability. With respect to auto accidents, while exposure both in imagination and in vivo is useful, Kuch's (1989) experience is that in vivo (real-life) exposure is the more robust procedure, as many patients are not psychologically minded and/or find it difficult to concentrate on imaginary stimuli.

Kuch's (1989) exposure paradigm treats traumatized passengers and drivers somewhat separately. With passengers, in vivo exposure of driving fears follows the same procedure as exposure therapy for fear of heights. The patient is placed in the phobic situation and instructed to pay close attention to the phobic stimuli with as little interruption as possible until the urge to flee or avoid has faded.

Therapeutic momentum is maintained by beginning self-exposure as soon after clinican-guided exposure as possible. A positive experience is encouraging and provides the first break in the vicious cycle of phobic avoidance and "fear of fear." The patient should aim to complete the exposure program within one month. Twelve hours of prolonged self-exposure in two- to three-hour sessions in the norm in this model. Kuch (1989) recommends postponing the treatment process with candidates who are resistant or who "do not have the time," but, in the meantime, to offer supportive therapy. This lessens the chance of treatment failure and its consequent demoralizing effect. Therapists' attitudes to distress are also important during this kind of process, which requires firmness and determination from both sides.

Because driving itself may not provide sufficient exposure to all relevant internal stimuli, *imaginal flooding* may be added to in vivo exposure when patients are preoccupied with accidents and injury. Imaginal flooding in an office setting can be made more realistic by audiotapes of squealing tires, canned odors, or other sensory aids, although this is rarely used in routine clinical practice. Covert avoiders should imagine the "worst possible situation" until anxiety fades (Kuch, 1989).

Another, perhaps less theatrical form of imaginal flooding involves encouraging the patient to simply tell the story of the trauma, while the therapist focuses the patient's attention on as many sensory details, thoughts, impressions, affective states, and physical sensations as possible at each part of the trauma narrative (Best & Ribbe, 1995). The therapist should have the patient tell her entire trauma story slowly, in minute detail, reporting every aspect of her experience, including affective states and physical sensations. The patient must be encouraged to stay with the fear-producing memories in order to not reinforce an avoidance response.

In Kuch's (1989) model, exposure treatment of traumatically phobic drivers is more complex than that of passengers, because safe driving is also an active skill. Before tackling the role of driver, desensitization to the role of passenger should be accomplished, because intense subjective distress may interfere with self-control. As noted above, however, in my experience some control-oriented patients actually find the passenger role more anxiety-provoking and virtually insist upon taking the wheel right away.

Instructions for drivers should include the kinds of exposure hierarchies described in standard behavior therapy protocols (Wolpe, 1973). Kuch (1989) recommends practicing in empty parking lots, on deserted country roads, or in cars parked with the engine idling. Formal courses in "skid control" and the like offer good opportunities for exposure as well as skill training. Related vehicle operation experiences such as downhill skiing, water-skiing, and snowmobiling allow exposure to heights, skidding, and speed. Single components of a driving phobia may thus be desensitized separately.

Noncompliance with self-exposure instructions may occur for a variety of reasons. Kuch's (1989) patients typically do not accept and work through the same degree of discomfort when asked to practice exposure on their own as when in the encouraging company of a therapist (therapists will recognize this as a generic problem with all kinds of therapeutic homework). Possible remedies include less demanding homework tasks and therapist-assisted exposure.

As noted above, postconcussion syndrome, whiplash, chronic pain, dizziness, and impaired equilibrium often occur along with PTSD and phobias following car accidents. Kuch (1989) observes that exposure therapies may be ineffective with patients suffering from episodic dizziness and unsteadiness. Typically, these patients report feeling as if everything around them is shifting, and often grab onto something to steady themselves. Some walk with the aid of a cane. This symptom is commonly seen after cervical whiplash injuries and may occur during an anxiety episode or without any provocation. It resembles otoneurological dizziness, but even extensive tests are usually negative. The sensation is aggravated by changes in head position and seems highly sensitive to stress. When it is present in its purest form, patients will drive on good days and avoid driving on dizzy days, thereby showing an avoidance pattern that is less stable and more situation-specific than in typical phobias.

In many of these cases, proper diagnosis and treatment of the underlying physical problem (postconcussion syndrome, middle ear pathology) often cures the "psychological" disorder. Therapeutic approaches include physical rehabilitation, balance training, and the judicious use of medication.

BUS ACCIDENTS

Bus, train, and other mass transportation accidents share some features with passenger car crashes in terms of injury effects, but in other ways may be more similar to disasters (see Chapter 7) because they typically involve a larger number of people, may require complex and protracted rescue efforts, and may be the subject of media attention.

Watts (1995) reported the case of a touring coach carrying members of a senior citizens social club that skidded off an embankment in Australia. The coach rolled several times before finally crashing into a tree. Eleven people were killed and 38 injured. Among the most distressing features of this accident for the survivors were seeing bodies and people dying, sustaining physical injuries, and being trapped in the bus, although the traumatic effects of the latter abated over time.

Delayed traumatic reactions to the accident also occurred. Both intrusive and avoidant phenomena were common. The horror of being surrounded by the deceased seemed to reinforce the narrowness of the survivors' escape from death. Many voiced the concern that "I'll never be the same again." Loss of function due to physical injury, even if slight, increased the burden of coping, particularly for those survivors who lived alone. Fifteen subjects reported that they had experienced another severely distressing event prior to the accident, apparently increasing their vulnerability to the traumatic effect of the bus accident.

Winje and Ulvik (1995) describe the case of a Swedish school bus carrying 23 children and 11 adult passengers that crashed into a tunnel wall in Norway. Twelve children and four parents died, and 18 of the passengers survived.

The authors describe a particular crisis intervention strategy with these survivors, intended to minimize overprotective avoidance and help the relatives confront and actively cope with the tragedy. This adaptation process was facilitated through stimulation of cognitive processing (information), emotional catharsis (exposure), sharing experiences (social contact), goal-directed behavior (active participation), and existential processing (religious rituals). The main confronting elements were detailed information about the accident, a visit to the accident site, contact with the other families, staying at the injured person's bedside, information about the causes of death, and viewing of the deceased.

The creation of a group community among relatives and victims can have important practical and psychological consequences. One strategy for fostering group cohesion is to take control of practical supportive functions, such as transport, accommodations, and information. This can facilitate close social contact and positive helping relationships even in very heterogeneous groups. To achieve this, on arrival at the hospital in Norway, each family was assigned to two support persons from the hospital staff who became the family's regular contact during their entire stay in Norway.

To counteract the potential additional traumatization of families by garish and inaccurate media portrayals of the accident, correct and detailed information was delivered to the relatives about the scene of the accident, the geography of the area, and the rescue work itself. In addition, the reactions of the adult and child survivors was normalized by educating them about the typical crisis reactions of adults and children who go through these kinds of experiences (see also Chapter 7).

In what might be considered a somewhat unorthodox move, helicopter trips were arranged for the relatives to visit the canyon to see where the accident happened. The importance of this closure experience is seen by the fact that 27 (73 percent) of the respondents wanted to see the site of the accident in order to understand what had happened. Of the 19 persons who participated in the trip, none regretted the visit. The visitors placed flowers at the tunnel wall and a Swedish church minister held a short service at the site.

The relatives of the deceased were advised to sit by the bedsides of the injured survivors as much as possible. They also participated in some of the daily routines of the injured patients and assisted in the emotional care of their children. Follow-up assessments indicated that these interactions had been a great source of comfort and support for injured survivors and bereaved families alike.

Initially, the relatives of the deceased were psychically numbed; however, they demanded quite early on to know what injuries their deceased loved ones had suffered and under what conditions they had died. Follow-up assessments showed that most relatives were grateful for such information from the coroner, even though much of this information must have been exceedingly unpleasant.

In a related vein, both clinical experience and widespread cultural practice have shown that viewing the deceased has great significance for the grieving process, if it occurs under suitable conditions, for example, not in the morgue itself. Therefore, a more formal, respectful viewing was arranged. The support personnel offered to see the deceased before the families, and the families discovered that their fantasies about how the deceased looked were far worse than reality. In cases where the injuries were in fact too disfiguring, it was recommended that the relatives view only the hands of the deceased. Each family was accompanied to the open casket by their support person, as tranquil organ music filled the chapel. The relatives kissed, patted, or touched the deceased, and it was recommended that the families bring personal items to place in the casket. All the participants felt they benefited from this respectful mourning ritual.

Winje and Ulvik (1995) point out that a cardinal symptom of crisis reaction is the strong feeling of unreality. This mental state, initially protective in an overwhelming situation, may be transformed into maladaptive passivity through the helpers' overprotection of the traumatized persons. Their psychosocial support program for the bus passengers' families helped them to confront the stressful situation and counteract passivity. Overall, the confrontational elements of the program turned out not to be overwhelming for the relatives, and this was due largely to the organizing of a group community that created mutual support. Thus, the combination of reality-confrontation and emotional support seemed to make a significant contribution in the crisis intervention services.

As a postscript to this case, the authors note that on the first anniversary of the accident, most of the families traveled to the accident site in Norway for a commemorative ceremony. At the request of the relatives, meetings were arranged between the families and the police, the rescue teams, and the hospital staff. The anniversary visit to the place where the accident took place shows that the families were ready, willing, and able to confront reality once more as part of the closure process of their grieving and coping (Winje & Ulvik, 1995).

RAILWAY ACCIDENTS

Other than cars and buses, most passenger surface transportation occurs by rail. Indeed, as noted in Chapter 1, railway accidents have a venerable place in the history of traumatology. But most of the older literature and much of the new has dealt with traumatized passengers. What kind of psychic specters haunt the dreams of railway personnel who are involved in such fatal accidents?

Because of the terrain of Northern Europe, much transportation there is by rail, rather than by automobile, and so, not surprisingly, much of the recent literature on railway accidents comes from that part of the industrialized world. One study (Malt, Hoivik, & Blikra, 1993) involved 117 Swedish and Norwegian train drivers who had been selected for this kind of work precisely because of their good physical and psychological health. These train drivers had all been involved in accidents where a pedestrian was killed on the tracks, most commonly in suicide attempts. In virtually all cases, the victim had leaped onto the track too suddenly for the speeding train to stop in time, and the driver had watched help-lessly as his engine bore down on the hapless pedestrian.

Because of the mass and momentum of the huge train engine, none of the drivers was physically injured or indeed received so much as a jolt from the impact with the victim, so physical injury was not a factor. However, more than half of the drivers reported posttraumatic symptoms of intrusive imagery within the first 24 hours after the accident. "Pictures of the accident situation keep popping into my mind," was the most frequent complaint.

Just as important, however, very few of these drivers—selected, re-member, because of their good overall physical condition and psychologi-cal stability—developed enduring, hardcore PTSD symptoms. In a day or so, most had recovered from the experience and were back at work. Those who did develop persistent stress reactions turned out to have other psychological, family, or social problems at the time of the accident that were complicating their reaction to the train fatality. For a few drivers, the accident appeared to have special psychodynamic meaning. In one case, the driver was undergoing a period of rather bitter domestic conflict and—just his luck—his train killed a woman of about the same age as his wife.

A follow-up study of these train drivers (Karlehagen, Malt, Hoff, Tibell, Herrstromer, Hildingson, & Leymann, 1993) confirmed that drivers who remained on sick leave one month after the accident were those with the strongest anxiety reactions, psychosomatic disorders, and intrusive symptomatology. These drivers had been in difficult life situations at the time of the accident, and in many cases they had been involved in a number of prior, nonfatal accidents or had endured other stressful experiences. The present train fatality could thus be seen as the prover-bial last straw. Interestingly, as in the first study, the single most important factor determining the outcome of these traumatic disability cases was the personal, psychodynamic meaning of the accident. For example, a middle-aged driver was having conflicts with his adolescent son. During that time, it happened that a distraught teenager threw himself in front of this driver's train. Therapists working with such patients should always be sensitive to both the general traumatizing effect of the accident, as well as the patient's idiosyncratic psychodynamic reaction.

AIRLINE ACCIDENTS

A few weeks before finishing this book, I was listening to a radio commentator discuss how, in the wake of the recent Valujet and TWA crashes, many passengers were now reviewing airline accident statistics to determine the "safest" carriers to fly on. The commentator pointed out that since the base rate of airline accidents is so low overall, picking a flight based on which airline has had the fewest crashes is like choosing a department store based on which retail chain has had the fewest building collapses. These things do happen, but so rarely, the commentator reassuringly intoned, that we should stop worrying and just keep flying.

Feel better? Neither do I.

For we terrestrially evolved human beings, there's still something viscerally alien and unearthly about hurtling through the sky in a tin can at hundreds of miles per hour, cut off—more so than the remotest ship at sea—from physical contact with solid ground. Unless we hit it.

Even more than bus and train crashes, airline accidents have all the features of a transportation accident and a technological mass disaster (see also Chapter 7), including survivor anger and a sense of futility that human error may have resulted in the occurrence of a potentially preventable tragedy (Marks, Yule, & de Silva, 1995). Airline personnel who survive may have to cope with the additional stress of working in an environment of blame and recrimination.

Marks et al. (1995) describe the case of a commercial jetliner with 118 passengers and eight crew members that crash-landed shortly after takeoff due to failure of one of the engines. Thirty-nine passengers died in the crash and eight more later died of their injuries. Of the 79 surviving passengers, 74 suffered serious physical injuries.

During interviews after the accident, all crew members reported having developed a fear of flying as well as of being a passenger on other modes of transportation. Most reported uncertainty surrounding their future career prospects due to their physical injuries and flying phobias. All survivors had accepted psychological help arranged by the airline after the crash but generally felt that the company had been unsupportive and had made no real effort to understand the stress they were experiencing. At follow-up, five had left their original employer and had accepted jobs with different airlines.

The overall level of PTSD pathology at 18 months was remarkably high. The three subjects who had reported the highest overall levels of symptomatology were the three most senior members of the crew, with the most responsibility on board. They had also suffered severe physical injuries. Compared to other crew members, these senior staff reported having felt more responsible for others but helpless during the crash, and they suffered more feelings of survivor guilt. Their rational knowledge that, as cabin crew, they had no realistic chance of actually preventing the tragedy did not stop them from experiencing emotional waves of remorse. Part of the guilt came from their failure, due to their own injuries, to help the passengers after the crash, which suggests that both factors—responsibility and personal injury—contributed to their higher posttraumatic stress severity than their lower-ranking colleagues.

The persistence of disabling psychological symptoms and disability for as long as 18 months may at least partly reflect a lack of proper treatment. While the crew members received some company-sponsored "counseling," it was clear that the most appropriate kind of posttraumatic therapy was not received. It seemed evident that early and appropriate treatment might well have prevented the persistence of severe psychological symptoms 18 months after the event.

A further complicating factor was the crew's feeling that they had not been sympathetically treated by their employers. Their anger at the way they were being handled poisoned their attitude toward the counseling arranged by the employers, which was apparently seen as simply trying to mollify the situation. The crew felt that the airline management had no understanding of what they had been through and had assumed that because they were members of the staff, they should be able to cope with minimal distress. They were also made to feel like "unpleasant reminders" to the airline of an event that the company wished to sweep under the rug in order to avoid bad publicity.

Even convicted criminals aren't allowed to be gratuitously taunted and reviled. Unfortunately, the situation described in Marks et al.'s (1995) study is all too familiar in my practice, as I see case after case of workers in all types of professions shunned and alienated after job-related trauma because their sufferings either cost the company money or cause embarrassment, or both. The irony is that solid prevention efforts plus early, effective, and sympathetic handling of work-related traumatic disability syndromes virtually always saves money and reflects well on the company in terms of public relations and good will (Albrecht, 1996; Susskind & Field, 1996; see also Chapter 9). Hopefully, more companies will get the message and offer their injured and traumatized employees the kind of psychotherapeutic services that truly aid in healing and recovery.

Chapter 7

OUT OF NOWHERE

Natural and Technological Disasters

We learn geology the morning after the earthquake.

—Ralph Waldo Emerson

In my clinical practice, I typically see patients who have been individually traumatized in assaults, work injuries, or traffic accidents. But
the experience of 1992's Hurricane Andrew in the South Florida area
acquainted many local clinicans firsthand with the traumatic effects of
disasters that affect whole groups of people. Many of these reactions
correspond to what we know from the general literature on traumatic
disasters that occur in earthquakes, shipwrecks, fires, floods, industrial
accidents, and terrorist bombings.

THE NATURE OF DISASTERS AND
THE DISASTER RESPONSE

Characteristics of Disasters

The word *disaster* is derived from the Latin *dis* ("against") and *astrum*
("stars")—hence, "The stars are against you." The difference between
an "accident" and a "disaster" may be one of degree. In a disaster the

basic social structures are affected sufficiently to threaten the existence and functioning of the community. Unlike in a accident, where outside resources are quickly mobilized to help the victims, in a disaster the scale of need often exceeds the resources available, at least in the immediate community (Eranen & Liebkind, 1993).

As a rough classification, disasters may be divided into two broad categories. As the name implies, *natural disasters* are those that are product of errant nature: hurricanes, floods, avalanches, wildfires, earthquakes. *Technological disasters* involve the misworks of man: shipwrecks, plane crashes, building collapses, toxic spills, nuclear reactor leaks. In some cases, the dividing line is not so clear. If a freak rainstorm swells a reservoir and causes a dam to burst, or if a seismic tremor cracks the casing on a nuclear power plant, is that disaster natural or technological or both?

Definitional distinctions aside, major disasters possess a number of characteristics that put them clearly in the category of shared traumatic events (Abueg, Drescher, & Kubany, 1994; Aldwin, 1994). First, there is often little or no warning that the event is about to occur, such as in an earthquake or bridge collapse. Even when supposedly adequate warning is available, as with a hurricane that is tracked for days, people often display a stupefying capacity for denial and minimization. Thus, by the time the threat is unmistakably clear, it's often too late.

Second, disasters generally occur in a relatively short time frame. By the time the full extent of the threat is realized, the worst may be over, yet the aftermath must be dealt with.

Third, disasters typically involve extreme danger, including loss of life. At the very least, people lose something of value, whether it's their home, treasured keepsakes, their livelihood, friends or family members, not to mention their sense of a secure and predictable world.

Fourth, both natural and technological disasters provide very little chance for people to exert any kind of meaningful personal control. Helplessness magnifies the traumatic effect of disasters. Conversely, engaging in rescue or relief efforts—doing *something* other than sitting around waiting for the next boom to fall—is typically associated with significantly lower levels of psychological trauma, even if the efforts are exerted after the peak of the disaster itself.

Finally, disasters happen to many people simultaneously. It's not unusual for disaster victims to feel like the whole world is coming to an end. As described below, this provides an opportunity for both cooperative support and divisive conflict. On the positive side, the fact that many community members share similar trauma experiences may facilitate therapeutic disclosure of fearful thoughts and feelings regarding the trauma. In addition, the community may pull together and provide a higher than usual level of social support for victims, which may be therapeutic to those most in need.

The Disaster Response: Clinical Features

Some observers note that the behavioral and psychological responses seen in disasters frequently have a predictable structure and time course (Ursano, Fullerton, Bhartiya, & Kao, 1995). For most individuals, posttraumatic psychiatric symptoms are transitory. For others, however, the effects of a disaster linger long after the event, rekindled by new experiences that remind the person of the past traumatic event.

Even relatively circumscribed disasters can have long-range effects. Victims of the 1972 Buffalo Creek dam collapse experienced anxiety, depression, and posttraumatic stress symptoms as long as 14 years after the event. Many of these PTSD syndromes were similar to those seen in traumatized Vietnam veterans (Green, Lindy, Grace, & Leonard, 1992). Control and support were important moderating variables. Loss of control as a stressor and intrusive thoughts about that stressor appear to be associated with traumatic disability long after the disaster event. Studies of conditioned emotional responses suggest that reliving memories of a disaster experience can generate substantial affect and physiological arousal (Baum & Fleming, 1993).

The severity of a disaster is perhaps the single best predictor of both the probability and the frequency of postdisaster psychological disability (Abueg et al., 1994; Green, 1991; Ursano, Fullerton, & Norwood, 1995), with studies suggesting that 10 to 30 percent of highly exposed individuals develop PTSD. The greatest risk is for persons exposed to life threat, grotesque scenes or activities (e.g., handling human remains), or similar situations evoking intense, overwhelming revulsion or fear. Intrusive thoughts and memories seem to be the most frequently reported PTSD symptoms following natural disasters, with avoidance symptoms— feelings of numbness, social withdrawal, and shunning of trauma-related situations or reminders—tending to be less common (Abueg et al., 1994).

PTSD per se is not the only psychological disorder associated with disasters (Ursano et al., 1995). Major depression, generalized anxiety disorder, adjustment disorder, and substance abuse have also been diagnosed in individuals exposed to a disaster. Grief reactions are common after all disasters. Single parents may be at a high risk for developing psychological disorders, since they often have few resources to start with and they commonly lose some of these already-meager social supports after a disaster. Over time, when resources remain limited and employment and postdisaster financial resources are scarce in the community, there is often a sharp increase in domestic violence and child abuse.

Indeed, hostility, with its disrupting effect on family and community, is all too common following disasters (Ursano et al., 1995). Although in some cases reemerging anger can be a sign of a return to normal (i.e., it is again safe to be angry and express one's losses, disappointments, and needs), in others hostility should remind the care provider to assess the risks of family violence and substance abuse.

Anger as a reaction to bereavement in the aftermath of a disaster—especially a man-made one—may be complicated by the desire to apportion blame and responsibility (Solomon & Thompson, 1995). The anger may be free-floating and unfocused, when there is no clear target of blame or responsibility, and may be displaced onto rescue workers, medical personnel, community officials, or anyone deemed responsible for the disaster event or failure of helping services (Lindemann, 1944; Raphael, 1986). This type of response was seen after the 1996 crash of TWA flight 800, where relatives of the doomed passengers blamed officials for "not doing enough."

Even in purely natural disasters, the sense of unfairness and existential outrage may be displaced onto human targets of opportunity. For example, in the aftermath of the Mount St. Helens eruption, where "blaming" the volcano was clearly pointless, many victims directed their anger at identification and rescue teams, government officials, and insurance companies (Murphy, 1984). Attribution of responsibility and blame seems to be one way of coping with the helplessness of many disaster situations by implying at least potential preventability and controllability of future events (Raphael, 1986; Walster, 1966).

The issue of culpability and controllability is a complex one, however. In some cases, blaming another person for an accident may be associated with poorer recovery (Janoff-Bulman & Wortman, 1977). Indeed, residents of Three Mile Island who accepted responsibility for their disaster-related reactions seemed to have had fewer stress-related difficulties than those who blamed others. Yet a study of burn patients (Kiecolt-Glaser & Williams, 1987) found that self-blame was associated with greater pain and depression, as well as poorer compliance with treatment. The poor coping of those who blame others may be related to the issue of justice. When the circumstances of an accident are particularly unfair, coping may be especially difficult and blaming may represent the only remaining ego-cohesive defense against total psychological decompensation (Janoff-Bulman & Wortman, 1977).

An investigation into the long-term reactions of survivors of several kinds of technological disasters (Solomon & Thompson, 1995) found that psychological distress persisted for many years in the form of intrusion and avoidance symptoms, generalized anxiety and depression, somatic complaints, and social dysfunction. This was accompanied by very high levels of specifically targeted anger, strong fears of other disasters happening again, firmly held ideas of who was to blame, and a widespread perception that justice was not done. Anger was felt mostly towards those who were seen as responsible for the event itself, but was also directed towards the media and the legal system. The anger was intense, focused, and long-lasting, persisting as long as 18 years postincident.

One model of the disaster response (Freedy, Shaw, Jarrell, & Masters, 1992; Hobfoll, 1989) suggests that loss of material resources (home, household items, money) and personal and social resources (feelings of control, family stability, time) can create psychological and physical distress, because these losses leave victims with fewer coping options to reestablish their lives. Lower socioeconomic groups may be more vulnerable to resource loss, coping difficulties, and psychological distress, since they have fewer available resources prior to the disaster; on the other hand, they may have "less to lose." Accordingly, many disaster experts emphasize the practical necessity of replenishing diminished or lost material resources as a means of lessening psychological distress and enhancing coping.

One study (Sattler, Sattler, Kaiser, Hamby, Adams, Love, Winkler, Abu-Ukkaz, Watts, & Beatty, 1995) examined of the effects of 1992's Hurricane Andrew on South Florida residents, many of whom were of low socioeconomic status before the storm. Many survivors were found living in public shelters without the material resources needed to reestablish their lives. About one-quarter of these shelter residents showed significant depression, and one-third met criteria for PTSD, including loss of interest in daily activities, difficulty sleeping, changes in appetite, emotional numbness, heightened irritability, anxiety, headaches, and difficulty concentrating. These findings reinforce the vital importance of providing material relief resources as quickly as possible after a disaster. Both Maslow (1968) and common sense are right: material needs precede psychological needs. You just can't do very effective psychotherapy with hungry, dirty, and exhausted people.

The psychosocial response to a civil disaster, the 1992 Los Angeles riots, was studied by Hanson, Kilpatrick, Freedy, and Saunders (1995). Here again, a combination of stressor severity and loss of material resources seemed to predict the degree of posttraumatic stress. In addition to direct exposure to violence, the residents of South Central Los Angeles experienced significant disruption of services and destruction of neighborhood establishments. Not surprisingly, higher rates of PTSD sequelae (e.g., reexperiencing, avoidance, and arousal) and subthreshold symptoms of PTSD were found among subjects who reported having directly experienced riot-related violence or destruction, compared with those who were more removed or secondarily affected.

Postdisaster chronic sleep disturbances are common clinical problems that may require treatment. Sleep difficulties can be due to anxiety related to current disaster events (e.g., fear of earthquake aftershocks) or to an underlying psychological disorder such as depression or PTSD. Physical injury increases the risk of postdisaster psychological disability by evoking ongoing retraumatization (pain and disability) and persistent reminders of the effects of the traumatic event (e.g., disfigurement). Similarly, often overlooked after a disaster are neuropsychological syndromes attributable to head trauma and metabolic disturbances following crush injuries, burns, exposure to toxins, and the like (Miller, 1993a, 1993b, 1995; Ursano et al., 1995). Indeed, postconcussion syndrome after head trauma and PTSD share many features and are frequently misdiagnosed (Miller, 1993a; see also Chapters 1 and 3).

Phases of the Disaster Response

Although all generalizations must be taken with the proverbial grain of salt, research and clinical study have shown that in many disasters, people's responses often follow a predictable course (Cohen, Culp, & Genser, 1987; Weiner, 1992).

In the immediate *phase of impact*, the victims experience a growing fear as the impending threat becomes known. This may pass over into paralyzing terror as the full realization of the danger unfolds. In many cases, numbing depersonalization, a kind of psychic anesthesia, permits the person to "go on automatic," partially ignore his pain and fear, and take some constructive action during the disaster.

The impact phase shades over into the *phase of heroism*, in which disaster victims make intense and valiant efforts to protect and save whomever and whatever they can. They often work feverishly, nonstop, for hours or even days at a time, propelled by grit and adrenalin, sometimes valorously distinguishing themselves in ways they never thought possible. However, if the emergency lasts too long, exhaustion, frustration, and disappointment eventually overcome them, especially if their brave efforts have been in vain.

After the acute danger has subsided, the survivors peek out from their bunkers, and the *honeymoon phase* begins, typically lasting days to weeks. The survivors survey the damage, exchange reminiscences and "war stories," and generally share in the elation of having survived the ordeal.

A veritable carnival atmosphere may prevail as survivors pat each other on the back, share remaining snacks and drinks, and look forward to imminent rescue, recovery, and rebuilding.

But all too often the reprieve doesn't come soon enough. Or it is half-hearted, disorganized, misapplied—too little, too late. The survivors, waiting and waiting for the relief they feel they've earned, become disillusioned and bitter in this next *phase of disappointment.* The communal spirit begins to fray as survivors bicker over dwindling resources. Tempers flare, people sicken, and many survivors sink into depression.

Hopefully, however, not for too long. In the *phase of reorganization,* the survivors come to realize that recovery is in their own hands. They begin to rally around the task of rebuilding their lives, or at least remaining as comfortable as possible until real help can arrive. Some remaining animosity and resentment may sully this renewed spirit of cooperation, but mostly the survivors gamely hold on and look toward the future. In many of these cases, the posttraumatic stress reaction may be delayed for months until it is "safe" to let down one's guard, to drop the numbed psychological survival mode and allow one's true feelings to surface.

Individual Responses to Disasters

Whether the disaster is natural or technological may affect the victims' appraisal of, and psychological response to, the catastrophic event (Baum, 1987; Baum & Fleming, 1993; Baum, Fleming, & Singer, 1983). Realistically, we don't expect to have control, certainly not complete control, over the forces of nature. So as tragic as the results of floods and earthquakes may be, perhaps we're better able to resign ourselves in a philosophical, will-of-God kind of way. But disasters caused by human folly or neglect are different. Here we often feel that there's been a violation of the trust we implicitly place in those who are supposed to protect us, a loss of control made all the more frightening by the idea that even matters we clever humans are supposed to have well in hand can sometimes elude our grasp and blow up in our faces.

For example, residents who discovered they'd been living on radon-saturated land reported overall lower stress levels than those who discovered that their homes were built over a toxic landfill—this, despite a greater perceived health risk from the radon vs. the toxic chemicals (Baum & Fleming, 1993). Radon is natural and when the homes were built, the risk was not yet understood. But people put the chemicals in the ground and the builders should have known better than to place houses over a toxic dump. In this case, blame and betrayal add emotional poison to the noxious brew of callously dumped chemicals and uncaringly constructed homes.

Moreover, unlike the slow, steady contamination of radonized houses, most natural disasters tend to come and go, to have a beginning, a middle, and an end. You're either drowned in the flood or you're not; you're either buried in the avalanche or you aren't; your home and heirlooms are either swallowed up in the earthquake or wildfire or mudslide or they escape. But certain types of technological disasters, most significantly toxic spills and nuclear leaks, contaminate not just the present but the forseeable future, even unto the generations. The frightening prospect of possible future cancer or genetic damage extend the time period of potential trauma into virtual infinity. There can be no relaxation of vigilance, no rest, no end.

Research confirms this. Studies of people exposed to the Three Mile Island nuclear disaster or found to be living near toxic landfills reported particularly high rates of somatic distress, anxiety, and depression (Baum & Fleming, 1993). On cognitive testing, these subjects did particularly poorly on tasks requiring concentration and persistence. They also showed increases in blood pressure, higher levels of circulating stress hormones, changes in immune functioning, and persisting posttraumatic stress symptoms, such as hyperarousal, intrusion, and avoidance. These changes were still present up to six years after the accident.

Feelings of uncertainty, helplessness, and loss of control appeared to be the most important mediators of stress among toxic landfill area residents. On the other hand, those Three Mile Island area residents who had more social support, perceived themselves to be more in control, or had more adaptive coping styles showed overall lower levels of stress. By the end of the decade, most of the problems had finally faded for virtually all of the residents.

In most disasters, only a minority of victims show a persistent, severe, dysfunctional PTSD pattern. Most victims of even the most severe stressors are usually able to cope with the circumstances and move on with few lasting effects. Individual differences in appraisal, response strength, characterological assets, and other relevant factors appear to contribute to how intense or long a stressful episode will be, or whether it is experienced as stressful at all. Together, the power of a stressful experience, its duration, and the vulnerabilities and sources of strength that people bring to each situation will determine the degree to which disaster stress or any stress affects physical and psychological functioning (Baum et al., 1983; see also Chapters 1 and 12).

But even disasters caused by callous neglect or incompetence may be easier for victims to deal with than destruction emanating from the direct intention to do evil. A study of survivors of the 1993 New York World Trade Center terrorist bombing (Difede, Apfeldorf, Cloitre, Spielman, & Perry, 1997) showed that the most distressing aspect of their ordeal was the shattering of their fundamental beliefs about themselves (invulnerability, immortality), the world (predictability, controllability, safety), and other people (trust, safety, isolation) that had previously shaped their lives. Many were angry that their fabric of belief in a just world had been rudely shredded. All felt isolated, in that others did not understand their ordeal. Concerns about death and questions about the meaning and purpose of their lives haunted many survivors. Subjects who had suffered previous traumas experienced a recrudescence of symptoms from those past events, along with the current traumatic reactions. Several subjects moved out of the area "to start over."

One universal risk factor for more severe reactions to disasters appears to be exposure to death and the presence of dead bodies. One component of this is the raw intensity of the exposure, for example, sights, smells, and sounds of the wounded and dying, distance from the bodies, or actual physical contact with the dead. Personalization and identification with the dead victims—"that could have been me"—appears to be a particular risk factor for later psychological disability. Subjects directly exposed to the dead have been found to subsequently show aversion to eating meat and compulsive handwashing; in most cases, these symptoms abated after several months (Lindy, Grace, & Green, 1981; McCarroll, Ursano, & Fullerton, 1993, 1995; Raphael, 1986; Ursano & McCarroll, 1990; Ursano et al., 1995).

Sometimes, the most traumatically stressful aspect of a disaster is the legal wrangling that ensues as victims and their families seek compensation, justice, or just some straight answers (Underwood & Liu, 1996). In the case of USAir flight 405, which crashed and burned during takeoff at New York's La Guardia Airport in March 1992, one survivor reported that lawyers for the airline and its insurance company actually argued that her emotional trauma stemmed not from the disaster itself but from dysfunctional family relationships during childhood, and they introduced counseling records from her divorce 14 years earlier to buttress their claim. It is sad and outrageous that survivors of such trauma can be made to endure retraumatization of this sort; hopefully, the judicial system will address these excesses.

Finally, psychological resiliency is an important, if uncommon, postdisaster response. The effects of traumatic events are not exclusively bad. For some people, trauma and loss facilitate a move toward growth and health, although, as noted elsewhere in this book, such salubrious effects of trauma of any type should be regarded as a gift, not an expectation (see Chapters 2 and 12).

CLINICAL INTERVENTION IN DISASTERS

Physical Care and Safety

We mental health clinicians like to think of ourselves as specializing in "psychological" forms of treatment, but, as noted above, what disaster victims often need first is down-to-earth, practical provision of basic services. Somebody's got to help stack the sandbags and hand out the sandwiches before we can even think of getting survivors to pay attention to our stress management lectures and coping skills groups. One way to look at this is to remember that in times of disaster physical care *is* psychological care, and initial postdisaster interventions must focus on establishing safety, providing nourishment and medical care, and affording protection from the elements (Kinston & Rosser, 1974; Ursano et al., 1995).

Information and Education

Once disaster survivors feel they're out of immediate danger, once they've been fed, clothed, bandaged, and sheltered, then they usually want answers. Lack of accurate information is itself potentially traumatic, and may be physically harmful if wild rumors result in panic or deprivation of services (Pitcher & Poland, 1992). Key points of information to be provided include the nature and effects of the disaster event itself and the progress of any ongoing or forthcoming response and relief efforts.

Moving to the psychological realm, victims of disaster appear to benefit from basic, understandable education about the onset and course of posttraumatic symptoms. In natural disasters, victims need to be warned of the resurgence of symptoms in the presence of disaster reminders: earthquakes are often followed by aftershocks; floods and storms rise and fall in intensity and vary in duration and geographic location. After the period of greatest impact, rain, wind, and aftershocks may act as vivid reminders of the original life-threatening experiences, and these reminders have been shown to be associated with increased severity of posttraumatic symptoms (Abueg et al., 1994).

It is important to reestablish communication networks in the disaster community as soon as possible. Newspapers, official bulletins, television, and especially radio can provide information as well as emotional help. Rumor management is an important task of community leaders and an area in which mental health personnel can assist. Fears of loss and separation should be addressed by establishing reliable communications, including casualty identification and notification procedures. Basic information should be provided about sanitation and injury care (Ursano et al., 1995).

Community Responses

For many mental health workers, disaster psychology requires a shift from the traditional focus on psychopathology. Ursano et al. (1995) have adapted preventive medicine's epidemiological model in infectious disease and toxicology as a paradigm for disaster intervention. This model includes determining the individual's level of exposure to emotion-laden stimuli, such as gruesome scenes or the experience of having family members killed or injured. It also involves identifying individuals at higher risk for illness and monitoring behavioral and psychological responses over both the short and long term.

Mental health consultation to the community can facilitate recovery and limit disability following a catastrophic event (Pitcher & Poland, 1992; Ursano et al., 1995). In the wake of a disaster, the mental health consultant attempts to identify high-risk groups and behaviors, foster recovery from acute stress, decrease the prevalence of serious disorders, and generally minimize pain and suffering. Both acute and long-term effects of the disaster must be considered. Initial interventions include consultation to the disaster community's leaders, teachers, and care providers to maximize their understanding of the responses to trauma and disaster.

Because disaster victims rarely present to traditional mental health services—indeed, even severely disturbed survivors of Hurricane Andrew felt that seeing a mental health counselor would be a further humiliation (Sattler et al., 1995)—psychological care must be organized around outreach programs into the community. Identifying high-risk groups is thus one of the most important aspects of disaster consultation (Pitcher & Poland, 1992; Ursano et al., 1995).

The disaster consultation team in the affected community must integrate smoothly into the disaster environment at a time when outsiders are often experienced as intrusive. A consultation team can be seen as "wanting something" from, or "getting off on," an environment in which resources are already stretched to the limit and survivors feel multiply stigmatized. Indeed, one of the more shameful aspects of the Hurricane Andrew experience related to me by survivors was the regular procession of "disaster tourists" who would wend their way down the interstate to view the devastated areas and its occupants, as if it were some kind of disaster theme park. In cases like these, liaison with primary care providers and disaster workers is critical for effective psychological intervention. The consultants must be knowledgeable of the culture and customs of the groups they wish to help (Sattler et al., 1995; Ursano et al., 1995).

Critical Incident Stress Debriefing

Critical Incident Stress Debriefing (CISD) is covered more comprehensively in Chapter 10 in connection with treating traumatized disaster relief and rescue workers and other emergency service and law enforcement personnel. In its application to disaster victims themselves, it serves as a form of structured, nonthreatening group crisis intervention in which each group member is allowed to tell the story of his disaster experience and express emotions in a supportive atmosphere.

The formal phases of a debriefing include an *introductory phase* in which the goals and purposes of the group are spelled out; a *fact phase* where each participant describes his own experience of the event; a *thought phase* in which each participant describes what "was going through my mind" cognitively during the event; a *reaction phase* in which the members express what they felt emotionally or describe what was the "worst part" of the event; a *symptom phase* in which members describe the various psychophysiological reactions (pounding heart, sleeplessness, etc.) that they may be experiencing postincident; a *teaching phase* in which the group leader educates the participants as to the nature of stress symptoms and the course of recovery; and a final *closure phase*, in which any unfinished business is discussed and the members provide each other with mutual support for the future.

Various modes of debriefing have been described in the literature on disaster relief (Abueg et al., 1994; Mitchell, 1988; Mitchell & Everly, 1996). The central tasks common to all these approaches is the disclosure of the individual's story. From a behavioral perspective, conditioned avoidance is minimized through healthy reexposure or extinction of feared cues in the context of the trauma. Feelings of safety are reclaimed most powerfully through the support inherent in group debriefings. Communal debriefings also permit the modification and enhancement of each individual's story to accommodate some shared reality representing the experience of the trauma. Personalization, or feeling as if one has been singled out or targeted by fate, can be minimized by the shared group debriefing experience. See Chapter 10 for a step-by-step description of the debriefing process.

Psychotherapy

What most mental health professionals think of as traditional psychotherapy usually plays its main postdisaster role after basic safety and comfort needs have been met, the rescue efforts completed or well underway, or even later, when the survivor has salvaged what he can, settled the insurance claims, and moved to a different locale. Now with the opportunity for reflection and the process of rebuilding a life, the full impact of the trauma may come flooding back, in the kind of "delayed reaction" described in Chapter 1.

In other cases, the trauma memories, or their emotional charge, remain choked off from consciousness, and the patient reacts to disaster cues and reminders with disturbing somatic symptoms or uncharacteristic deterioration in behavior. In these latter cases, the traumatic experience and the patient's reaction to it may first have to be elicited and uncovered by careful probing on the part of the clinician. Such contextually conditioned fear cues can best be obtained through careful questioning regarding the disaster victim's experiences at the height of the traumatic experience. By simply asking what the victim saw, heard, felt, touched, or tasted, the clinician opens additional channels of information and facilitates additional storytelling. Proprioceptive and kinesthetic cues can draw forth intense elaborations of the disaster experience, such as being crushed, pinned, or confined (Abueg et al., 1994). The careful and skillful use of assistive techniques, such as relaxation, hypnosis, and EMDR, may be helpful in individual cases.

Guilt may be a pervasive theme following disasters. The therapist must help the survivor explore such themes as feeling he or she did not do enough, made a mistake during the recovery phase, or somehow was responsible for some unfortunate consequence. Once the history of these events is pieced together, information on what to expect, cognitive-behavioral restructuring, and skill-building in desensitization to feared imagery can be implemented. In this regard, therapists can assist patients in modifying distorted attributions, e.g., "It's all my fault—if only I had insisted that we not go away that weekend, we wouldn't have been caught in the landslide (flood/plane crash/building explosion) and my wife (child/parent/friend) would still be alive" (Abueg et al., 1994; Ursano et al., 1995).

One important goal of psychotherapy that is basic to all trauma therapy is increasing the disaster victim's sense of controllability and predictability. In this sense, disaster psychotherapy follows the basic guidelines of trauma therapy described in Chapter 2. As noted there, the construction of meaning from adversity is an active process that appears to affect the outcome of the traumatic experience and recovery. The meaning of a disaster to any one person emerges from the interaction of the his past history, present context, and physiological state. The ascribed meaning will then direct individual behaviors of what to do, what to fix, and whom or what to blame. Remember that the "meaning" of any given traumatic event is dynamic, not static: it changes over time as the individual's psychosocial context changes (Abueg et al., 1994; Ursano et al., 1995; Ursano, Kao, & Fullerton, 1992; Ursano & McCarroll, 1990).

Disaster Psychotherapy with Children and Families

As much as they affect adults, disasters can also have a profound impact on the psychosocial functioning of children and family groups (Abueg et al., 1994; Johnson, 1989; Nader & Pynoos, 1992; Pynoos & Nader, 1988; Pitcher & Poland, 1992; Vernberg & Vogel, 1993). For example, dramatic increases in illness, domestic violence, alcohol abuse, and utilization of family mental health resources followed the eruption of Mount St. Helens (Adams & Adams, 1984). If family functioning of adult caretakers is impaired, it is likely that children will also be directly and indirectly traumatized.

Often, during and following a disaster, community leaders and teachers notice how eerily quiet the children are, and may be thankful, given the adults' own level of distress, that these children seem to be "coping" so well. However, the inhibition of children's normal spontaneous activity is usually an indicator of a great deal of underlying stress. In other cases, children's distress is more evident, showing clinging, crying, and behavioral regression. In addition, the distress of parents, teachers, and other adults is usually picked up on by the children and increases their own fear and disorientation. Accordingly, interventions with parents and families should be directed at assisting the child to regain a sense of safety, validating the child's emotional reactions rather than discouraging or minimizing them, anticipating and providing additional support during times of heightened distress (such as anniversaries of the event), and minimizing secondary stresses (Johnson, 1989; Pitcher & Poland, 1992; Ursano et al., 1995).

The stresses on families, particularly the persistent postdisaster problems of lost income, employment, and housing, result in increased feelings of powerlessness and loss of control, which often lead to increased rates of child and spouse abuse. This is why the provision of information, education, and basic services, though not usually thought of as "therapy" itself, is often an indispensable part of improving the mental health of families after a disaster (Ursano et al., 1995).

The death or serious injury of a child in a disaster carries particular meaning and portends high risk for a severe traumatic stress response. Following an Australian rail accident and the 1988 Armenian earthquake, the worst bereavement responses were seen among parents who lost children (Singh & Raphael, 1981). Child victims of trauma universally evoke powerful emotional reactions and generally create disturbing memories for witnesses, including rescuers (Ursano et al., 1995; see also Chapter 10).

Several large-group, mostly school-based, postdisaster interventions for children and adolescents have been reviewed by Abueg et al. (1994). Stewart, Hardin, Weinrich, McGeorge, Lopez, and Pesut (1992) describe an intervention in the wake of Hurricane Hugo that used a single, extended group therapy format to lower disaster-related distress and to enhance social support among students. The intervention incorporated physical and group-enhancing activities, including a didactic portion that explained the relationship between unmet needs and stress and also attempted to normalize stress-related symptoms.

Abueg et al. (1994) also cite Weinberg's (1990) large-group intervention program for adolescents to deal with the grief and loss issues following such school traumas as accidents or suicides. Students meet in the familiar, supportive atmosphere of a large school assembly. They are provided didactic information and encouragement with regard to healthy grief responses and adaptive coping efforts. Students showing unusually strong, negative emotional reactions and those who attempt to leave the meeting are met with one-on-one by counselors and are encouraged where appropriate to participate in small-group sessions. In many respects, this intervention follows a CISD-type model, as described above.

A school-based approach more explicitly modeled on the CISD protocol is described by Johnson (1989). This adaptation for children and adolescents involves a post-crisis group debriefing that incorporates an *introductory phase*, in which the goals and purposes of the group are spelled out; a *fact phase*, where the children each describe what happened to them in the disaster; a *feeling phase*, in which the children may express the emotions and reactions they have had to the crisis; a *teaching phase*, in which the group leader educates the children as to the nature of stress symptoms and the course of recovery; and a *closure phase*, in which the children are encouraged to develop some plan of action to facilitate improved coping in the future.

Johnson (1989) emphasizes that the group's sense of security and normal routine needs to be reestablished at the conclusion of the debriefing. Even class debriefings, designed to help students adjust in a familiar setting and structure, are themselves upsetting. To the extent possible, a sense of continuity should be provided by a return to some semblance of a normal schedule of activities. After the debriefing process has fulfilled its therapeutic purpose, the leader lets the students know that the time has come to resume a normal routine.

Another CISD model of intervention for use in the schools is presented by Ritter (1994). This approach encourages schools to act proactively to establish a working relationship with CISD teams in the local community, instead of waiting for a disaster to occur and then trying to play catch-up by throwing something together. Ritter (1994) also recommends the careful credentialing of CISD mental health team members to assure that they have the proper experience for this type of clinical work.

Schools have effectively utilized CISD team resources in connection with student suicides, homicides, hostage incidents, natural and man-made disasters, motor vehicle deaths, and sports event deaths. Protocols for the effective use of CISD-type resources require flexibility, coopera-tion, and coordination of local and regional debriefing resources. They may also require additional expenditures to coordinate different groups and individuals and bring them all up to the appropriate level of knowl-edge and skill on such topics as the CISD process, trauma, death and dying, and grief responses (Ritter, 1994).

Harris (1991) describes a family-based crisis intervention model de-signed for use within one week following a disaster. Initial sessions are designed to elicit open expression of feelings and the development of rapport with the therapist. Cognitive restructuring is used when appro-priate to correct distortions and irrational thinking on the part of the family members. Next, issues requiring immediate attention are identi-fied. Communication skills are taught and social support systems are mobilized within and outside the family. The family is then encouraged to take concrete, positive problem-solving action to create a sense of movement and progress toward goals.

Vernberg and Vogel (1993) describe a disaster-intervention protocol that divides intervention strategies into four phases. The *predisaster phase* primarily involves incorporating mental health services in local or regional disaster plans. Interventions in the immediate *impact phase* of the disaster include ensuring support for help providers at affected sites, gathering and disseminating accurate information, and making initial contact with children who have been affected by the traumatic disaster events.

Short-term adaptation phase interventions include classroom strategies that allow emotional expression and cognitive processing of the traumatic events through group discussions, drawing, play therapy and other appro-priate outlets. Interventions during this phase also include family ap-proaches, such as providing information and education, absenteeism out-reach, and brief family therapy. During this phase individual modalities, such as one-on-one debriefing, individual psychotherapy, and pharmacological approaches, may be used where appropriate. Finally, *long-term adjustment-phase* interventions include more extensive individual and family psychotherapy, as well as the use of rituals and memorials.

Throughout—as in most of the other well-run intervention programs in this category—there is an emphasis on providing the maximum degree of adaptive recovery and normalization with a minimum of therapeutic intrusion and overload, while at the same time identifying those at-risk children and families at each stage who may require more intensive and extensive treatment and support.

Community Responses

By definition, most disasters are community events, and there is much that community leaders can do to offer support and increase therapeutic and social morale.

Symbols are an important part of the recovery process. Commendations and awards to rescue workers and to those who have distinguished themselves are important components of the community recovery process. Memorials to the victims of the disaster are part of the healing process and should be encouraged. Leaders are powerful symbols in and of themselves. Leaders should be encouraged to express their own grief in order to lead the community in recognizing the appropriateness of constructive mourning (Ursano et al., 1995).

The recognition of a disaster by outside authorities, such as the governor or president, is also an important part of recovery. When a community is recognized and its distress acknowledged, its members often feel less alone and more in communion with the world at large. These outside support networks offer the hope of additional resources as well as emotional support. The mental health consultant, who may at first feel like an outsider, fills some of these same functions, serving as an indicator of the larger world's concern, providing hope for the return to "normal" life, and allowing a brief respite from the ongoing issues of disaster stress and recovery (Ursano et al., 1995).

By their sheer scope, disasters clearly exceed the ability of any one group of professional responders to control and ameliorate the total situation. Psychotherapists and mental health consultants can best contribute to disaster recovery efforts by recognizing the importance of concrete support, providing appropriate debriefing and other therapeutic interventions, and serving as a resource for "helping the helpers" (see Chapter 10). In their proper postdisaster role, mental health clinicians can have a profound healing impact, not just on individuals but on whole populations and communities, often making the difference between mere hardscrabble survival and healthy, foward-moving recovery.

Chapter 8

THE EVIL THAT MEN DO

Criminal Assault and Crime Victim Trauma

The real significance of crime is in its being a
breach of faith with the community of mankind.

—Joseph Conrad

Certain traumas do more than injure us: they violate our sense of
security and stability, yank the existential ground right out from
under our feet. More than most traumas, violence perpetrated by
other people robs us of our sense that the world can ever be a safe
place again. The suddenness, randomness, and fundamental unfairness
of such attacks can overwhelm victims with helplessness and despair.
As difficult as it may be to bear the traumas of injury and loss that
occur in accidents and mishaps, far more wrenching are the wounds
that occur at the deliberate hands of our fellow human beings, that
result from the callous and malicious depredations of others. Assaults,
rapes, forcible robberies, and even petty but frightening harassments
and threats nick, dent, and occasionally pierce the psychic shell of
security we all envelop ourselves in to get through the day. Violent
crimes shatter us in mind, body, and soul.

In some populations, as much as 40 to 70 percent of individuals have
been exposed to crime-related traumas sufficient to meet PTSD diagnostic criteria, and many individuals have been multiply exposed to such
extreme stressors (Breslau, Davis, Andreski, & Peterson, 1991; Norris,
1992; Resnick, Kilpatrick, Dansky, Saunders, & Best, 1993). Except for
rape, men appear to be assaulted under the same kinds of situations as
women, but it may be more difficult for a man to report an assault for

fear of shame, ridicule, or disbelief (Saunders, Kilpatrick, Resnick, & Tidwell, 1989).

TYPES OF CRIMINAL VIOLENCE AND CRIMINAL TRAUMA

Criminal Assault

The U.S. Department of Justice estimates that rapes, robberies, and assaults account for 2.2 million injuries and more than 700,000 hospital days annually. Annual costs (in 1987 dollars) due to medical bills, mental health bills, and lost productivity are estimated to exceed 6.1 billion. Indeed, for many Americans today, violent crime is *the* overriding social and political issue (see also Chapter 9). The bad guys seem to have gotten more brazen, while the rest of us cower helplessly, feeling vicimized not just by the criminals but by the justice system that is supposed to protect us (Bidinotto, 1996; Kirwin, 1997).

One of my patients, a middle-aged woman, was walking to her car in the parking lot of a shopping mall at dusk. Laden with packages, she didn't see the tall figure in the dark green hooded sweatshirt until too late. "Give it up, bitch" was all she heard before the assailant pushed her to the ground and warned her not to look up or he'd shoot her dead. Rifling through her belongings, he apparently wasn't satisfied with the yield and, out of frustration or sheer meanness, put his foot on the prostrate woman's cheek and proceeded to grind her face into the pavement for several minutes, telling her over and over again that she would be killed. Then, as quickly as he appeared, he abruptly fled. The police came, but the assailant was never apprehended.

"My whole life is ruined," the woman later told me. She can no longer go to shopping malls, and seeing dark green clothing of any kind produces terrifying flashbacks of the assault. Although she suffered only minor lacerations and abrasions on her cheek, she experiences bouts of excruciating facial pain. She has been worked up neurologically for trigeminal neuralgia, but all standard medical tests have been negative. Sleep is almost impossible due to nightmares of being chased and attacked by "wild animals." Sometimes at night she hears the phrase, "Give it up bitch" playing repeatedly in her head like a stuck tape loop. She gets headaches and night sweats, and has lost more than 30 pounds.

Another patient, a young male gym teacher in a rough high school, tried to break up a fight during a basketball game and was stabbed for his efforts. He hasn't been back on the basketball court yet, and even ball games on TV disturb him. Another patient was beaten by overzealous bouncers in a bar and sustained a closed head injury plus a posttraumatic stress syndrome characterized by intrusive recollections of the event and frightening dreams. A third patient, a male mugging victim who was hit on the head with a baseball bat, relates that "I wake up every night hearing my head crack."

In addition to PTSD, other diagnosable psychiatric syndromes may be seen following criminal assault. Depression, anxiety, and substance abuse are common psychological disorders found in victims of robbery, rape, and burglary (Falsetti & Resnick, 1995; Frank & Stewart, 1984; Hough, 1985), and a high proportion of panic attacks trace their onset to some traumatically stressful experience (Uhde, Boulenger, Roy-Byrne, Geraci, Vittone, & Post, 1985). In follow-up study, approximately 50 percent of crime-induced PTSD cases were found to persist in a chronic course after three months (Rothbaum, Foa, Riggs, Murdock, & Walsh, 1992). Clinical experience suggests that such traumatic effects may persist in some form for far longer—years, decades, or a lifetime.

Crime can affect those not directly assaulted or killed. When a family member has been murdered, surviving family members may suffer from intrusive images of what they imagine the scene of their loved one's death to have been, even if—perhaps especially if—they were not present at the time of the death (Falsetti & Resnick, 1995; Schlosser, 1997). Criminal assault survivors may be scapegoated and blamed for their attack by friends and family members seeking to distance themselves from the contagious taint of vulnerability that crime victims are all too often imbued with.

Abduction and Torture

Anyone who has been tortured remains tortured.

—Jean Amery

Perhaps the most extreme form of violence that one human being can perpetrate upon another is abduction and torture. These acts typically take place in a political context or as part of a civil crime, such as a botched robbery, attempted extortion, sadistic sex crime, or revenge. Treatment of hostages can range from gracious to atrocious and may sometimes vary between these two extremes within the same event. The duration of captivity may range from minutes to years, but in most civilian crime settings, hostage crises are typically resolved within hours or days (Frederick, 1994; Rosenberg, 1997).

One of my patients, a middle-aged businessman, was abducted from the underground parking garage of his office building by criminals who mistook him for an errant gang member who'd skipped with a large sum of their money. He was thrown into the back of a van and taken to a remote motel room, where he was beaten and tortured for several days before finally being dumped unconscious onto a deserted street where he was found and taken to a local hospital. He claimed to have virtually no memory of the ordeal itself, aside from a few frightening dream-like images. In addition, his overall short-term memory and concentration were seriously impaired.

One of the differential diagnostic dilemmas in this case was figuring out how much of this patient's well-documented cognitive impairment was due to head trauma sustained in the beatings and how much to extreme psychological numbing. Happily, this man was able to obtain a degree of justice in seeing his attackers prosecuted, which aided greatly in his integrating the trauma and getting on with his life. However, he will always carry a certain edgy wariness about him, and he now tries never to go anywhere alone. Underground parking is out of the question.

It is hardly surprising that kidnapping, with or without actual physical violence, can produce severe posttraumatic stress reactions. Yet many hostages manage to survive their ordeals relatively intact, some even emerging somewhat seasoned and ennobled by their experience. Several factors seem to be associated with better outcomes after hostage situations, including: (1) age over 40; (2) a belief in one's own inner strength of self; (3) reflective thoughts of loved ones; (4) faith in a higher power; (5) continuing hope that the captivity will end favorably; (6) using one's powers of reasoning and planning to figure out possible plans for escape or release; (7) physical or mental exercise; (8) appropriate expression of anger, where feasible; and (9) ability to focus attention and become task-oriented (Frederick, 1994).

Crime and the Social Environment

DSM-IV (APA, 1994) recognizes that posttraumatic stress reactions can occur in persons who observe terrible events happening to others, even if they are not directly affected. This includes witnessing crimes of violence or threats of violence to others. Indeed, certain segments of the population may be exposed to traumatically stressful events on a fairly regular basis, for example, residents of crime-ridden and socioeconomically depressed inner-city neighborhoods.

Breslau and Davis (1992) and Breslau et al. (1991) studied over one thousand young adults from a large health maintenance organization in inner-city Detroit and found that many of these residents showed classic signs and symptoms of PTSD. Precipitating events included the standard traumatic events of sudden injuries, serious accidents, physical assaults, and rape. But also important was the traumatic effect of having one's life threatened without actually being physically hurt, getting news of the death or injury of a close friend or relative, narrowly escaping injury in an assault or accident, or having one's home destroyed in a fire. Overall, almost half of this sample of young inner-city adults reported experiencing potentially traumatic events and about a quarter of them developed full-blown PTSD.

Many of the young adults with PTSD continued to experience symptoms for a year or longer. These chronic PTSD sufferers were more likely than those whose symptoms resolved sooner to show hyperreactivity to stimuli that symbolized the traumatic event, as well as interpersonal numbing. They were also more likely to report greater anxiety, depression, poor concentration, and medical complaints. Women were found to be more susceptible to PTSD than men, and subjects who were poorly educated, were outgoing and impulsive, had a history of early conduct problems, and came from families with psychiatric and substance abuse histories were more likely to experience traumatically stressful events. This makes sense: people who are more impulsive and disturbed to begin with tend to take greater risks and more often find themselves in trouble-prone situations where they may be victimized and traumatized. Thus, in many cases, criminal activity may be as much related to the impulsivity and maladaptive lifestyle that leads to traumatic events in the first place as it is to the stress syndromes that result from those events; a similar relationship has been noted for impulsive antisociality and traumatic brain injury (Miller, 1987, 1988, 1989, 1990, 1992a, 1994a, 1994b, 1994c, 1997a; see Chapter 3).

Real Crime versus Fear of Crime

Now, some more bad news: Fear of crime may be hazardous to your health. Increasingly, social scientists are finding that the sheer overload of crime and disaster stories on television, especially on local television newscasts, is giving the public a warped view of reality and contributing to a type of media-induced trauma known as "*mean world syndrome*" (Budiansky, Gregory, Schmidt, & Bierck, 1996). Since most of the general public have little direct experience with crime, our beliefs about crime and the criminal justice system are largely based on what we see on TV and read in the papers, where sensational and violent crimes are often overrepresented.

Political scientist Robert Putnam of Harvard University has observed that the rise of television in the 1950s led to a "civic disengagement" of Americans around 1960. Television watching may breed pessimism and apathy. The mean world syndrome makes us paranoid about our neighbors and cynical about society and human nature in general (Budiansky et al., 1996). Just as importantly, if falsely exaggerating the extent of the crime problem contributes to a deterioration of mental health in individuals or groups, are news services liable for damages by engaging in what would amount to journalistic malpractice? Stay tuned.

TREATMENT OF CRIME-INDUCED TRAUMATIC STRESS SYNDROMES

Again, respecting the individuality of each patient and his or her unique situation, this chapter offers some therapeutic guidelines that can be applied to crime victims of different types.

Self-Help

As with trauma patients generally, often the best immediate help is the most practical and self-empowering. Much aid to crime victims is not what would ordinarily be considered "therapeutic" from a strictly clinical point of view; rather, it involves directing patients to self-help groups and support organizations (Brown, 1993). If patients can't find a good local group, have them contact the various local, state, and national victims' rights organizations that pertain to their specific needs. If they are unsure of which group to contact, they can call one of the two national umbrella victims' rights groups: the National Organization for Victim Assistance (NOVA) and the National Victims Center. Often the therapist may have to assist the patient in accessing this help—you may even have to (with permission) make the call yourself on the patient's behalf.

Workers in the victim services field offer certain general advice for survivors of a murdered family member (Brown, 1993). Ordinarily, it takes about 18 to 24 months just to stabilize after the death of a family member, and the worst part may be a "delayed reaction" that occurs several months after the murder, when the psychic novocaine has worn off. Paradoxically, this is just the time when others may be expecting the patient to be "getting over it."

When people ask the patient how she's doing, encourage her to answer honestly, albeit diplomatically, and not to always just say "fine." Within certain limits, such as casual greetings, patients needn't be afraid to let others—especially close friends and family members—know how they really feel. The line between forthright self-disclosure and immoderate spewing is often a delicate and shifting one, however, and therapists may have to assist patients in role-playing appropriate responses to questions by others. Also, patients need to know when they can self-protectively decline to elaborate on their emotional states in response to questions that may have less benign motivations behind them, i.e., from people who are "getting off on" the patient's ordeal.

In many cases, talking with a true friend or with others who have been there and survived can be at least as helpful as formal psychotherapy. Patients should let their emotions emerge at their own pace. They should be reassured that it's okay to feel a little sorry for themselves, as long as this doesn't interfere with adaptive coping efforts. They should try not to let themselves be thrown by other people telling them "how well you're handling it" (Brown, 1993).

Victim Support Services and the Criminal Justice System

Victim services, in one form or another, now exist in all 50 states, but budgetary considerations typically restrict the range of services offered. The victims most frequently targeted first for assistance programs are sexual assault victims, domestic violence victims, and children. The National Organization for Victim Assistance (NOVA) has developed a generic model of victim services that contains three major components: (1) emergency response at the time of the crisis; (2) victim stabilization in the days following the trauma; and (3) resource mobilization in the aftermath of the crime (Young, 1988).

All too commonly, attitudes and beliefs regarding the criminal justice system are sorely challenged following violent crime experiences. In response to this, a movement promoting the establishment of rights for crime victims has developed during the last two decades (Freedy, Resnick, Kilpatrick, Dansky, & Tidwell, 1994). Victims and family members may find the legal maze intimidating. Interacting with criminal justice representatives may become a traumatic reminder of the painful and humiliating crime experience. If the perpetrator is known to the victim, as in the typical case of sexual assault, the victim may fear revenge if charges are pursued. Victims often fear the social stigma associated with media reporting, being questioned and disbelieved, and having temporarily lost personal control. Even when victims decide to press charges, ideal images of swift justice can quickly dissolve as legal proceedings drag on for months or years.

Studies have shown that the prevalence of PTSD is higher among victims who wade through the criminal justice system than among crime victims in general (Freedy et al., 1994). Crime victims most likely to develop PTSD are those who have suffered violent crimes, such as physical or sexual assault, or homicide of a loved one, or who were in fear for their life or serious injury during the crime incident. However, support services for victims, including psychological counseling, are typically meager. A prevalent attitude among law enforcement seems to be that solving cases is paramount, with the needs of the victim only an afterthought.

However, direct clinical experience (Freedy et al., 1994) demonstrates that more humane treatment of victims and their families can foster optimum cooperation with the criminal justice system, which in turn may facilitate an increase in the number of crimes being reported and otherwise lead to quicker and more successful closure of cases and prosecution of offenders.

Freedy et al. (1994) examined the prevalence of PTSD and victim service utilization among crime victims and family members recently involved in the criminal justice system. About one-half of the participants met PTSD diagnostic criteria during their lifetime. Females were overrepresented among victims of more violent crimes, such as homicide and sexual assault. Victims of these more violent crimes—who sustained physical injuries, who perceived that they would be seriously injured, and who perceived their lives to be threatened—were more likely to suffer from PTSD than victims without these characteristics. While most subjects believed the criminal justice system should provide a range of victim services, including counseling and psychotherapy, most reported inadequate access to services. The results imply that crime victims involved in the criminal justice system are at risk for developing PTSD, which is rarely addressed by mental health professionals due to inadequate access to health care services.

Young (1988) has provided a model for victim assistance in criminal proceedings. The majority of victims never see their perpetrators and typically receive little information or consideration surrounding bail proceedings, pretrial hearings, plea bargains, trial proceedings, or sentencing. In most states, victims are even barred from observing the trial proceedings, except from the witness stand. All this is further demoralizing to victims who believe that it is "their" case that is being prosecuted.

Prosecutor-based *victim/witness programs*, in part spurred by legislative *victims' bills of rights* in some jurisdictions, now inform victims of an arrest, seek their opinion at bail hearings, inform them of the prosecutor's decision as to what charges, if any, to file, and provide the victim with practical information about the procedures, language, and general philosophy of the criminal justice system. However, such "bills of rights" are not self-executing, and victims may need help in accessing appropriate resources.

Therapists and others must be prepared to help crime victims face the frustrations and indignities of the criminal trial system. This includes pretrial appearances and court appearances, where the victim must face her assailant and withstand the sometimes withering cross-examination by defense attorneys. In homicide cases, the family must often sit there and hear the slain family member shamed and vilified. Young (1988) recommends that the victim/witness's counselor be especially available during the trial and perhaps even accompany her to court.

With regard to sentencing, victims should be encouraged to file a *request for restitution* to be included in the proposed sentence, as well as a *victim impact statement* presented in person, in writing, or both. Such a statement is now allowed in most states; in some states the victim also has the right to give an opinion about what constitutes an appropriate sentence.

After the sentencing, mental health services may become even more important. Many victims and their families essentially put their lives on hold while they pursue justice through prosecution and conviction. It is common for victims to return from a sentencing hearing, even if it went their way, feeling depressed, drained, and isolated. Also, murder convictions involving the death penalty or a lengthy sentence will almost certainly be appealed. A growing number of states now give victims an opportunity to express their opinions at offenders' parole hearings.

Victims may wish to pursue legal recourse through the civil courts after the criminal case has concluded. This can include damage suits against offenders, as well as lawsuits against third parties who failed in meeting a duty to prevent the crime. Referrals to appropriate legal resources should be made, and therapists should feel no shame about directing patients to such legal resources, as long as the referrals don't constitute a conflict of interest. If such legal action is taken, victims may need continued support through that process in much the same way as they received it during the criminal trial (Young, 1988).

PSYCHOTHERAPY OF CRIME VICTIMS

Early treatments for crime victims were based on crisis theory and focused on helping victims deal with the immediate aftermath of victimization. More recently, as PTSD has become recognized as a primary disorder following victimization, the treatment of crime victims has focused on alleviating the reexperiencing, avoidance, and arousal symptoms of PTSD (Falsetti & Resnick, 1995). Furthermore, there is a need to develop treatments to address the concomitant problems of substance abuse, depression, and panic disorder.

Obtaining Help and Self-Help

Even indigent patients should not assume they can't afford any kind of therapy. If not covered by insurance, the Victim Compensation program in the patient's state may pay for some form of counseling, which is now explicitly covered in state victim compensation programs as a condition of receiving a federal grant under the Victims of Crime Act of 1984. Also, patients should seek out support groups in their community. The victim/witness coordinator, religious leader, or local counseling agency may know of a good volunteer organization or reduced-fee therapy sessions the patient can join or attend (Brown, 1993; Young, 1988).

Crisis Intervention and Emergency Psychological Aid

For most crime victims whose lives were relatively stable before the crime, the first intervention should consist of crisis intervention-type brief therapy. The goal should be to help the patient cope with the impact of the crime itself and find ways to deal with the aftereffects, such as overwhelming loss, dealing with friends and family, and handling work, child care, and other responsibilities. At the end of this phase of therapy, the patient should have some sense of empowerment—although her life has been altered by the event, she can cope with what has happened and can reasonably face what lies ahead (Brown, 1993).

In general, crisis intervention is an active and direct approach that is by its very nature short-term (Gilliland & James, 1993), Information is provided about the likely course of reactions and these reactions are normalized to assure victims that they are not "going crazy." Victims are encouraged to talk about what happened and to express their feelings about it. Patient concerns, such as the personal meaning of the crime, whom to tell, and concerns about others' reactions, should also be addressed. Basic resources, such as food and shelter, should be inventoried, and necessary community resources should be accessed and mobilized. For example, a robbery victim may need help with paying bills and obtaining food. A victim advocate can provide such services as contacting utility companies to delay payment without penalty and locating food through local food banks or churches.

Crisis intervention also involves clarifying and reinforcing adaptive coping mechanisms. Social support should be assessed and mobilized as well. The need for referral to other services, including more intensive mental health or medical services, should be assessed. Since this may be the only contact many victims have with any mental health services, crisis intervention continues to provide an important link for referral to more comprehensive services when needed. In addition, the victim may need information about what to expect in the legal process.

Two of the most common questions that crime victims ask are "How could he do that to me?" and "Why me?" (Clark, 1988). Being victimized evokes a range or emotions, including fear, shame, guilt, helplessness, powerlessness, and anger. Crime tears victims' lives apart and leaves them feeling out of control. Ironically, it destroys their basic sense of trust in other people at just the time they need people most.

Clark (1988) offers some recommendations for how law enforcement and emergency services personnel can best deal with crime victims on scene. I have found that these recommendations also readily apply to the work of mental health professionals dealing with crime victims on scene, in emergency rooms, at police stations, and at sites of workplace violence (Miller, 1997b; see also Chapters 9, 10, and 11).

The responder's first concern is to see that serious injuries get treated. How you approach patients during and beyond this stage can have a significant impact on their subsequent level of cooperation and overall psychological recovery. Clark (1988) offers several common-sense guidelines for emergency reponders that, for the most part, differ little from the way crisis intervention mental health professionals should deal with patients in acute distress.

First, introduce yourself to the patient and bystanders—even if you are in uniform, have a picture ID tag, or "look like a doctor," the victim may be too distraught to understand who you are. You may need to repeat the introduction several times. Remember that victims still in shock may respond to you as if you are the criminal, especially if you arrived quickly on the scene.

Avoid statements such as "What were you doing out alone at this time of night?" or "Why did you let him into the house?" These not only needlessly upset the patient, but also erodes trust, making further treatment attempts extremely difficult. Avoid platitudes such as "It's okay" or "Everything will be all right," which will doubtless sound hollow and insincere to a victim whose world has just been shattered. Better are

concrete supportive statements such as "We're here to treat your injuries" or "We're going to take you to a safe hospital."

Although less a problem with mental health than with law enforcement
personnel, it is important to avoid statements or actions indicating to the
patient that you think she should "Stop crying and act like an adult."
People don't act the way they normally do when they have been victimized. Many crime victims revert to childlike behavior after the incident.
Rather, simple, nonjudgmental statements such as "I can understand
why you're upset" or "What can I do to help?" can ameliorate the
patient's distress.

For medical treatment personnel, explain what you're doing, especially
when you are touching the patient or doing an invasive or otherwise
intimate procedure, such as putting in an IV, applying a breathing mask,
or cutting away clothing. If possible, let the victim help you treat her if
she wants. This may be as simple as having her hold a bandage on her
arm or letting her undo her own clothing, but it can offer a much-needed
quick restoration of a sense of control in a situation where the victim is
otherwise reeling in a state of helpless disorientation.

Also related to restoration of control, respect the victim's wishes, whenever reasonable. If, for example, the victim wants a family member or
friend to remain in the room or on scene during examination and treatment, let that person stay. Don't take offense if the patient refuses to
let you touch, treat, or even talk to her: you may look, act, speak, smell,
or have the same name as the assailant. Patients are often unable to
express their fears and may just flail or shout, "Get away from me!"
Perhaps another member of the emergency medical or mental health
team can treat the patient more comfortably.

Listen to the victim if she wants to talk. Again, it's the mental health
clinician's essential role to listen, but emergency medical or law enforcement personnel may not consider empathic listening to be part of their
job description. Yet even the most hardboiled detective or medic should
understand that a sympathetic, nonjudgmental responder can do much
to restore the crime victim's trust and confidence and thereby facilitate
all aspects of the case. At this stage, don't press for more details than
necessary for purposes of immediate treatment; crime victims will inevitably be forced to tell their stories again and again, especially if they
become involved in the criminal justice system. At the same time, it's
important to let victims express their emotions if they just have to "get
it all out" (Clark, 1988).

Psychotherapy

Once the immediate crisis has passed, the patient is confronted with the
process of working through the traumatic victimization and trying to get

on with her life. In addition to the general guidelines for trauma therapy offered in Chapter 2, the following are some therapeutic recommendations specifically applicable to crime victims and their families.

EXPOSURE THERAPY AND DESENSITIZATION. Falsetti and Resnick (1995) describe an application of *prolonged imaginal exposure therapy* to the treatment of violent crime victims. Although not without its critics, this type of approach has proven effective in treating PTSD in Vietnam veterans, and more recently it has been applied to rape victims with PTSD (Foa, Rothbaum, Riggs, & Murdoch, 1991). One of the primary goals of exposure therapy is to confront the feared stimuli in imagination so that fear and anxiety decrease. This is similar to watching a scary movie over and over: at first it may be quite frightening, but by the tenth or twentieth viewing it is, if anything, innocuously boring. Analogously, a repetitively replayed frightening memory becomes less intimidating as it is recounted numerous times in an objectively safe environment.

In this treatment model, patients are also asked to confront fear cues that are not dangerous in themselves but that may have been paired with danger at the time of the traumatic event. In vivo exposure to fear cues is used to extinguish the fear associated with these stimuli. This involves exposure to objects or situations in real life. In the case of one woman who was raped in a parking garage, in vivo exposure entailed sitting in a parking garage with her therapist. She would monitor her anxiety, which decreased as she was able to learn that it was not the parking garage itself that was dangerous but, much more specifically and restrictedly, her assailant (Foa et al., 1991).

Despite the success of prolonged exposure treatment, it has been recommended that this modality be used with caution to guard against the potential for severe adverse complications, including precipitation of panic disorder, exacerbation of depression, relapse of alcohol abuse, and hypersensitization and retraumatization (Pitman, Altman, Greenwald, Longpre, Macklin, Poire, & Steketee, 1991). In addition, flooding used alone has received criticism because it does not address faulty cognitions and fails to enhance the development of coping skills.

Foa, Hearst-Ikeda, and Perry (1995) have developed a *clinical intervention brief prevention program* for treating complicated PTSD reactions in victims of sexual and nonsexual assault. The program consists of four weekly meetings, two hours each, of cognitive-behavioral therapy. The program is not characterized as "therapy," per se, but is described to the assault victim as a four-meeting program that aims at facilitating her recovery by teaching stress-management strategies that she may use as needed.

The program consists of techniques that Foa et al. (1991) have found effective for alleviating chronic PTSD in assault victims. These include: (1) education about the common reactions to assault; (2) breathing and relaxation training; (3) reliving the assault by imaginal exposure; (4) confronting feared, but safe situations (in vivo exposure); and (5) cognitive restructuring.

Meeting 1 is devoted to information-gathering, education, and an overview of the program. The therapist evaluates the victim's PTSD symptoms, presents an overview of the program, and describes the agenda of the meeting. The normal reactions to assault are discussed to educate the victim about posttrauma reactions and to normalize them. During this discussion, the therapist notes any trauma-related cognitive distortions or, irrational beliefs in the patient's view of the world or about herself. Next, the therapist and the victim construct a list of situations and people that are objectively safe but that she has been avoiding since the assault.

Meeting 2 begins with a discussion of the past week's problems. In the first part of this meeting, the information collected in the introductory meeting about avoided situations and people is rank-ordered according to the degree of anxiety each scene evokes. Next, a rationale for imaginal exposure to memories of the assault, i.e., reliving the trauma, is presented in terms of putting "unfinished business" into proper perspective by repeatedly "beating the memory to death" until it loses its power to scare and hurt.

The patient is helped to contruct a hierarchical list of feared situations. Instruction is then provided in deep breathing and muscle relaxation, and the relaxation procedure is audiotaped, so the patient can listen to the tape and practice relaxation at home. Next, the victim is instructed to close her eyes and relive the assault "as if it were happening now," and this narrative is also audiotaped. Every ten minutes, a reading is taken of the patient's fear regarding the relived assault memory. During the reliving exercise, the therapist makes notes of cognitive distortions that the victim expresses about the dangerousness of the world and her perceived helplessness. After the reliving exercise, there is a discussion of these distorted, exaggerated, or irrational beliefs.

At the end of the session, the therapist suggests that the patient use the audiotape to relive the traumatic experience several times during the ensuing week and to confront a few of the situations each day from the list that has been created in the beginning of the session.

Meeting 3 begins with a review and discussion of the previous week's homework. Next follow 45 minutes of imaginal exposure to memories of the assault. The remainder of the session is devoted to cognitive restructuring, starting with a rationale for the technique and a description of common cognitive distortions, such as global unpredictability and uncontrollability, negative self-views, fears and expectations for the future, and beliefs about the world and its inhabitants.

The therapist helps the patient to identify distorted cognitive assumptions about the dangerousness of the world and her coping abilities. Homework assignments focus on daily, audiotape-assisted repetition of imaginal exposure and on continuing to confront feared situations. The patient is instructed to use a daily diary to record her negative thoughts, distressing feelings, and cognitive distortions three times daily. Finally, she is reminded to continue to use the relaxation and breathing skills when she notices herself becoming anxious.

Meeting 4 begins with the homework review. Imaginal exposure to assault memories is followed by cognitive therapy that includes a discussion of the thoughts and feelings that were recorded in the daily diary. The therapist reviews the skills the patient has learned during the program, the progress she has made, and the schedule of follow-up sessions.

Foa et al. (1995) studied the efficacy of this brief prevention program with ten recent female victims of sexual and nonsexual assault. Two months postassault, victims who had undergone the cognitive-behavioral prevention program had significantly less severe PTSD symptoms than victims in the assessment control condition. Five and a half months postassault, victims in the brief prevention group were significantly less depressed than victims in the control group, and had significantly less severe reexperiencing symptoms. The prevention program was also effective in reducing depression.

Foa and colleagues (Foa et al., 1995; Foa & Kozak, 1986; Foa & Riggs, 1993) hypothesize that the behavioral prevention program enables victims to repeatedly relive the traumatic memories, thus activating the trauma structure and its emotional component. By the end of the session, the emotional response to the traumatic memories decreases for most victims, thus signaling habituation within a session. Repeated reliving produces a long-term decrease in emotional responding, i.e., habituation between sessions.

The victim's mistaken view of herself as totally incompetent and helpless is also addressed in the prevention program in two ways. First, the victim realizes that she can confront the traumatic memories and tolerate the resulting emotional activation. This realization helps modify her perception of herself as a weak, inadequate person. Second, she acquires specific effective techniques for coping with anxiety, such as relaxation and cognitive restructuring. The experience of being able to successfully control her anxiety provides evidence that contradicts the victim's perception of being inadequate, thus enhancing her perception of self-competence.

An extension of this approach was recently studied by Echeburua, de Corral, Zubizarreta, and Sarasua (1997), who compared self-exposure and cognitive restructuring with progressive relaxation training in the treatment of adult rape victims and adult victims of childhood sexual abuse. In contrast to Foa et al. (1991), Echeburua et al. (1997) used an exposure technique that addressed the stimuli the patients tended to avoid and was applied to intrusive thoughts more than to traumatic memories. The cognitive restructuring technique focused on (1) normalizing the stress reaction to sexual assault; (2) modifying guilt and other negative thoughts about the rape; and (3) putting the experience in a positive perspective by emphasizing adaptive coping skills and hope for the future.

Results showed that the self-exposure and cognitive restructuring modalities were far superior to progressive relaxation in reducing traumatic stress symptoms in these sexual assault survivors immediately and at 12-month follow-up. In fact, the authors report a startling 100 percent success rate at 12 months for their cognitive behavioral treatment program (Echeburua et al., 1997).

With appropriate modifications, these kinds of cognitive-behavioral treatment approaches can be used for other types of crime victims, as well as victims of disasters and automobile accidents. As noted above, the key elements appear to be the instillation of hope, control, and empowerment by the progressive mastery of practical coping skills and the reconceptualizing of the self as an active, competent agent in directing one's own life.

EMDR AND CRIME-RELATED TRAUMA.   Kleinknecht and Morgan (1992) describe the application of EMDR to treat a case of PTSD in a patient shot during a burglary. The authors relate that the initial traumatic scene of the shooting was desensitized "within about three minutes," with complete resolution of PTSD symptoms. Treatment success is described in terms of the patient's being unable to generate a coherent image of the shooting scene, which appears to characterize the treatment modality as repressive, rather than desensitizing or integrative. In addition, during the eye movement procedure, two prior traumas from earlier in the patient's life were reportedly recalled and were resolved as well. The therapeutic gains were sustained over an eight-month follow-up.

Whereas reports of such rapid and complete cures of trauma-related PTSD would seem to strain clinical credulity, apparently some select patients are peculiarly susceptible to the suggestive elements of EMDR (see Chapter 2). For such patients, these kinds of approaches may have significant clinical utility, at least in the short-term, although further follow-up study with larger populations is clearly called for.

PSYCHOTHERAPY OF BEREAVEMENT AFTER HOMICIDE. Few family victimizations are as ferociously tragic as the death of a loved one by homicide (Schlosser, 1997). Rage, horror, and despair all comingle as the survivors struggle for understanding and a sense of justice—indeed, for a reason to go on, to "keep fighting," as several have put it, as living itself has now become a battle. While a number of authors have tangentially touched upon the therapeutic issues of family member homicide survivors, this topic has been extensively addressed by Rynearson (1988, 1994, 1996; Rynearson & McCreery, 1993), and this section is based largely on his work, along with my own clinical observations.

Unlike a death that is preceded by a serious prolonged illness, in which family members may show the greatest degree of emotional distress *before* the actual demise, bereavement by sudden and unpredictable death is frequently more painful and prolonged because of the absence of anticipatory bereavement. There is no advance notice, no time to prepare, to "put affairs in order." In addition, unlike even sudden accidental death, a murder is both violent and transgressive, a brutal, purposeful assault forced on an unwilling, helpless, and innocent victim. It is also often a widely publicized event, placing the bereaved family members at the center of social and media scrutiny. The bereaved are forced to cope with the demanding processes of investigation, apprehension, trial, sentencing, and media intrusion, which necessarily divert attention and energy from the primary tasks of mourning and recovery.

Posttraumatic stress reactions to a family member's murder can take several forms (Rynearson, 1994) affecting emotions, cognition, and behavior:

Emotion: In addition to the feelings commonly associated with bereavement (sadness, anxiety, and guilt), there are wrenching emotions that are specifically related to the violence of the homicide death. A pervasive fear creeps in with the first awareness of the murder and can linger for years. A deep and justifiable anger toward the killer alternately smolders and flares as the trial meanders along. Even after sentencing, this anger might diminish after one or two years, but it often never disappears entirely.

Cognition: The presence of intrusive, repetitive images of the violent homicidal dying may appear in the form of flashbacks. The images often focus on the terror and helplessness the victim presumably felt during the last minutes of his or her life. Memory and concentration may be impaired. Vivid recurring nightmares of the murder are common, as are dreams and conscious fantasies in which the bereaved survivor is murdering the murderer.

Behavior: Up to a year or more following the homicide there is heightened anticipation and protective avoidance of violence, including hypervigilance and startle reactions. The individual's usual range of territorial and affiliative behaviors becomes constricted as the home is turned into a protective fortress, strangers are avoided, and unfamiliar surroundings are circumvented. There is a preoccupying need for the physical proximity and palpable assurance of safety of the remaining family members, and survivors may compulsively "check on" these family members. Behaviors directed toward retribution are also common, beginning with cooperative efforts with law enforcement in the murder investigation, later evolving into direct involvement, and sometimes into obsessive preoccupation with "solving" the case and seeking justice.

Victimization: The posttraumatic stress reaction that follows physical assault or threat of assault is often accompanied by a residual attitude of resignation and/or rage. Victims commonly experience humiliation, isolation, feelings of worthlessness, compensatory hatred, and obsessions with revenge. Individuals who are bereaved through homicide commonly identify with victims of other crimes.

Grotesque death imagery: By any account, murder is a nasty business that sometimes involves excessive brutalization, torture, and disfigurement. Even if they have not witnessed the murder directly or viewed the body, individuals who have lost a family member through homicide may experience intense and frightening death imagery. The very nature of their psychological attachment forces survivors to work through an internalized fantasy of grotesque dying.

I've observed that, for some survivors, body identification is the worst part of the whole ordeal of homicidal bereavement, while for others the actual sight of the deceased provides a strange sort of reassuring confirmation that the murder victim's death agonies may have actually fallen short of the survivor's imagined horrors, and even if not, that the physical presence of the body means that the suffering is at least over.

Despair: The very fact of homicidal dying dispels our comforting illusion of protection from violence and inhumanity. Death in such cases is not "fair" or "normal" and it does not conform with the life plan that was anticipated for the deceased in the course of the natural rhythms of living, growing, maturing, and dying. No amount of explanation or retribution can ever completely mend the cracked protective emotional bubble of safety.

Rynearson (1988, 1996) offers a set of recommendations for treatment of families of homicidal bereavement, especially involving a murdered child, which are presented here with some of my own clinical observations.

In the beginning phases of treatment, beware of pushing the cathartic narrative too quickly. Many bereaved patients adopt an unnatural flippancy or hyperrational attitude in the early aftermath of homicidal bereavement, which observers may mistake for unconcern or callousness. This typically represents a massive defense mechanism and, especially in the early stages, some patients cope better with an avoidance posture, which should provisionally be respected by the therapist. There is nothing to be gained from dramatic displays of emotional agony: this will happen soon enough. The therapist should take his cue from the patient's history (where this can be elicited) of dealing with traumatic events in the past. The judicious use of antianxiety, antidepressant, and hypnotic medication, as well as cognitive-behavioral stress management techniques, may help quell vicious cycles of arousal and withdrawal. As noted in Chapter 2, learning to modulate one's own arousal level is often the first step toward regaining a sufficiently secure sense of control to allow expressive psychotherapy to take place.

At some point, the therapeutic narrative begins to flow. Psychotherapy of the homicidally bereaved patient combines many of the features of individual PTSD therapy and family therapy modalities described in Chapter 2. Before being able to discuss the traumatic death, the patient and the therapist must first establish a basic alliance that promises sufficient support and security to accomodate and assimilate what has happened. This security rests upon the nonverbal capacity to modulate intense fear and divert one's mind from horrifying imagery. At this point, the therapist uses a number of techniques to strengthen pacification (relaxation strategies) and partition (cognitive strategies), in line with protocols outlined in Chapter 2.

Inquiry about the patient's private perception of death is another important assessment task. Nihilism and despair are common early responses, and often the only antidote is the development of a sustaining spiritual or philosophical belief system that can buffer the disintegratory effects of the homicide. Therapeutic measures may involve exploring the patient's general concepts of death and meaning in life and encouraging participation in religious rituals, pastoral retreats, or investment and commitment to caring for others. Photos and mementos of the deceased can also serve as comforting images. For example, therapist and patient can review family albums together, thus evoking nurturing, comforting imagery to counterbalance the horrifying grotesque imagery of the homicide. Similar activities include writing about the deceased, drawing pictures, or creating a scrapbook, as long as these don't become the focus of unhealthy, obsessive preoccupation.

Once the psychological coping mechanisms of self-calming and distancing from the homicide event are strengthened, therapy can begin to confront the traumatic imagery more directly. Less verbally expressive patients may be asked to draw their perception of the death scene, which can then be directly viewed and shared by the therapist. (This type of drawing exercise is very effective with traumatized children and adolescents, not just with traumatic bereavement but more generally in trauma work; see James, 1989.) Efforts by the patient to place herself within the reenactment drawing allows a beginning of abstract distancing instead of mute avoidance. In these exercises, patients often portray themselves beside the deceased, defending, protecting, or rescuing the victim.

At this point, the patient has hopefully gained sufficient autonomy from the homicide trauma bereavement to begin addressing less immediate issues, such as self-esteem enhancement, dealing with survivor guilt, working through of previous vulnerabilities, and any complexities or ambivalencies in her relationship with the deceased (Rynearson, 1996).

Special problems arise when a child is killed by another family member, confronting the entire family with the dilemmas of identification, divided loyalties, belief, and trust. Intrafamily killing accounts for 25 percent of homicides and often occurs in families with a long history of dramatic dysfunction. In these cases, not only do all the family members identify with the victim, but they are identified with the murderer as well. These families need specialized, skilled intervention, and even with this care the prognosis for a positive family outcome remains guarded—as it probably was before the homicide (Rynearson, 1994, 1996; Schlossen, 1997).

When the child has disappeared, the acceptance of homicidal death cannot begin until the body is found or the family tires of searching—and many families never stop. When the murder remains unsolved, as it does in 28 percent of homicides, the bereaved are left with an internalized traumatic dying that remains unbuffered by solution, punishment, retribution, or redemption (Rynearson, 1994, 1996; Schlosser, 1997).

When the family is ready, the therapist should encourage participation in appropriate support groups, such as Compassionate Friends, Parents of Murdered Children, and the like. When traumatically bereaved patients tell us that "you can't possibly believe what we're going through," they're right, we can't—unless we've lived through it ourselves. That doesn't rule out our being therapeutically effective, just as therapists who successfully treat terminally ill patients, learning disabled children, or schizophrenics need not have these syndromes themselves. But a group of peers is a powerful therapeutic adjunct for almost any kind traumatic disability syndrome (Miller, 1992b); often, in fact, meaningful psychotherapy cannot be wholly successful without such in-group comradeship. In the case of bereavement by murder, the support group members who have survived the horror share an immediate resonance and empathy with the specific aftereffects of homicide, and embody the hopeful promise of recovery for new members. The group can also guide new members through the uncharted experiences of public scrutiny with press and television and the investigative and judicial ordeal to come.

Recently, Temple (1997) has described a treatment approach with siblings of inner-city homicide victims. He notes that, in addition to the usual traumatic bereavement issues, siblings of murder victims often struggle with urges and social pressures toward retaliation, thereby putting themselves and others at increased risk for violent death. Older siblings may be plagued by guilt for "not looking out for" the younger brother or sister, and this may further fuel the impulse toward self-justifying revenge.

The treatment goals of Temple's (1997) program, called *contextual therapy*, include: (1) rapid restoration of family functioning following the homicide; (2) prevention of retaliatory violence by family members of the deceased; and (3) encouraging the family members to develop future plans based on honoring the memory of the murdered family member. These goals are achieved by quickly and effectively connecting the involved families to as wide a range of practical and supportive services as possible and by encouraging them to support one another. In addition, psychotherapy with siblings focuses on deriving some meaning or lesson from the deceased's life and death, and on honoring the deceased's memory by both symbolic artifacts (e.g., a scrapbook or photo album) and behaviors (e.g., establishing a productive direction in life, becoming active in antiviolence programs).

In addition, the contextual therapy program concretizes the therapeutic gains by awarding therapeutic "Certificates of Healing" to siblings who have shown courage and dedication in confronting their feelings and developing ways to positively honor the memories of their murdered family member. The program reportedly continues to enjoy great therapeutic success in the inner-city neighborhoods of Kansas City, Missouri, where it originated. Long-range follow-up studies of this valuable program are eagerly anticipated by those of us in the trauma field.

In general, therapists need to remind themselves of the limited therapeutic goals in most cases of this type: don't expect families to totally "work through" the trauma of a murdered loved one; don't tell them they'll "get over it." They won't. The bereaved will always maintain an attachment to the dead child, and it would be a mistaken therapeutic objective to insist on decathexis. Instead, it is hoped that the bereaved will learn to maintain involvement with others, while always retaining an internalized relationship with the slain child's image. The therapist's job is, first, to keep the family members from destroying themselves and each other, and second, to restore some semblance of meaning and purpose in their lives that allows them to remain productive, functioning members of their community. Often, the crucial first step is to get the family members to believe in one simple fact: "You can live through this." In the best cases, family members may "grow" from such a horrendous experience, but such cases are the blessed exceptions. Many families do well just to survive.

Working with bereaved families of homicide victims or individual survivors of criminal assault often makes the therapist an accidental tourist of the foulest, dankest grottos of the human spirit, only occasionally penetrated by thin, lifesaving shafts of light and fresh air. Therapists who can keep their own guiding rays from being sucked into the black hole of cynicism and despair, who can beat back their impending burnout by creatively diversifying their practices and updating their assessment and treatment skills, and who know when and how to get their own support represent vital allies of the forces of law and justice against the everyday barbarisms that corrode our civilization.

Chapter 9

KILLER JOBS

Workplace Violence—
Prevention, Response, and Recovery

Violence does even justice unjustly.

—Thomas Carlyle

Labor disgraces no man, but occasionally men
disgrace labor.

—Ulysses S. Grant

We hear it on the news so often, it's almost a stale joke:

A disgruntled [pick one: postal worker, law client, store customer, hospital patient, factory worker, Workers Comp claimant] stormed into his place of business yesterday, killing six people, before turning the gun on himself. Film at 11.

Often, this lead story is followed by interviews with coworkers or neighbors, who invariably comment something like: "He was always a little strange, y'know, quiet. Kept to himself a lot, didn't get along with too many people, but came in and did his job. Didn't seem the *violent* type, though."

In other cases: "I knew it was just a matter of time till something like this happened. That guy was bad news, a ticking bomb, and there were no precautions at all. We tried to tell management, but they just got annoyed, called us paranoid, and told us not to stir up trouble. When he finally snapped, we were sitting ducks."

It may be a stale joke, but if you're going to work tomorrow, stop laughing.

This chapter will address the role that mental health clinicians can play in collaborating with corporate executives, supervisory managers, and rank-and-file personnel in preventing, responding to, and helping employees recover from workplace violence. Most of the traumas described in these chapters strike suddenly and without warning or control; correspondingly, the clinical emphasis is on treating victims, survivors, and their families *after the fact*. However, in virtually no other area covered by this book is education, training, and prevention so important in foreseeing and planning for emergencies as in the area of workplace violence. Consequently, special attention is given to what companies can do *ahead of time* to reduce the risk of this kind of tragedy.

WORKPLACE VIOLENCE: DEMOGRAPHICS AND CHARACTERISTICS

The Grim Statistics

The 1994 National Institute of Occupational Safety and Health (NIOSH) report (cited in Labig, 1995) found that homicide is the second leading cause of death in the workplace. Murder was the number one killer of women and the third cause of death for men, after motor vehicle accidents and machine-related fatalities. A total of 7,603 Americans were slain on the job in the last decade, 1,004 in 1992 alone. In 1992, robberies accounted for 822 deaths, business disputes for 87, personal disputes for 39, and law enforcement line-of-duty deaths for 56. The large majority of workplace homicides are committed by firearms (Labig, 1995; Simon, 1996). According to the U.S. Department of Labor, over 1,000 people were murdered in the workplace in 1993, with an estimated 111,000 sublethal violent workplace incidents (Mantell & Albrecht, 1994).

In a 1993 survey conducted by the Society for Human Resource Management, 75 percent of violent workplace incidents were fistfights, 17 percent were shootings, 7.5 percent were stabbings, 6 percent were rapes and other sexual assaults, and less than 1 percent were bombings and explosions (Simon, 1996). Employees are about twice as likely to die from homicide as from a fall, four times more likely than from electrocution, and five times more likely than from a plane crash (Kinney, 1995).

In addition to every workplace homicide, there may be a dozen suicides, occurring on or off the job, that are related to work stress or work-related disorders (Labig, 1995; Simon, 1996). Indeed, suicide in the workplace may be a trend that will increase over the next several years (Kinney, 1995). Suicides also may occur as the concluding event of a single or mass homicide by a disturbed worker.

Costs of Workplace Violence

In 1993, workplace violence cost American business approximately $4.2 billion, estimating (conservatively) that each significant episode runs upwards of $250,000 in lost work time, employee medical benefits, and legal expenses (Mantell & Albrecht, 1994). Additional costs of workplace violence include replacing lost employees and retraining new ones, decreased productivity and diversion of management resources from other productive business, increased insurance premiums, increased security costs, bad publicity and lost business, and expensive litigation costs (Kinney, 1995).

In terms of the human costs, 88 percent of workers polled say that they are psychologically affected by the threat of workplace violence, 62 percent say their work life is disrupted, 23 percent are physically injured or sick, and only seven percent report no negative effect. A 1994 Gallup poll reported that fully two-thirds of the American people do not feel safe at their jobs (Labig, 1995).

Victims of Workplace Violence

According to NIOSH, in the 1980s, 80 percent of workplace violence victims were male, but 41 percent of female deaths on the job were caused by homicide. Eighty-three percent of workplace violence victims are Caucasian, 10 percent are black, 3 percent Hispanic, and 3 percent Asian.

According to Bureau of Justice statistics and other studies, the riskiest occupations for all different forms of physical injury are recreational workers, bartenders, liquor store salespersons, taxicab drivers, retail sales clerks, food service workers, police officers, parking attendants, gas station attendants, auto mechanics, security guards, social workers, grocery store and jewelry store cashiers, bus drivers, firefighters, and service station attendants (Flannery, 1995; Simon, 1996). Service and sales workers have the most work-related homicides, especially if they work alone and/or at night, followed by executives, administrators, and managers. Thirty-six percent of victims are in retailing, 17 percent in service industries, and 11 percent in public administration, including law enforcement (Kinney, 1995; Labig, 1995).

Nonlethal Workplace Violence

While the chances of being murdered on the job are still remote for the average worker, other nonlethal but quite dangerous forms of violence occur regularly. In addition, perpetrators who turn deadly often engage in threats and harassing behaviors before their actions escalate to killing, emphasizing the need for early boundary-setting and other preventive interventions (Kinney, 1995).

A 1992–1993 survey by the Northwestern National Life Insurance Company concluded that verbal abuse and harassment can be even more destructive to employee morale and productivity than physical assault. The reason is that, while employees who fistfight are likely to be assertively disciplined, "mere" verbal threats, curses, and snide remarks typically aren't taken as seriously, until something dramatic happens (Kinney, 1995; Labig, 1995). Nonlethal violence can also take the form of sabotage against company property, as well as sexual harassment (Schouten, 1996; Simon, 1996).

Reasons for Workplace Violence

Compiled from the reports of victims, in one study the attackers' perceived "reasons" for their workplace violence included irrational behavior, i.e., no comprehensible reason (26 percent), being dissatisfied with service (19 percent), interpersonal conflict (15 percent), being upset with having been disciplined (12 percent), criminal behavior (10 percent), personal problems (8 percent), being fired or laid off (two percent), prejudice (1 percent), and "unknown causes" (7 percent) (Labig, 1995). In another study, the leading motives found for workplace violence included personality conflicts (38 percent), family and marital problems (15 percent), drug or alcohol abuse (10 percent), nonspecific stress (7.5 percent), firings or layoffs (7 percent), and violent criminal history (2 percent) (Simon, 1996).

In reviewing these numbers, what's striking is the high proportion of violent acts in the workplace that occur for "no good reason," i.e., are irrational and even incomprehensible. The average working stiff, who would never resort to violence himself, might nevertheless understand or even empathize with someone who, having exhausted all acceptable channels of grievance, flies off the handle after suffering brutal unfairness or discrimination at the hands of a coworker or supervisor. But the sheer number of outright mean and crazy "reasons" for workplace violence suggests that a large number of very dangerous, unstable people are out there doing many of the jobs we all depend on.

Policies and Procedures

Despite the alarming growth of workplace violence as an occupational problem, denial still appears to be the coping method of choice among American employers. Only a quarter of companies surveyed offer formal training to employees at any level in dealing with workplace violence, and only 11 percent offer training to all employees (Labig, 1995).

It doesn't have to be this way. By responding forthrightly to the problem, the retail trade, which had accounted for more than one-third of workplace violence deaths, experienced a 46 percent decrease in the rate of homicide over the past decade (Stout, Jenkins, & Pizatella, 1996). Corporations are people-driven, and companies cannot function productively if their employees feel threatened, abused, or frightened. Violence prevention ultimately can be thought of as an insurance policy or productivity measure that most organizations can't afford to ignore if they want to succeed and prosper (Kinney, 1995).

ROLE OF THE MENTAL HEALTH PROFESSIONAL IN WORKPLACE VIOLENCE

Psychologist-Company Relationship

A current controversy regarding mental health clinicians who serve corporations, school systems, law enforcement, and emergency service organizations is whether these practitioners should be part of an in-house Employee Assistance or Human Resources team or play an outside, objective consultant role (see also Chapter 10).

According to the in-house model (e.g., Mantell & Albrecht, 1994), the company psychologist establishes an ongoing relationship with the firm and participates in the preemployment screening, helps with the hiring process, is involved in the human resource training programs for the first-line supervisors, middle managers, and top executives, and is available to provide individual and group counseling at all levels throughout the organization. The bond with the firm makes it easier for the psychologist to intervene before, during, or after potential workplace violence episodes, so ultimately, if an incident occurs, he will be there to help everybody in the organization recover.

The free-lance, or consultancy model (e.g., Slaikeu, 1996) sees the mental health clinician as a resource that can be called upon by many different companies at different times, as needed. The lack of formal reporting relationship to any one firm gives the clinician a certain objectivity when mediating disputes, provides a setting for confidential counseling, and affords the clinician wide latitude in constructively criticizing company policies or individual actions. This non-"hired gun" approach to corporate mental health services gives the company only slightly less control over the process and outcome, but may facilitate genuine change for the better. Utilized by skilled, responsible clinicians who are sensitive to the needs of their individual corporate clients, either approach is valuable.

Qualifications

While Employee Assistance Programs (EAPs) have historically focused on treatment of substance abuse and family problems, other services now becoming important include workplace violence prevention and critical incident stress debriefing (White, McDuff, Schwartz, Tiegel, & Judge, 1996). One problem in this age of slapped-together managed care "provider panels" is that some EAP practitioners may be inadequately trained and qualified to diagnose violence and aggression. It is possible that employees may become even more disturbed, angry, and abusive if they are subjected to incompetent or inappropriate evaluation or treatment. Employers who fail to check the credentials and experience of their providers may be setting themselves up for serious liability issues (Kinney, 1995; Lowman, 1993; Mantell & Albrecht, 1994; Sperry, 1996; Yandrick, 1996).

Intervention—Prevention

After the evaluation of a potentially dangerous employee, there are several options, including recommending voluntary counseling, mandatory counseling with treatment monitoring, use of graded disciplinary measures, or in extreme cases, instituting termination procedures (Grote, 1995; Kinney, 1995).

If the employer decides he wants to salvage an employee, he should make this clear to the psychologist. The employer should be informed of the minimum essential psychological and other personal information he needs to make an informed business decision about the disposition of the employee. Specifically, the employer will want to know if a problem or condition can be diagnosed, what the course of treatment will be, and when the employee can be expected to return to work (Kinney, 1995).

In general, mental health professionals must be available to promptly offer emergency services to employees. In addition, employers should insist that mental health professionals relay any warnings of violence that may be communicated by the employee (Kinney, 1995), although I recommend you check the local laws and rules about reporting requirements in your jurisdiction.

Intervention in the Aftermath of Violence

Skilled mental health professionals trained in crisis intervention strive to provide a highly supportive environment and offer a sense of safety and control to the survivors of a workplace violence incident. Clinicians teach coping skills, conduct critical incident stress debriefings as needed, and help victims identify their feelings and release stress by talking to an uninvolved yet empathic third party about the event. Cumulative experience in the crisis intervention field has demonstrated that with quality mental health services and support from friends, family, coworkers, and professionals, recovery is usually complete within six months (Flannery, 1995; Kinney, 1995; Mantell & Albrecht, 1994).

Training

In addition to direct clinical services, the staff or consulting mental health professional can also be helpful in reducing the risk of violence by training all employees and managers in the sensitive areas of cultural diversity, sexual harassment, domestic violence, grievance procedures, stress management, and effective conflict-resolution skills (Crawley, 1992; Flannery, 1995; Kinney, 1995; O'Brien, 1992).

Supervisory personnel should have ongoing training. Managers should routinely review strategies for dealing with difficult employees, develop skills in communication and defusing potential conflicts, revise formulations of threat management teams and action plans, and be given training in observing the signs of potential loss of control, increasing substance use, and other potentially dangerous situations. Managers should also be trained in grievance procedures, conflict resolution and dispute mediation, and in humane practices of discipline and termination (Crawley, 1992; Flannery, 1995; Grote, 1995; Kinney, 1995; O'Brien, 1992; Slaikeu, 1996; Yandrick, 1996).

The remainder of this chapter will consider these roles of the mental health clinician in more detail.

THE WORKPLACE VIOLENCE CYCLE

Accounting for individual variations, there appears to be a certain predictable pattern in the evolution of many workplace violence incidents (Kinney, 1995; Labig, 1995).

The cycle typically begins when the individual encounters an event (actual or perceived) that he experiences as stressful. This may be a single overwhelming event or a capping event to a cumulative series of stressors—the "straw that breaks the camel's back." The person reacts to this event cognitively and emotionally, based on his predisposing personality and life experiences. In the typical workplace violence perpetrator, this often involves persecutory ideation, projection of blame, and violent revenge fantasies. As thoughts and emotions stew, the individual isolates himself from the input of others and enters a mode of self-protection and self-justification in which a violent act may come to be perceived as "the only way out." Attention then turns to determining the actual means of responding to this perceived threat. The operational plan may be executed impulsively and at once, or may undergo numerous revisions. The next step is the violent act itself, which may occur any time from hours to months following the final perceived injustice.

PSYCHOSOCIAL FACTORS IN WORKPLACE VIOLENCE

Demographics

Behavioral and business forecasters seem to agree that the next generation of workers will be less mature, with poorer social skills, little experience in conflict resolution and mediation, reduced trust in older generations, deficits in attention span, poorer self-discipline, and higher rates of violence. Teenagers watch an average of 18 hours of TV a week and see more graphic and glamorized violence in the media than ever before in history; in the first half of the 1990s, murders by teens more than doubled (Kinney, 1995).

Cultural Factors

Some authorities view workplace violence as a spillover from the streets into the workplace of the violence that is generally spreading through the country. For the past 20 years people have been bombarded by the egocentric message that all personal problems are caused by "society."

Individuals are not responsible for their actions and all blame is externalized. At the same time, there has been a breakdown in traditionally
stabilizing institutions such as family, home, church, school, and community. Some workplace violence perpetrators have been quite blunt in
stating that they want to "strike back" and hurt as many people as
they can, no matter who those people are (Kinney, 1995; Labig, 1995;
Simon, 1996).

The Media

Glamorized violence is a staple of the entertainment media. For their
part, the news media have also recently taken an enormous interest
in workplace violence, but unfortunately, they often misinterpret and
misrepresent such events and the reasons behind them. In straining for
simplistic conclusions or lurid angles, the media typically talk with a
perpetrator's friends or co-workers, who may share his agenda and objectives or may spin their own bizarre interpretations of what happened
and why. The all-too common conclusion of this sound-bite journalism
is that the lethal perpetrator is either a "nut case" or else engaged in a
crusade of righteous retribution against an unfair or even darkly conspiratorial employer. This may lead marginally disturbed viewers to "justify"
their own future acts of violence (Kinney, 1995).

Changed Workplace and Work Ethic

Changes in the American workplace itself have created a fertile environment for breeding discontent and potential violence. Levels of stress
accumulate in many work settings as survivors of downsized corporations
are made to take on extra work and fill multiple jobs. For the terminated,
anger and hopelessness mount at the inability to replace lost jobs with
new positions with equal pay and benefits. The sense of long-term
common corporate purpose that may once have existed between managers and the rank-and-file has largely disappeared. The newly emerging
young workforce is ill-equipped for the world of work, work culture, and
work ethic. Most teenagers are introduced to work in low-skill jobs
with minimal mentoring, which may increase frustration. High turnover
encouraged by poor management reinforces the impression that everyday
work is for "chumps" and further denigrates authority. Managers and
supervisors are increasingly unable or unwilling to use effective discipline. The new, changed culture of resentment and entitlement in the
workplace says, "This company *owes* me something, and if I don't get

it, I'm gonna take it the hard way" (Kinney, 1995; Mantell & Albrecht, 1994).

"Sick" workplaces have several characteristics, including chronic labor-management disputes; frequent grievances filed by employees; large numbers of injury claims, especially psychological injury and occupational stress; understaffing and/or excessive demands for overtime; high number of stressed personnel; and an authoritarian management style (Kinney, 1995).

Work, Identity, and the Meaning of Life

Simon (1996) points out that satisfying work affords more than an income; it provides stability, direction, security, a sense of achievement, self-worth, camaraderie, and a feeling of belonging. For most individuals, losing a job is a traumatic event, but one that they eventually accept and resolve by picking up the pieces, going forward, and searching for new opportunities. But for a small minority of vulnerable personalities, job loss—especially if perceived as "unfair"—is a devastating blow to the psyche, a narcissistic mortal wound.

Positive identification with one's vocational role is a normal, even healthy, trait, as part of a matrix of overlapping identity systems that include family, friends, religious beliefs, and other roles. But some people's entire identity and sense of worth are inextricably tied up with their jobs. For such people, job loss becomes a devastating personal failure in life rather than a disappointing but survivable event. Such a blow is all the more acute when overemphasis on work has crowded out relationships and other resources that might have been called upon to support the employee through the crisis. If the situation is further compounded by financial difficulties, health problems, family friction, lack of personal support, or setbacks in other areas of life, mental deterioration, demoralization, and desabilization may be accelerated and the person may feel bereft of options (Simon, 1996).

Job Loss and the Workplace Violence Cycle

For some people, the loss of a job reverberates with hidden vulnerabilities rooted in their past. Fueled by such a history of narcissistic wounds, job loss may trigger an overwhelming rage that seems out of proportion to the current loss. Blame is externalized, and vengence brews as the worker begins to think, "I'll show them they can't do this to me and get away with ruining my life." For some, the intolerability of the job loss leads to hopeless suicidality with a retaliatory tinge: "If they can screw me, I can screw them back—big time. Why should other people go on having what they want and enjoying themselves, when I can't? I may be going out, but I'm not going out alone." The idea percolates in the perpertrator's mind that after he's gone, his Ramboesque exploits will be reported to millions of people around the world—his name will be a household word. Far from meekly slinking away, defeated and unnoticed, our "hero" will leave this world in a blaze of horror and glory—just like in the movies (Flannery, 1995; Kinney, 1995; Labig, 1995; Mantell & Albrecht, 1994; Simon, 1996).

WORKPLACE VIOLENCE
PERPETRATORS

It is important that clinicians operating in corporate and industrial settings know something about the kinds of perpetrators who commit violent workplace crimes. The behavior, personality, and psychopathology of different species of workplace violence perpetrators are described below.

Robberies and Other Crime

Strangers typically commit most robberies; sometimes, these criminals have some grudge against the business (Flannery, 1995; Labig, 1995). By far the majority of murders on the job are committed by strangers. Certain factors increase the risk of an employee's being killed in the workplace by a robber, including exchanging money with the public, guarding valuable property, working late-night or early morning hours, working in high-crime areas, and working in community settings (Labig, 1995).

Customers

Occasionally, an angry customer may lose control during an altercation and assault an employee. Or the customer may nurse the grudge and come back later to commit violence (Flannery, 1995; Kinney, 1995). In medical and mental health settings, "customers" also mean patients (see Chapter 11).

Domestic Violence

Violence may be committed on the job by spouses and lovers involved in domestic disputes. Or those infatuated with a particular employee may stalk or harass her at work (Labig, 1995; Meloy, 1997).

The Disgruntled Worker

This is the "classic" perpetrator of workplace violence, the one that makes the headlines when the event is dramatic or unexpected. As Flannery (1995) points out, the term *disgruntled* connotes mere ill-humor or discontent that doesn't begin to describe the state of rage and psychological disorganization characterizing most perpetrators of serious workplace violence.

The typical fired disgruntled employee is less likely to be terminated for being incompetent to do his duties than for being unable to get along with other people on the job. He usually has particular problems with supervisors. Often, the employee's colleagues have an intuitive sense that this person is dangerous, or "bad news" (Flannery, 1995). In many cases, there is a spectrum of disgruntled worker actions, ranging from nonviolent to extremely lethal. Often, early levels of acting-out are tolerated in a problem worker, and this reinforces the escalation of intimidation and violence. Mantell and Albrecht (1994) have identified several levels of disgruntled employee activity:

The *covert employee* engages in silent, hidden, or behind-the-scenes activities that serve to disrupt the workplace, including small-scale sabotage, vandalism, anonymous "poison pen" letters, threatening faxes and e-mail, and suspicious phone messages. At this level, the threats tend to be indirect, anonymous, and verbal or nonverbal, and any physical damage is aimed against inanimate objects. The worker at this stage is satisfied to be a silent saboteur.

The *fence-sitter* straddles the border between covert activities and actual violence. At this level, the threats are more verbally direct and the damage is more intrusive and destructive to office equipment or other employees' personal property. The perpetrator may target someone in the company for particular verbal lashings, but overt physical attacks against people have usually not yet occurred.

The *overt employee* ups the ante, so that the risk of this person's attacking other workers is now high. Activities at this stage may include injurious physical assaults, as well as extreme forms of sabotage and vandalism, often aimed at some tangible symbol of the target company.

The *dangerous employee* is potentially homicidal and may be psychotic and armed. Activities include direct threats, confrontations, and armed aggression. The signs of impending escalation have usually been apparent well in advance of the overt acts.

The Mentally Disordered Perpetrator
(a.k.a. The "Psycho")

This is the other most common "classic" workplace violence perpetrator stereotype, often overlapping with the "disgruntled worker" category, and most commonly representing a combination of paranoia and depression (Simon, 1996). Mantell and Albrecht (1994) delineate several types of paranoid violent workers:

Perpetrators with *paranoid personality disorder* are characterized by a longstanding set of maladaptive behaviors grounded in misinterpreting the words, actions, and motives of others as threatening, demeaning, or exploitive. They may be quite outspoken in their complaints, often filing numerous grievances and lawsuits before resorting to violence.

Workers with *delusional paranoid disorders* may be excellent, punctual, reliable workers, and have few if any performance or conduct problems, as long as work does not involve their systemized delusions; these are the so-called silent paranoids. However, their inner mental life is typically a melange of hyperlogical conspiratorial theories, and they are always plotting and outthinking their "enemies," careful, however, not to tip their hand.

Paranoid schizophrenics are severely disturbed and show a range of psychotic symptoms during the active phase of their illness, including disorganized thinking and hallucinations; indeed, their sheer level of pathology may make them relatively easy to spot.

Aside from paranoia, other medical, neuropsychological, and psychiatric disorders in workplace violence perpetrators include the following (Flannery, 1995; Mantell & Albrecht, 1994):

Organic personality disorders due to brain injury, strokes, dementia, or substance abuse effects may be associated with violent outbursts and may be preceded by impairment in memory, concentration, reasoning, or planning that affects job performance.

Workers with *temporal lobe epilepsy* may rarely show aggressive outbursts associated with seizure activity. These tend to be short and circumscribed and to occur in a state of relative disorientation and unawareness, followed by amnesia for the event.

Intermittent explosive disorder is characterized by sudden outbursts of rage upon minimal provocation and may be associated with subclinical abnormal brain wave activity. The rage attacks are typically impulsive and unplanned and are perceived by the perpetrator himself as uncontrollable, although consciousness is retained, memory for the event is variable, and remorse is often expressed at "losing control."

Alcohol and drug abuse can potentiate violence from almost any other source. In so-called *pathological intoxication*, even small amounts of alcohol can trigger intermittent explosive rage attacks, and the two syndromes often go together.

Workers who have themselves been victims of violence may experience wartime, civilian, or developmental *posttraumatic stress disorder*.

They thus bring their hypersensitivity and hair-trigger reactivity to the jobsite, where seemingly minor jibes and hassles can "set them off."

Workers with *antisocial personality disorder* are likely to have a long wake of employment, financial, legal, and personal troubles behind them. They are motivated exclusively by self-interest and will qualmlessly utilize any means necessary, including violence and intimidation, to get what they want. They are also usually quite impulsive and nonreflective and may thus compound their workplace troubles through poor judgment and thoughtless actions.

Workers with *borderline personality disorder* will typically experience drastic mood swings, mercurial personal attachments, and extremely intense emotional reactions. Having idealized a particular job setting, supervisor, or workmate, the borderline employee may be plunged into rageful despair by a subsequent rebuff or disappointment, real or perceived. The thirst for vindication and restoration of self-worth becomes an all-consuming passion and may include destructive or violent acts.

Impulsive violence against others and against the self often go together, and the sense of hopelessness that is part of *depression* may facilitate aggressive acting-out if the demoralized worker feels he has "nothing to lose" and decides to take others to the grave with him.

RISK FACTORS AND WARNING SIGNS OF WORKPLACE VIOLENCE

Mental health clinicians should help managers and supervisors identify certain risk factors in the hiring process and in later disciplinary actions (Kinney, 1995; Labig, 1995; Mantell & Albrecht, 1994; Simon, 1996).

Predicting the Risk for Workplace Violence

Demographic risk factors include male sex, young age (under 40), low socioeconomic status, and single status. Personal risk factors include past history of assaultive or other violent behavior; indeed, the most reliable risk factor for future violence is past violence. This includes nonwork violence (domestic violence, military misconduct). It also includes verbal threats, and the combination of current threats and past violence history is an especially ominous sign. If the present context is similar to past situations and environment where violence has occurred, the chances of imminent violence increase dramatically. Workers at risk for violence often have a history of other employment problems, such as unstable, migratory job history, multiple complaints about work stresses and working conditions, frequent overreaction to changes of policy or personnel, chronic labor-management disputes, and often a string of prior unresolved physical and emotional injury claims.

High-risk workers often single out certain coworkers or supervisors as their sources of persecution, and these may later become the targets of harassment or violence. There may be a specific motive and plan behind the aggression, and this may have been communicated in gripe sessions to other workers or kept a tightly guarded secret. High-risk workers also frequently possess the means and methods for violent actions, such as firearms and other weapons. They are often fascinated with military or law enforcement culture and paraphernalia (cop shows, gun magazines) and show excessive interest in media reports of violence (news clippings, scrapbooks), especially workplace violence.

Psychological risk factors for workplace violence include low intelligence and poor conceptual reasoning ability, undiagnosed or inadequately treated medical or neurological disorders, an impulsive and nonrational cognitive style, poor control of anger and temper, few if any healthy outlets for frustration and nervous energy, low self-esteem, an all-or-nothing tendency to completely disown or endorse violent or other socially unacceptable feelings, a tendency to externalize blame for all the bad things that happen to them ("It's not my fault, they set me up again"), one or more diagnosable psychiatric or personality disorders, a history of childhood physical abuse or witnessing family violence, current alcohol or drug problems, current unstable family life (which can be a source of stress, as well as indicating a volatile temperament), and perhaps subtle or overt pleas for help of some kind.

While some workers with stable personality disorders may be able to maintain acceptable work records for years, the worker undergoing an acute crisis will usually not be able to keep his distress secret for very long, and coworkers and supervisors will notice something wrong. The relationship between psychological disturbance and work disruption often occurs in a vicious cycle, where declining performance brings managerial criticism, which provokes further anger and deterioration in work, alienation of coworker support ("Those suckups—now they're *all* out to get me"), and so on. If the opportunity to intervene administratively or therapeutically is lost, the downward spiral continues until violence is seen as "the only way out" (Mantell & Albrecht, 1994; Labig, 1995; Simon, 1996).

Just as important, but frequently overlooked, are a number of "anti-risk factors" that may inhibit violent acting-out in workers under stress (Kinney, 1995; Labig, 1995). These include a reasonably rational, reflective, future-oriented cognitive style, an emotionally stable personality, a repertoire of good coping skills, a history of handling aversity in an adaptive way, no violent or antisocial history, no alcohol or drug abuse problems, good overall work history, a stable and secure family life, no major financial difficulties, and varied outside interests in hobbies, friendships, religious, and community groups. Of course, these traits define the overall characteristics of good workers in general—indeed, of good citizens as a whole (see Chapter 12).

Warning Signs of Impending Workplace Violence

There are, of course, no absolute predictors, but some guidelines and recommendations can be offered (Labig, 1995; Mantell & Albrecht, 1994; Simon, 1996).

Since threats are often a prelude to violence, all threatening statements and gestures should be taken seriously. Verbal threats may range from an actual stated intention to kill someone ("I'm gonna blow that sonofabitch away"), to persistent indirect threats against a coworker or supervisor ("You'll be sorry" "He deserves whatever's coming to him"), to veiled threats in the form of preoccupation or commiseration with related current events ("Now I know how that restaurant shooter felt").

Escalating potential for workplace violence may also be nonverbal and indirect, such as incoming reports by coworkers of being "spooked" or intimidated by the worker's presence or actions; increasing insubordination, confrontation, and challenging authority of company policies; crossing behavioral boundaries at work by misusing company phones and equipment or bothering other employees; becoming increasingly agitated, irritable, unreliable, excuse-making, and outwardly-blaming; and showing marked job performance decline, such as attendance problems, decreased work quality and productivity, increased work accidents, belligerently alienating customers, and being a source of embarrassment to the company.

Even if job performance per se is not inordinately affected, there may be significant changes in the worker's mood, behavior, or personality that may signal the potential for violence. These include withdrawal or secretive behavior, change in personal grooming habits, mood swings or flattening of mood, evidence of irrational or bizarre thinking, changes in daily schedules, obsession or preoccupation with a particular person or event, especially a recent violent event, increased time on the gun range, evidence of increased substance abuse problems, evidence of sleep disturbances, and general loss of interest and confidence in life or work, especially making "terminal plans," such as selling off possessions or making statements about settling affairs or evening scores (Labig, 1995; Mantell & Albrecht, 1994; Simon, 1996).

WORKPLACE VIOLENCE: PREVENTION

In addition to direct clinical services, the mental health professional can play an important administrative role in helping companies design workplace violence prevention programs, training the staff, setting up the teams, and supervising the practical exercises and drills. So as not to stray too far from this book's emphasis on psychotherapy, only an overview of these programmatic topics will be provided here; the details of such programs are covered extensively in this chapter's references.

Clear Policies

Companies that are serious about preventing violence should have clear, strong, fair, consistent, written policies against harassment, effective grievance procedures, good security programs, a supportive work environment that gives employees adequate control over their work, open and trusting communication, and training in resolving conflicts through team building and negotiation skills. Organizations must have a clearly stated policy of *zero tolerance for violence.* This should be contextualized as a safety issue, the same as with rules about fire prevention or storm emergency drills. Company policies should state clearly that any form or manner of threatening remark or gesture in the workplace is unacceptable and that anyone who engages in such behavior will face disciplinary action, including possible removal from his job. All threats should be thoroughly investigated. Having official rules makes enforcement objective and impersonal (Flannery, 1995; Kinney, 1995; Labig, 1995; Simon, 1996).

Plans should be in place that specify how threats are to be reported and to whom, as well as a protocol for investigating threats. Other policy and procedure items include security measures, disciplinary and grievance procedures, and services available for dispute mediation, conflict resolution, stress management, safety training, and other administrative and mental health services.

Safe Hiring

As a general, if deceptively simple-sounding rule, the best way to avoid workplace violence is not to hire violent workers. The mental health clinician can assist companies in the hiring process by playing an active or advisory role in application review and background checks, interviewing the prospective employee, administering psychometric tests and

other psychological screening measures, and identifying potential problem employees (Kinney, 1995; Labig, 1995; Mantell & Albrecht, 1994).

Safe Discipline

The ideal goal of any discipline program is to strike a balance between
a too heavy-handed and austere approach that presents management as
a bunch of unreasonable hard-asses and a too lax approach that gives
employees the impression of wishy-washyness and lack of control in
the organization.

Mantell and Albrecht (1994) and Grote (1995) endorse a model that
relies on collaboration. By identifying areas of agreement and disagree-
ment, looking for alternatives, thinking creatively, and eventually finding
solutions that have the full support and commitment of all parties, a
human resources manager is more likely to do his best to prevent the
creation of tension that may spark workplace violence.

"DISCIPLINE WITHOUT PUNISHMENT." The model of *discipline without
punishment* (DWP), developed by Grote (1995) and Grote and Harvey
(1983), begins by treating each worker like an adult human being worthy
of respect and conducts the discipline procedure on a mature and professional level. In fact, this overall approach is emblematic of good employer-
worker relations more generally and may serve as one useful model for
mental health clinicians to use in helping to shape corporate policy.

The focus of the DWP disciplinary procedure is not on the "bad
employee" but on the problem to be solved, and the responsibility is
placed squarely on the shoulders of the employee. The manager or
supervisor models mature problem-solving behavior by keeping the tone
of the meeting calm, professional, and focused. In this system, the discipline process, at least in the early stages, is less like punishment and
more like coaching.

The DWP model relies on a five-step approach. Step one is to identify
the problem to be addressed by determining the desired job performance
and the specific features of the employee's actual performance that devi-
ate from this standard. Step two is to analyze the impact of the problem,
determine the consequences of the problem, and determine the appropriate action(s) to be taken. Step three is to address the problem with
the employee, gaining the employee's commitment to change, discussing
alternate solutions, and deciding what specific actions the employee will
take. Step four is to document the disciplinary/coaching procedure by
describing the problem, the history, and the discussion that took place.
Step five is to follow up by determining if the problem has been solved,

reinforcing improvement, and taking any additional action required (Grote, 1995; Grote & Harvey, 1983).

ROLE OF THE SUPERVISOR/MANAGER.   The supervisor's role can be conceptualized broadly as including observation of the work environment, listening to what the employees are telling him, mediating low-level disputes, communicating between upper management and line workers, referring employees for mental health services as needed, and acting as a barometer of thought and feeling in the work environment as a whole. Supervisors should *not* "play shrink" or try to psychoanalyze employees, and should use common sense when meeting with potentially dangerous employees. They should not make threats they can't back up or that are not part of the formal disciplinary procedure (Kinney, 1995).

THE MENTAL HEALTH PROFESSIONAL'S ROLE IN DISCIPLINE.   If the company has an in-house psychologist, he should be brought into the disciplinary meeting as either a facilitator or intermediary who can guide the process in a safe and fair manner. Other companies may want to hire independent, free-lance mental health professionals specifically trained in this type of workplace mediation on an as-needed basis. By serving as a trained observer in any potentially difficult disciplinary meeting, the mental health clinician can intervene to lower the emotional temperature of the meeting room and safely deal with the employee's conflicts, concerns, anger, and paranoia.

Safe Termination

Mental health clinicians can advise or participate in termination procedures. As with discipline, termination can be clear and firm without being inhumane.

TERMINATION GUIDELINES.   Normally, the best person to terminate an employee is the manager or supervisor who has had the best relationship with that worker. A termination should, of course, include a systematic process of documentation. The key to effective termination is to make it as clear as possible to the person that this action is for a specific reason, rather than for general "attitude" or personal reasons (Grote, 1995; Labich, 1996; Mantell & Albrecht, 1994).

In an uncomplicated, or "cool," termination, the company's own policies may dictate a variety of moves, including the opportunity for the employee to finish half-done work, receive severance pay, or get insurance benefit protection for a specified time period. In a hostile, or "hot," termination, the disturbed or disgruntled employee should be asked to leave immediately. Don't allow the terminated employee time to stew, either by delaying the inevitable or allowing him to hang around and poison the workplace atmosphere with negative talk or dangerous behavior.

Terminations should be done at the beginning or end of the shift. In the case of the employee who leaves in anger, don't allow him easy access to the building. The employee should be told not to return to the work area. Have a strict badge policy in place and enforce it. Again, the employee should be treated with reasonable respect, but should understand in no uncertain terms—by the presence of security or police, if necessary—that the termination action is final and will be backed up. The employee should also be informed of any counseling or other services offered by the company for the transition period. Providing continued medical and mental health benefits to help the fired employee over the hump may be an important measure in avoiding a tragedy (Flannery, 1995; Labig, 1995; Mantell & Albrecht, 1994).

THE MENTAL HEALTH PROFESSIONAL'S ROLE IN TERMINATION.   Using the psychologist or other trained mental health professional as a buffer between the supervisor and the disturbed employee may help defuse a potentially violent termination. When the employee is uncooperative and termination looks like the only alternative, the psychologist may work as a mediator and go-between and help explain the risk of termination to the employee. He may explain the choices the employee must make or be fired. The meeting with the psychologist can take place on company grounds or at an office away from the company (Labig, 1995; Mantell & Albrecht, 1994).

By foreshadowing the coming events, the psychologist can lessen the impact, prepare the employee for what it to come, and deal with feelings of fear, depression, or anger right on the spot. If the highly disturbed employee refuses to cooperate with the termination proceedings, company security or the local police may have to be called in to escort the employee off the premises (Mantell & Albrecht, 1994). Even in this process, the mental health clinician may help keep an emotionally simmering situation from boiling over into overt violence.

DEBRIEFING REMAINING EMPLOYEES.   After a termination, the remaining employees will want to know what happened. On an individual basis,- company representatives should make themselves available to anyone who would like to sit down and discuss why the terminated employee is no longer with the company. It's not management's obligation to offer rationalizations or justifications as to why an employee was terminated, and the purpose of the debriefing is not to gossip about the terminated employee. Address comments to the concerns voiced by the remaining workers about their roles and responsibilities, and lay the groundwork for more effective communication in the future. Importantly, management should control wild rumors and let the workers know that, if they have a problem with another employee, they can bring it up without fear of recrimination from their bosses (Mantell & Albrecht, 1994).

WORKPLACE VIOLENCE: RESPONSE TO EMERGENCIES

Sometimes, despite the best efforts at prevention, a dangerous situation begins to brew and a violent incident becomes a distinct possibility. Or the incident just begins abruptly, even explosively, and personnel have to respond. What do they do? The answer to that question depends on how thorough the preincident violence response plan and training have been. Here, the mental health professional can be instrumental in helping companies design violence response policies and protocols, identifying clear staff roles and chain of command, and providing ongoing education and training in violence response techniques, such as the following.

Warning Signs of Impending Violence

Red flags that an employee may be on the verge of losing control include disorganized physical appearance or dress, tense facial expression, glazed eyes, inappropriate use of dark glasses, evidence of substance abuse, severe agitation, verbal argumentativeness, verbal threats, especially to specific persons, and threat of weapons (Flannery, 1995).

Defusing Potentially Dangerous Situations

A potential workplace violence crisis can be thought of as occurring in several stages (Caraulia & Steiger, 1997; Labig, 1995), each with its own recommendations for defusing-type interventions.

In the *anxiety phase*, the response that is most needed is support. The focus of the intervention should be on how the employee feels and what his concerns are. This involves rapport building and active listening, the mainstay of crisis intervention as a whole.

In the *defensive phase*, the employee comes to feel increasingly trapped and out of options. The response needed here is a directive one in which the employee is shown a safe and dignified way out of the danger zone. Helpful techniques involve self-control, redirecting anger, calming body language, giving limited choices, and gently but firmly setting limits.

In the *acting-out phase*, the employee has lost at least some control. The response needed is professional control and containment. The focus is on the employee's immediate behavior, setting clear and reasonable limits, and using calming techniques. If talk is unproductive, physical restraint by security or law enforcement may be required.

In the *tension-reduction phase*, the crisis has passed and the employee should be ready to accept help in reducing his level of tension. Assuming no serious harm was committed and the employee is not actually in custody, the appropriate response is a therapeutic type of rapport that is caring, helpful, understanding, and calm. Reinforcing a controlled and face-saving ending to the violent episode is often the best insurance that it won't be repeated.

Handling a Violent Episode

When the situation looks like it is not being defused adequately, the intervener's level of awareness should increase accordingly. Pay attention to the environment and to potential dangers and think about possible outside assistance. The following general guidelines (Caraulia & Steiger, 1997; Gilliland & James, 1993; Labig, 1995) should be combined with your own clinical judgment and common sense and be supplemented by appropriate training.

Initial Action. If possible, don't become isolated with potentially violent persons in the first place, unless you have made sure that security precautions have been taken to prevent or limit a violent outburst. If things begin to get out of hand, casually interrupt the interview to call and request something, while actually calling for help. Here's where your planning comes in handy if you have a prearranged signal for just such an emergency. Some authorities recommend telling the subject you are going or calling for help in order to maintain credibility in the interaction and because this may actually reassure some subjects who are feeling out of control. Assess the situation and use your judgment.

Body Language. Don't engage in behaviors that could be interpreted as aggressive or threatening, such as moving too close, staring, pointing, or displaying provocative facial expressions or postures. Try to stand at an angle facing the subject—not directly in front and certainly not behind him, both of which are likely to be perceived as threatening. Remember the general rule of standing "two quick steps" away from the subject. If possible, the intervener should ask if he can sit down, as this will constitute a less threatening figure. Then encourage the subject to be seated as well. Always move slowly and keep your hands where they can be seen.

Communication Style. Keep the subject engaged in conversation about his feelings or about a specific problem, but avoid "egging him on." Keep the conversation going, pace it, and modulate your voice. Don't shout, put a sharp edge on responses, or use threats. Conversely, don't mumble, speak hesitantly, or use so low a tone of voice that the subject has trouble understanding you, which may be irritating. Give the subject undivided attention and use empathic listening skills, such as simple restatement of the subject's concerns. Use common sense and your own clinical judgment, but generally don't attempt to reason with a subject who is under the influence of drugs or alcohol or is clearly irrational or psychotic. When in doubt, shut up: use silence while the subject talks, as the more energy and adrenalin he uses up, the sooner he will fatigue and the easier it will be to control the situation. However, avoid seeming like you're ignoring the subject.

Communication Content. Don't argue, give orders, or disagree when not absolutely necessary. Don't push your own importance or authority or blather on in an officious, know-it-all manner. Conversely, don't be overly placating or patronizing and don't condescend by using childish responses that are cynical, satirical, or insulting. Be careful with even well-intentioned humor, which may be misinterpreted as mocking or dismissive under stressful circumstances. Don't make promises you can't keep, except possibly to buy time in emergency situations. Avoid complex "why" and "what" inquiries that put the subject on the defensive; rather, use simple, direct, closed-ended questions. Calmly and concretely explain the consequences of further violent behavior without provocation or condemnation. Set limits, but give choices between two alternatives, such as sitting down or walking outside for a smoke. Try to de-escalate slowly, moving from alternative to alternative.

Scene Control. Don't allow a number of interveners to interact simultaneously with the subject in multiple dialogues, as this can be confusing and irritating. Have one intervener take charge. If this person is clearly rejected by the subject, try to find someone who can establish better rapport. Other security or support staff should remain at a discrete distance and wait calmly and silently unless or until they are needed to intervene physically. Any physical restraint or take-down procedures should be carried out by personnel with specialized training in this area. Don't allow an "audience" to gather around the subject, cheer him on, insult him, or shout at him from a distance. Anyone who has no business being there should leave immediately. If professional negotiators or law enforcement show up on scene, brief them as thoroughly as possible and let them take charge.

Guns and Weapons

If the perpetrator wields a firearm (Dubin, 1995; Flannery, 1995), the intervener should acknowledge the weapon with a neutral and obvious remark, e.g., "I see the gun." Maintain your distance, keep your hands visible, and move slowly. Never tell the perpetrator to drop the gun or attempt to grab it, as he may have another weapon concealed or may simply overpower you. As rapport develops, if the perpetrator appears ambivalent about using the weapon, request that he point it away while you talk. Appeal to his sense of competence and control: To avoid an "accident," ask if he will at least decock the gun (revolver) or put the safety catch on (semiauto).

If the perpetrator seems willing to surrender the weapon, don't ask him to hand it over, but rather have him unload it, place it down in a safe, neutral corner, and back away. Some authorities recommend that the intervener then slowly pick up the gun and neutralize it, being careful not to point it at the perpetrator, as this may give him an "excuse" to pull another concealed weapon or otherwise attack you. Where feasible, to avoid being baited into "going for" the gun, I would recommend that after the perpetrator has put it down safely, ask him to calmly walk out of the room with you, leaving the weapon behind.

Although by no means a hard and fast rule, the more time that passes without the perpetrator's actually firing the gun, the lower the likelihood of its actually being used. Initially, however, the intervener should comply with whatever reasonable and safe demands the armed perpetrator may make and take special care to avoid agitating him further. Continue to talk to the perpetrator, reasonably empathize with the perceived grievance or his feelings about it, and acknowledge that he is in control. The intervener should appear calm and not intimidating, confrontational, or argumentative. The intervener should encourage the armed perpetrator to talk out his concerns, and should employ the relevant defusing strategies discussed above until the crisis is, hopefully, safely and successfully resolved.

WORKPLACE VIOLENCE RECOVERY

Sometimes the worst occurs, and a violent incident stuns and horrifies the workplace and everyone in it. People may be killed, others wounded, some held hostage, and many traumatized. It is in the aftermath of such a dramatic episode that the trauma therapist typically makes his or her most important contribution to the recovery of the affected personnel.

Workplace Violence Response Patterns and Syndromes

Individuals affected by workplace traumatic events may include injured employees, employees remote from the scene, witnesses, first responders such as police or paramedics, family members, stakeholders such as suppliers or customers that knew the victims, or any others connected to the trauma (Kinney, 1995).

Employees can be conceptualized as falling into three general groups following a trauma (Kinney, 1995). First, a few individuals will recover quickly, seemingly without the assistance of any type of mental health intervention. Sometimes these seemingly stoic souls are internalizing their pain and grief, only to maladaptively unleash their emotions at a later date. A second group will require modest counseling, usually on an outpatient basis, in order to regain their previous level of confidence, security, and safety. Finally, a third group will develop serious psychological disorders that may require more extensive therapy or clinical services.

Some authorities (Flannery, 1995; Mantell & Albrecht, 1994) have identified three basic stages of reaction in the aftermath of a workplace violence incident, which appear to bear some similarity to the stages of response to disasters (see Chapter 7).

Stage one of the workplace violence response consists of *shock, disbelief, and denial*. This stage begins immediately after the incident and may last anywhere from minutes to months. In severe trauma cases, people wander about aimlessly, stunned and dazed by the event they just experienced. This reaction usually dissipates over time, shading into the remaining stages.

Stage two consists of a *cataclysm of emotions*. Here, the victims may run a gauntlet of different feelings as they try to come to terms with their experience. This stage can last for a few days or linger for years and can include feelings of vengeance directed against the perpetrator of the violence, anger against the company for failing to protect them, rage against God, fate, society, or the criminal justice system, and self-blame for failing to take the proper action, misperceiving the obscure warning signs, or just being in the wrong place at the wrong time. Survivors may experience fear and terror, suffer from phobias and panic attacks as they attempt to return to the workplace, and develop hypervigilance, intrusive imagery, withdrawal, sleep disorders, and health problems. They may experience grief, sorrow, survivor guilt, self-loathing, confusion, and depression as they return to the workplace and are reminded of fallen coworkers by worksite "grief anchors," such as a desk, workstation, locker, photos, nameplates, media accounts, anniversary dates, and so on.

Stage three consists of *reconstruction of equilibrium*. Here, the survivors have finally started to regain their emotional and mental balance. They have a new outlook, not just about what happened, but also about themselves and how they have coped and will continue to cope. There are still good days and bad days, but the movement is definitely in the direction of recovery.

When the serious psychological impact of the workplace violence event persists beyond one month, the employee victims often develop full-blown PTSD (Flannery, 1995). Physical symptoms include hypervigilance, exaggerated startle response, difficulty sleeping, impaired concentration and memory, and mood swings between anger and depression. Intrusive symptoms include recurring and distressing thoughts, emotions, memories, flashbacks, nightmares, and hyperreaction to stimuli that depict or symbolize the violent event. Avoidant symptoms include emotional numbing, diminished interest in significant activities, and avoidance of specific thoughts, feelings, activities or situations reminiscent of the violent episode.

As reviewed by Flannery (1995), PTSD symptoms seen in victims of workplace violence have their own particular rationale. Traumatic events destroy one's sense of reasonable mastery and personal control. Some victims assume a stance of overcontrol, trying to avoid ever being vulnerable again. Others try to regain control by blaming themselves for what happened. The implicit assumption is that if the victim did something to put himself in harm's way, then he can change this so that it will never happen again; blaming the company, supervisor, or coworkers is an analogous process. Still others give up completely and descend into drugs and alcohol. They seem to have developed the assumption that because they were unable to avert the violence at work, they are unable to control anything in their lives.

Disruption of caring attachments and basic human trust is related to the fact that workplace violence is perpetrated by other human beings. To make matters worse, other employees may distance themselves from the victims in order to avoid "contagion" or to search for some aspect of the victims' behavior that "caused" the violence. This reinforces employee victim withdrawal and produces a vicious cycle of alienation and recrimination.

A sense of meaningful purpose in life is disrupted in the wake of workplace violence. Victims do not feel safe, no longer regard daily life at work or home as predictable or controllable, and do not feel motivated to "carry on." The deliberate, conscious destruction of human life by others is frightening and demoralizing, and raises the existential problem of evil that must be addressed before the victims can once again begin to invest their time and energy in work, family, and recreational activities.

Several consequences of inadequately treated workplace violence trauma may be seen. Anxiety disorders may express themselves in the form of panic attacks, somatoform disorders, or chronic pain. Depressive states may be cripplingly severe, sometimes to the point of suicide. Addictive behavior may increase, as victims self-medicate to try to numb their anxiety and hypervigilance with alcohol, barbiturates, or benzodiazepines, relieve their depression with cocaine or amphetamines, or dampen their rage with opiates. Impulsive acting-out behavior may be seen in the form of sensation-seeking, risk-taking, gambling, compulsive sexuality, and eating disorders, as well violent behavior on the part of victims themselves; sharp increases in domestic violence are often observed following traumatic events of many types (Flannery, 1995).

Plans, Policies, and Procedures

The mental health professional can guide companies and institutions in proactively setting up policies and procedures for responding to the aftermath of a workplace violence incident. The plan should include the following elements.

MENTAL HEALTH MOBILIZATION.   In the best case, planning may have included a detailed drill with the company psychologist. In other instances, it simply means that the post-trauma specialist has become sufficiently familiar with the organization to know how to gather critical information and respond promptly and effectively at the time of a crisis. During the planning period, company representatives should be building confidence in the mental health clinician's ability to work constructively with company personnel during crisis and recovery (Kinney, 1995).

Company representatives should know how to contact their mental health professional immediately, and arrange for the clinician to meet first at the top levels of the organization for executive debriefings, and then schedule meetings with anyone in the organization who needs to talk about what happened. A critical incident debriefing area should be established for the responding mental health professionals. Optional debriefing services should be made available for all potential workplace violence victims outside of immediate survivors or employees. A follow-up schedule should be arranged for the clinician to return for further debriefings (Albrecht, 1996; Mantell & Albrecht, 1994; Simon, 1996).

MEDIA AND PUBLIC RELATIONS.   A specially designated media spokes-person should brief the media and, more importantly, shepherd them away from grieving employees, family members, and eyewitnesses. A firm, forthright, proactive, and sincere approach is preferable, from some-one in a high position within the organization or, alternatively, a qualified outside public relations spokeperson or firm. Companies should always be prepared to offer a concerned and honest answer to the question, "What is this company doing for the survivors?" (Albrecht, 1996; Man-tell & Albrecht, 1994; Susskind & Field, 1996).

EMPLOYEES AND FAMILIES.   Someone should be designated to notify the victims' families of the incident and be ready to offer them immediate support, counseling, and debriefing services. Personnel managers should arrange time off for grieving employees as appropriate. After the initial stages of the incident, the mental health clinician should help managers and supervisors find ways for the employees to memorialize the victims (Mantell & Albrecht, 1994; see also Chapters 8 and 10).

LAW ENFORCEMENT, PHYSICAL SECURITY, AND CLEANUP.   Someone should be designated to immediately check, protect, or restore the integ-rity of the company's data systems, computers, and files. A representative should be designated to work with local law enforcement. The crime scene should be kept intact until law enforcement has gone over the area. A cleanup crew for the site of the attack should be available, pending approval from law enforcement investigators. Exquisite sensitivity to surviving staff's strong feelings about "cleaning up the mess, like nothing happened" is essential, and such cleanup operations should be conducted in as respectful, even solemn, a manner as possible (Kinney, 1995; Man-tell & Albrecht, 1994).

LEGAL MEASURES.   In-house legal counsel or the company's outside law firm should be notified of the incident and asked to respond to the scene (Albrecht, 1996; Kinney, 1995; Mantell & Albrecht, 1994).

Critical Incident Debriefing and
Psychological Services

There are a number of steps that the traumatized company should take following a workplace violence crisis, and the mental health professional can be instrumental in guiding and implementing the psychological recovery process.

RESTORING ORDER: POSTTRAUMA CRISIS MANAGEMENT.   In the immediate aftermath of a workplace violence incident, available personnel must begin the process of accounting for slain, injured, and surviving employees while awaiting the arrival of a posttrauma professional service provider. Company officials must communicate the message that all personnel and family members will be provided the utmost care and concern. They must recognize that many of their employees are destabilized, demoralized, and disoriented, and that they are looking to company authorities to restore order and their sense of confidence and mental equilibrium. Failure to demonstrate constructive leadership following a crisis can have damaging effects on the company for months or years to come (Albrecht, 1996; Kinney, 1995). The following steps are designed to help affected companies express concern and restore order following a workplace violence trauma (Labig, 1995; Mantell & Albrecht, 1994).

1. Demonstrate concern and caring for those who have been harmed by the trauma. The clear message that employees and other organization stakeholders need to hear with certainty is that management is going to do everything humanly and administratively possible to care for those affected by the trauma.
2. Within the limits of security, open up communication channels and control rumors. Describe what actions the company is taking to assist in recovery and what measures are being developed to reduce the risk of this ever happening again.
3. Assess the organization's personnel and business requirements in order to restore business performance. Inform employees what it will take to get back to normal.
4. Following the immediate and short-term crisis interventions, arrange for the posttrauma mental health team to return to the workplace on a periodic basis to counsel and debrief employees as needed.

POSTTRAUMA INTERVENTIONS.   Although most authorities emphasize the advantage of early identification and treatment of workplace and other PTSD syndromes, many companies, agencies, and insurance carriers are still reluctant to make psychological referrals after a traumatic incident at work, fearing that such referrals will lead to expanded claims against them or "excessive" outlays for treatment and disability benefits. In fact, actual experience documents the exact opposite: prompt and appropriate psychological care of traumatized employees can reduce the number of stress claims and the amount of settlements, because it makes a positive statement about the commitment of management to employee well-being. Further, with proper intervention, the employee is less likely to develop costly substance abuse, chronic pain, somatization, or other traumatic disability syndromes (Albrecht, 1996; Everstine & Everstine, 1993; Flannery, 1995; Yandrick, 1996).

Brom and Kleber (1989), Everstine and Everstine (1993), and Flannery (1995) have independently developed their own preventive trauma treatment programs, the first in response to a rash of terrorist robberies at financial institutions in the Netherlands, the second to deal with American workplace accidents and violence, and the third to manage workplace violence in health care settings.

Brom and Kleber (1989) outline several principles of intervention that underlie their program. To avoid the potentially stigmatizing singling-out of individuals, assistance of traumatized employees is standardized and all involved personnel participate. Assistance is formulated as an official program within the organization, with a clear delineation of staff and responsibilities. Management assigns a skilled staff member or other clinician who is in charge of victim assistance, has no direct association with the career of the traumatized employees, and is not bound to report on the employees.

In this model, the clinician's function is solely to support the traumatized employees immediately after the event and in the longer-term recovery period. Organizations develop clear policies and procedures with regard to the temporary absence of traumatized employees and, if necessary, the transfer of an employee to another position within the organization without penalty or stigmatization.

Everstine and Everstine's (1993) program is similar. Treatment of traumatized employees is carried out by professionals with specialized training and experience. All employees are encouraged to participate, but those who are particularly resistant to the group process may be referred for individual therapy. The treatment services are individualized to meet the needs of the specific employee and job environment. Where return to the original worksite is not possible, retraining and reassignment are implemented.

According to this model, when a traumatic event occurs at the workplace, it is the responsibility of employers to take decisive steps to facilitate stabilization and recovery. For example, time should be set aside for employees to discuss and work through their reactions to the event. Employees should be given as much factual information as possible about the incident, as well as the condition of coworkers, to mitigate dangerous rumors and restore a sense of control. Employees who are in the hospital or recuperating at home need information and support as well, and efforts should be made to prevent them from being alienated from their fellow workers.

Workplace superstitions about "bad luck" often take the form of unaffected workers avoiding or actively ostracizing the trauma survivors for fear that the victims' ill fortune could "rub off" or because the victims are defensively regarded as somehow responsible for their fate. These potential sources of conflict may be defused in group meetings, restoring needed cohesion and workplace support (Everstine & Everstine, 1993).

Building on the work of Mitchell and Everly (1993, 1996), Flannery and colleagues (Flannery, 1995; Flannery, Fulton, Tausch, & DeLoffi, 1991; Flannery, Penk, Hanson, & Flannery, 1996) have designed a comprehensive, voluntary, peer-help, systems approach, called the *assaulted staff action program* (ASAP), for health care staff who are assaulted by patients at work. It provides a range of needed services, including individual critical incident debriefings (see also Chapter 8 and 10) of assaulted staff, debriefings of entire wards, a staff victims' support group, employee victim family debriefing and counseling, and referrals for follow-up psychotherapy as indicated. The ASAP team structure is comprised of 15 direct-care staff volunteers. The approach is psychoeducational, rather than conceptualized as formal clinical counseling or "psychotherapy," per se. The ASAP has three supervisors, and the ASAP team director is responsible for administering the entire program and for ensuring the quality of the services.

When combined with preincident training and stress management. The ASAP program has proven effective in ameliorating the psychological impact of patient assaults on employees and in significantly reducing the overall level of violence itself. In facilities where it has been applied, the program has proven to be cost-effective in terms of reduced staff turnover, less use of sick leave, fewer industrial accident claims, and less medical expense as overall assault rates have declined. Indeed, the authors point out, the costs associated with the entire program are less than that of one successful lawsuit.

Flannery (1995) recommends the following basic steps in implementing an organization's own ASAP: (1) develop administrative support for the program; (2) tailor the model for the individual facility; (3) recruit the team members; (4) train the team; (5) field the completed service.

Each step generally takes about one month, so teams can be online within about six months.

Based on several individual and group interventions I've carried out with survivors of workplace violence, I can't stress enough the importance of organizational support. In the worst case I can remember, a bank branch grudgingly arranged for a staff debriefing after a holdup, only because the service was mandated by their managed care contract. The branch managers clearly regarded the whole thing as a waste of time that cut into employees' work hours. The most uncomfortable back room in the storage and lunch area was found for the debriefing, which was frequently interrupted by people coming in and out to use the bathroom. Entering coworkers gawked at the seated debriefees and a few made audible sarcastic comments about "free time." Needless to say, the participants wanted the whole thing over with as quickly as possible, and little therapeutic work was accomplished.

The best case I can remember (in terms of company support) involved a hostage and shooting crisis perpetrated by a disturbed customer of a medium-sized investment firm, which resulted in two deaths and several injuries. Almost immediately, the firm's president suspended business as usual, arranged for temps to cover the basic needs of the company, offered his home to be used for almost round-the-clock debriefings, and provided food, beverages, and in a few cases, bed and board to employees who were too upset to drive home. He and the senior management staff offered any kind of help they could to survivors and their families, personally checked on proper funeral arrangements for the slain employees, visited the employees who were in the hospital, and generally shared in the grief and recovery of the members of their staff. Far more than any specific clinical services I could provide, this natural, unselfish, human response to tragedy within the ranks on the part of senior staff—the true definition of "leadership"—helped this firm to heal quickly and move on, always holding a place of respect for their slain comrades, but honoring their memories by productively continuing their work.

Workplace Violence Recovery: Follow-Up

Moving on and continuing to work productively is something every company must do in order to survive and succeed. It's obviously unrealistic to expect an organization to just "get over" a significant workplace violence incident. But even here, the mental health clinician can contribute to the long-term recovery of the company and its members through direct services and consultation.

ORGANIZATIONAL AND ADMINISTRATIVE POLICY.   Albrecht (1996) and Mantell and Albrecht (1994) suggest several measures companies can take to restore confidence after a workplace violence incident. This begins with messages from top management emphasizing the company's willingness to take responsibility, address the causes of the incident in a forthright manner, provide services for all who need them, and take every necessary step and reasonable action to see that something like this never happens again.

ROLE OF EXECUTIVES AND LEADERS.   The top officials in a company that has experienced a workplace violence incident should be ready and willing to give employees the time they need to grieve, mourn, and recover. At minimum, the leader's role is to bring in the law enforcement and mental health professionals and then stand back and let them do their jobs (Mantell & Albrecht, 1994).

POST-INCIDENT INVESTIGATIONS.   Questions asked during the incident "postmortem" may address the nature of the perpetrator; his relationship to the organization; his relationship with coworkers and supervisors; his history of disciplinary action or termination; his role as a customer; the actions that led to his dissatisfaction as a customer; any restraining orders and their enforcement; the workplace stressors that may have been involved; the domestic or other life stressors that may have been involved; financial pressures, drugs or alcohol, mental illness or personality disorders; any warning signs that should have been heeded; and the company's overall security and threat assessment procedures (Mantell & Albrecht, 1994).

In general, if there is any positive outcome that can emerge from a workplace violence incident, it is in the nature of what can be learned in order to reduce the chances of the same kind of tragedy happening again.

WORKPLACE VIOLENCE AND WOMEN

As more women join the workforce, they increasingly become the targets of violence. Certain special considerations affecting women on the job warrant this special section.

Demographics

Homicide is the number one cause of death for women in the workplace. Although the leading instrument of death on the job is firearms, women are six times more likely than men to be strangled to death. In the U.S., while only one out of five people murdered at work is a woman, 40 percent of women who die on the job will die from homicide, compared to 10 percent of men. In other words, while men are more likely to die from falls, electrocution, or other industrial accidents, women are more likely to die from workplace violence (Kinney, 1995; Simon, 1996).

Types of Workplace Violence Against Women

Women are susceptible to many different forms of workplace violence, including homicide, rape, other sexual assault, sexual abuse and harassment, gunshot wounds, stabbing, strangulation, physical beatings, verbal abuse, and psychological trauma. Women may be victimized because they appear more vulnerable or weaker than men. Both the number and the percentage of women who work outside the home have increased steadily throughout the 20th century. At the same time, divorce rates are high and single motherhood continues to increase. Many women are relegated to low-wage and low-status service or clerical jobs that place them on the front lines as cashiers, waitresses, etc., where workplace security measures are often meager or nonexistent. When violence does strike women, the repercussions are likely to impair the financial as well as the emotional well-being of their families (Kinney, 1995).

More women than men work in the retail industry, such as in convenience stores, and women in these settings often work alone and unprotected, at high risk of being injured or killed. Moreover, employees in these low-status positions are less likely to have the clout to persuade employers to take threats seriously. In some cases, workers who "make trouble" are simply fired so that the boss doesn't have to deal with those threats or with the person making the complaints. In addition, the entry of greater numbers of women into the workforce produces frequent emasculating resentment in insecure men, who may feel that their jobs or promotions have been unfairly "stolen" by women (Kinney, 1995; Simon, 1996).

Sexual Harassment and Domestic Violence

Sexual harassment has become perhaps the quintessential form of interpersonal workplace problem experienced by women. Sexual harassment itself can be a form of violence. Even verbal intimidation and harassment can inflict acute and longlasting psychological and emotional harm. In addition, sexual harassment is often a precursor of more overt forms of physical violence, such as assault, rape, or murder in the workplace (Kinney, 1995; Schouten, 1996).

Domestic disputes have become the third major source of conflict leading to homicide in the workplace. A sagging economy usually brings an increase in domestic violence as unemployed husbands or boyfriends threaten their wives or partners at work. Rejection of on-the-job suitors or workplace harassers often places these women at increased risk of violence at the hands of the spurned and jilted. When romances outside the workplace sour, the rejected male abuser may become a stalker, who usually knows where the woman works and generally has ready access to her place of employment. A common response of employers who are fed up with all the trouble is simple to fire the woman (Brownell, Tucker, Neville, & Imperial, 1996; Friedman, 1996; Hamberger & Holtzworth-Munroe, 1994; Kinney, 1995; Labig, 1995; Meloy, 1997; Walker, 1994).

How Women Can Protect Themselves

With regard to domestic violence spillover, sometimes police restraining orders work, and sometimes they just make matters worse. Much depends on the willingness of the local police to enforce them. Many domestic violence cases involve a victim who is struggling emotionally to let go of the abuser, which can prove to be quite frustrating for bosses and coworkers who are trying to be helpful, because all of their suggestions are rejected or misinterpreted by the ambivalent or frightened employee. People's privacy at work should of course be respected, but if they are going through messy domestic battles or, for that matter, other personal crises that affect their jobs and lives, they need to know that it is all right to confide in the right persons at work and that the proper protective or other assistive measures will be taken (Labig, 1995; Pierce & Aguinis, 1997).

Companies can take several steps to protect employees from stalkers (Flannery, 1995; Kinney, 1995; Meloy, 1997; Pierce & Aguinis, 1997). They should establish a policy of providing protective services to threatened employees. If possible, the threatened employee's office or work station should be relocated to a place unknown to the stalker, and the employee's work schedule altered to confuse the stalker. Descriptions or photographs of the stalker should be provided to receptionists, security officers, and other relevant personnel. Law enforcement can be encouraged to enforce restraining orders by forging links between company security and local police. If the threat is acute, employees at risk should be given time off. Silent alarms or buzzers should be placed at the threatened employee's work station, and security cameras should be deployed near entrances to the employee's work area. Security measures work best when they are coordinated and integrated.

With regard to sexual harassment, companies can take several effective measures (Kinney, 1995; Schouten, 1996). A serious sexual harassment policy should describe the specific conduct that constitutes harassment and state that such conduct is tolerated neither by the company nor by state or federal law. The policy should explain the employee's right to complain about sexual harassment without fear of retaliation and without having to directly confront the harasser, at least at the time of the initial complaint. The policy should have a grievance procedure that the harassed employee can follow, as well as sexual harassment hotlines for emergency situations; such hotlines are now required by law in at least 30 states.

In summary, employers must learn to take all threats to worker safety seriously and take action to deal with those threats. They must encourage all employees, men and women, to report any breaches of personal or company security. Violence prevention should be right up there with fire prevention as a corporate safety issue. Companies must have measures in place to deal with disciplinary matters, safe hiring and firing, escalating crises, ongoing emergencies, and aftermath effects. Most importantly, companies that encourage a fair and honorable corporate culture are more likely to earn the respect and loyalty of their employees and reduce the risk of avoidable tragedies. Working safe is working smart.

Chapter 10

HELPING THE HELPERS

*Psychotherapeutic Strategies
with Law Enforcement
and Emergency Services Personnel*

The noblest service comes from nameless hands.
And the best servant does his work unseen.

—Oliver Wendell Holmes

"I've seen dead bodies, fresh ones and ripe ones. I've scraped eyeballs off the bedroom wall in suicide shootings, I've investigated murder scenes you wouldn't believe. But this was different, this was a little kid, this could have been *my* kid. And there was no reason for it, just no reason."

This statement came from a veteran detective following the shooting death of a young child by his mentally handicapped brother who had been left unsupervised by the children's parents in the same house as an unsecured handgun. It wasn't the worst death the emergency responders had ever seen, it wasn't the grisliest, nor the most touch-and-go in terms of lifesaving attempts—the child had apparently died instantly from a .357 magnum bullet wound to the head. It wasn't even the first child death for several of the workers. The main traumatizing effect of this call was the sheer existential indigestibility of the death circumstances: an innocent victim, even an essentially innocent perpetrator set up by stupidly careless adults who should have known better—there was "just no reason."

Every time we dial 911, we expect that our emergency will be taken seriously and handled competently. The police will race to our burgled

215

office, the firefighters will douse our burning home, the ambulance crew will stabilize our injured loved one and whisk him to the nearest hospital. We take these expectations for granted because of the day-to-day skill and dedication of workers who serve the needs of law enforcement, emergency services, and public safety.

These "heroic helpers," as they have sometimes been called, are routinely exposed to special kinds of traumatic events and daily pressures that most civilians can only try to imagine. Indeed, the recent popularity of TV documentary cop and medic programs probably expresses both our fascination with the kind of work these professionals do and our fervent hopes that these rescuers will be there when we need them. To function effectively in their daily jobs, these helpers require a certain adaptively defensive steeliness of attitude, temperament, and training—attitudes that are sometimes perceived as coldness and callousness by the general public. Sometimes, however, the stress is just too much, and the very toughness that facilitates smooth functioning in their daily duties becomes an impediment to helpers seeking help for themselves.

This chapter describes the types of stresses and problems experienced by police officers, firefighters, paramedics, and other crisis workers—the "tough guys" and "tough gals" (Miller, 1995)—and outlines the psychotherapeutic strategies that may prove most effective in helping these emergency responders.

STRESS AND COPING IN LAW ENFORCEMENT AND EMERGENCY SERVICES

Although there is some overlap in services—e.g., police sometimes have to perform emergency first aid, and firefighters and paramedics are often cross-trained—there are certain issues that are specific to each group, and the present section will therefore consider each of them separately.

Police Officers

Even people who don't much like cops have to admit that theirs is a difficult, dangerous, and often thankless job. Police officers regularly deal with the most violent, impulsive, and predatory members of society, put their lives on the line, and confront miseries and horrors that the rest of us view from the sanitized distance of our newspapers and TV screens. In addition to the daily grind, officers are frequently the target of criticism and complaints by citizens, the media, the judicial system, opportunistic politicians, hostile attorneys, "do-gooder" clinicians and social service personnel, and their own administrators and law enforcement agencies (Blau, 1994).

PATROL OFFICERS.   Police officers generally carry out their sworn duties and responsibilities with dedication and valor, but some stresses are too much to bear, and every officer has his breaking point. For some, it may come in the form of a particular dramatic event, such as a gruesome accident or homicide, a vicious crime against a child, a close personal brush with death, the killing or wounding of a partner, the mistaken shooting of an innocent civilian, or an especially grisly accident or crime scene. For example, following the massacre at a San Diego McDonald's restaurant in which 21 people were gunned down, half the officers exposed to the aftermath of this mass killing developed full-blown posttraumatic stress disorder (PTSD), twice the rate for the department as a whole (McCafferty, McCafferty, & McCafferty, 1992).

For other officers, there may be no single major trauma, but the identified mental breakdown occurs under the cumulative weight of a number of more moderate stresses over the course of the officer's career. In either case, all too often the officer feels that the department doesn't support him and that there is nowhere else to vent his distress. So he bottles up his feelings, acts snappish with coworkers, superiors, civilians, and family members, and becomes hypersensitive to small annoyances on and off the job. As his isolation and feelings of alienation grow, his health and home life begin to deteriorate, work becomes a burden, and he may ultimately feel that he is losing his mind, or going "squirrelly."

Most police officers deal with both routine and exceptional stresses by using a variety of situationally adaptive coping and defense mechanisms, such as repression, displacement, isolation of feelings, humor—often seemingly callous or crass joking—and generally clamming up and toughing it out. Officers develop a closed society, an insular "cop culture" centering around what they refer to as *The Job*. Part of this closed-society credo is based on the shared belief that no civilian or outsider could possibly understand what they go through on a day-to-day basis. A smaller number of police officers spend most or all of their time with other cops, watch cops shows, read cop stories, and so on. *The Job* becomes their life and crowds out other activities and relationships (Blau, 1994).

Apparently, police pressures and their responses to them are remarkably similar in most Western societies where these have been observed. A study of Australian police officers (Evans, Coman, Stanley, & Burrows, 1993) found that most prefer problem-focused and direct action methods of coping rather than social support, self-blame, or wishful thinking. A study of Scottish constables (Alexander & Walker, 1994), found their coping methods to consist of displacement onto colleagues or the public, delegating work, taking sick leave, using psychotropic medication, seeking spiritual help, engaging in physical exercise, relaxing, smoking, eating, or using alcohol. A frequently reported coping method was talking things over with colleagues. However, in general, the report found that these constables generally are not very satisfied with the methods they use to counteract work-induced stress.

According to one estimate (Sewell, Ellison, & Hurrell, 1988), after a traumatically stressful incident, such as a shooting, approximately one-third of officers have minimal or no problems, another third have moderate problems, and the final third have severe problems affecting the officer, his family, and the department. Seventy percent of officers involved in a fatal line-of-duty shooting leave the force within seven years of the incident. Police are admitted to general hospitals in significantly higher numbers that the general population and have significantly higher rates of premature death, ranking third among occupations in death rates (Sewell et al., 1988). Interestingly, however, despite the popular notion of rampantly disturbed police marriages, the empirical evidence does not support a higher-than-average divorce rate for police officers (Borum & Philpot, 1993).

Up to two-thirds of police officers involved in shootings experience significant emotional reactions, which include a heightened sense of danger, flashbacks, intrusive imagery and thoughts, anger, guilt, sleep disturbances, withdrawal, depression, and other stress symptoms (Solomon, 1995; Solomon & Horn, 1986). But stressful incidents include more than shootings. By focusing too much on "the big one," police often overlook the cumulative effect of more common stressors, such as long overtime during disasters, dealing with child victims, attempting resuscitation on a victim who dies, or working a fatal accident where the officer knows the victim.

Emotional reactions of guilt, irrationally taking responsibility for events that were beyond control, and rage at being lucklessly involved in a miserable situation—"being at the wrong place at the wrong time"—are common themes to be worked through. Failure to resolve these issues often leads to a variety of maladaptive response patterns. Some officers begin to overreact to perceived or imagined threats, while others ignore clear danger signals. Some cops quit the force prematurely, while others become discipline problems or develop increased absenteeism, burnout, stress disorders, substance abuse, or a host of other personal problems that can interfere with functioning at home and on the job (Solomon, 1995).

Perhaps the most tragic form of police casualty is suicide (Hays, 1994; Seligmann, Holt, Chinni, & Roberts, 1994). Twice as many officers, about 300 annually, die by their own hand as are killed in the line of duty. In some localities, the suicide rate of police officers is more than double the rate for the surrounding population. In fact, the true totals may actually be even higher, since such deaths are sometimes underreported by fellow cops to avoid stigmatizing the deceased officers and to allow the families to collect benefits. Most victims are young patrolmen with no record of misconduct, and most shoot themselves off-duty. Often, problems involving alcohol or romantic hassles are the catalyst, and occupational availability of a weapon provides the ready means (physicians and pharmacists, with access to potentially lethal prescription drugs, have even higher suicide rates). Cops under stress are caught in the dilemma of risking confiscation of their guns, transfer to desk duty, promotional setbacks, or general loss of face if they report distress or request counseling.

HOMICIDE INVESTIGATORS.   Aside from the daily stresses of patrol cops, special pressures are experienced by higher-ranking officers, such as homicide detectives, who are involved in the investigation of particularly brutal crimes, such as multiple murders or serial killings (Sewell, 1993). The normally expected societal protective role of the police officer becomes even more pronounced at the same time as their responsibilities as public servants who protect individual rights become compounded by the pressures to solve the crime.

A multiple murder investigation forces an officer to confront stressors directly related to his projected role and image of showing unflagging strength in the face of adversity and frustration, responding competently and dispassionately to crises, and placing the needs and demands of the public above his personal feelings. Moreover, the sheer magnitude and shock effect of many mass murder scenes and the violence, mutilation, and sadistic brutality associated with many serial killings, sometimes involving children, often exceed the defense mechanisms and coping abilities of even the most seasoned and hardboiled investigator. Revulsion may be tinged with rage, all the more so when fellow officers have been killed or injured.

As the investigation drags on, the inability to solve the crime and close the case further frustrates and demoralizes the assigned officers and seems to mockingly emphasize the hollowness of society's notions of justice and fairness. All the more vexsome is when the killer is known but the existing evidence is insufficient to support an arrest or conviction. Frustrating in routine investigations, this becomes even more galling where the officers have witnessed the perpetrated violence and believe the suspect will kill again. The stress is further magnified when the failure to apprehend the bad guy is caused by human error, as when an officer's bungled actions or breach of procedure lead to suppression of evidence or testimony or when critical evidence is inadvertently lost, damaged, or destroyed.

Complicating all of the above, often in a spiraling vicious cycle, is the cumulative effect of fatigue, as the concentrated, intense, sustained effort to close the case results in case errors, poor work quality, and deterioration of home and workplace relationships. Fatigue also wears down the officer's normal defenses, rendering him or her even more vulnerable to stress and failure (Sewell, 1993).

UNDERCOVER COPS.   Probably the epitome of stressful law enforcement work involves undercover policing, the realities of which rarely resemble glamorous movie portrayals. Undercover work is grueling, often boring, frequently terrifying, and occasionally lethal, and individuals successful in such assignments need to have the right mix of narcissistic toughness and adaptive psychological resilience. Still, 16 percent of undercover officers in one study (MacLeod, 1995) suffered major psychological disturbance, including PTSD. These officers are even more likely than most to deny problems and attempt to tough it out until cumulative stress causes them to make careless mistakes, necessitating their reassignment to other duty, which is in itself demoralizing. In the worst cases, complete decompensation may occur, with psychotic symptomatology, substance abuse, or violence. Clearly, this particular population of dedicated "tough guys" is underserved by mental health.

Firefighters

Every child hears the story about brave firefighters battling blazes and rescuing hapless citizens from infernal doom. Firefighters routinely display exceptional skill and bravery in the performance of their duties, but as in any role that involves dealing with life-threatening emergencies, stress can take its toll. According to the National Commission on Fire Prevention and Control, firefighting is the single most hazardous occupation in the United States. Every day approximately 280 firefighters are killed or injured, and each year over 650 are forced to retire due to occupational illness, including psychological disability (Hildebrand, 1984a, 1984b).

In February 1983, a huge brush fire tore through a large tract of South Australia (McFarlane, 1988). Battling the blaze required the efforts of several thousand trained volunteer firefighters, many of whom were exposed to extreme danger. About half of the firefighters showed symptoms of PTSD within the first four months of the event, and two-thirds of these continued to show symptoms several years after. An interaction between premorbid history and the current stressor was seen, in that a firefighter was more likely to have persistent PTSD if (1) he had suffered one or more personal crises prior to the fire; (2) he had a history of prior treatment for mental disorder; (3) he showed evidence of neuroticism on psychological testing; or (4) he had a characteristic tendency to avoid thinking about negative experiences.

Even less dramatic experiences can produce cumulative stress effects over the course of a firefighter's career. In addition to fires, firefighters must periodically deal with crimes, suicides, accidents, medical emergencies, toxic spills, and bomb explosions. In a study of the Toronto Fire Department (DeAngelis, 1995), firefighters confronted an average of 3.91 such traumatic experiences per year. In the last year of the study, these included rescuing citizens from a deadly ammonia cloud, recovering a woman's severed head in an industrial accident, and dealing with various and sundry stabbings and suicides. Compared to a 1 percent rate for the general population, the prevalence rate of diagnosable PTSD for firefighters was 16.5 percent—1 percent higher than PTSD rates for Vietnam veterans. Personal injury on the job was also a factor in psychological disability, as was organizational stress with respect to the department, job demands, and promotion conflicts.

Several positive stress-buffers were identified in the Toronto study (DeAngelis, 1995). Firefighters who were able to discuss problems with peers and who felt that their supervisors backed them up were 40 percent less likely to develop PTSD than those who did not get such administrative support. Similarly, family support decreased firefighters' chances of developing PTSD by 40 percent. In addition, self-help support groups allowed firefighters to feel that they were not the only ones to have experienced these problems and to break the conspiracy of silence that typically characterizes firefighters' reactions to trauma.

Paramedics

In many areas, firefighters and paramedics are cross-trained, while in other jurisdictions they function as independent, autonomous departments. Within the medical field, the Emergency Medical Services (EMS) experience is somewhat unique (Becknell, 1995). Whereas most other branches of medicine practice in the relatively controlled, secure, sterile environment of the hospital, clinic, office, or even busy emergency room, paramedics find their victims in their homes, on the street, under wrecked cars, in demolished buildings. The deaths they witness are not the decorous, sedated passings of the hospital bed; rather, are often abrupt, messy, noisy, agonized, and undignified. Although their efforts may be capped by many heroic and lifesaving events, for many paramedics the succession of both everyday tragedies and occasional stark horrors can take a grim psychological and existential toll.

For paramedics, as for police officers and firefighters, a given call may be especially traumatic because it resonates with events from the crisis worker's personal history. Becknell (1995) relates the case of a paramedic who tried unsuccessfully to save the life a 43-year-old man who'd suffered a heart attack while working in his yard. Noticeably agitated after the call, the worker began to yell and curse about his inability to intubate the patient. As he continued talking, the content took a personal turn. It seemed his father had died several years earlier under similar circumstances. The worker had had many disagreements with his father and had not been able to make peace with him before he died. After nearly an hour of emotionally charged ventilation, he finally declared, "I feel like I just vomited my guts out."

One of my own patients, a paramedic who was referred for "disciplinary problems," had enjoyed an apparently unblemished performance record until the day he responded to what should have been a routine call, only to discover that the call was at his own home and the patient was his own mother. In the breach, his training kicked in and he was able to intubate and carry out life support, but there was nothing anybody could have done in the face of a massive heart attack, and his mother died at the scene. Since the incident, he had become irritable and perfunctory with coworkers and patients alike, leading to several fractious episodes, which resulted in his suspension and referral for mandatory counseling.

After a few sessions of psychotherapeutic reflection, he was able to grasp the connection between the traumatic event and his subsequent mood and behavior, and was then able to cathartically express his grief and remorse. If "I couldn't even save my own mother," what good was he as a paramedic? His anger at himself became projected onto his coworkers and the general public, leading to complaints and the suspension. A few more sessions were devoted to resolving these guilt and anger themes. Soon after, he was reinstated to active service, where he continues to perform his job well. In his favor were a relatively clear premorbid mental health history and the presence of a reasonably supportive department. More complex cases may require more extended treatment.

In dealing with death, paramedics use a number of coping strategies similar to those employed by other crisis workers (Palmer, 1983). These include desensitization processes that are actually part of some paramedic training, dark humor and crass joking, overuse of technical jargon and a special working language, cognitive compartmentalization and escape into the "scientific" aspects of paramedical work, and focusing on the condition of the patient, i.e., that the patient could not have been saved regardless of their efforts—"he/she was gone before we got there."

Once again, the strain sometimes becomes too much, and, like police officers and firefighters, some paramedics take their own lives, although precise suicide statistics for this population are sketchy. There are a number of reasons why paramedics commit suicide (Mitchell, 1987), including romantic troubles, major illness, death of a close family member, economic problems, job failure or failure to achieve career goals, humilation in the presence of peers, or boring retirement after an active career. The stresses are usually multiple, diverse, and cumulative, and only rarely do job-related factors alone lead to suicide. Again, there is the fear that requesting psychological help may lead to damaging fitness-for-duty ratings and other stigmatizing consequences.

Body Handlers and Survivor Rescuers

A plane goes down, a building is bombed, a fire razes a neighborhood, a flood drowns a town. After those who can be rescued have been taken to safety, somebody has got to go in and pick up the pieces—sometimes literally. Various groups of responders, such as police, firefighters, paramedics, military personnel, and sometimes civilian volunteers, may be called upon to retrieve and handle human remains or fatally injured survivors; therefore, this category of worker is treated in a separate section.

Rescue workers endure a double stress—the event itself plus their role as help providers—and many experience feelings of fear, anger, hatred, and resentment that interfere with effective functioning (Raphael, 1986). In many cases, close peer and administrative support can help ameliorate some of the emotionally disturbing effects of such unpleasant duty (Alexander, 1993; Alexander & Wells, 1991). However, in other circumstances, exposure to such grim visual, auditory, and olfactory images—charred corpses, screaming victims, scattered personal effects—may leave a powerful, lasting, traumatic impact.

In 1987, Northwest Airlines flight 255 out of Detroit crashed on takeoff (Davis & Breslau, 1994). Bodies and body parts were strewn over a large area, and police and rescue workers were sent in to remove the remains. Many of these officers had previously dealt with assaults, rapes, shootings, and various forms of violent death, but none of this could have prepared them for the scope of the carnage they encountered at the crash site. A number of the rescue workers were Vietnam veterans, and one man described the emotional scene as "like being on patrol." For some of these vets, the sight of dismembered human remains triggered PTSD flashbacks of decades-old combat experiences, while other workers continued to be plagued weeks later with persistent intrusive images of the crash scene.

In 1989, a United Airlines DC-10 carrying 296 passengers and crew was forced to crash-land after a midair explosion over Sioux City, Iowa. Rescuers had to handle dead passengers and remains, as well as trying to rescue survivors with all degrees of injury and in varying stages of dying. The wreckage was scattered over a marshy cornfield, making the rescue and recovery attempts especially difficult. Fullerton, McCarroll, Ursano, and Wright (1992) studied a group of firefighters participating in this mass-casualty air disaster rescue and another group consisting of a special firefighting unit performing more routine, but highly skilled rescue missions in New York City. Four characteristic responses were noted among both groups: (1) identification with the injured survivors and the dead; (2) feelings of helplessness and guilt at not being able to do more for the victims—that they "should" have been able to do more; (3) fear of the unknown; and (4) physiological reactions, such as extreme fatigue and exhaustion, intrusive images and smells, impaired sleep, and nightmares about the dead.

There is something inherently horrifying about encountering a dead human being, especially if we identify with the victim in some way, if he or she is "like us." The handling of human remains, or even the anticipation of having to do so, appears to produce one of the highest levels of stress among rescue workers (McCarroll, Ursano, Fullerton, Oates, Ventis, Friedman, Shean, & Wright, 1995; Ursano & McCarroll, 1990). This has been documented among rescuers who responded to the Jonestown mass suicide (Jones, 1985) and the more recent mass suicide of the Heaven's Gate cult in California. It was observed among the rescue and recovery personnel at Oklahoma City, and studied among military personnel assigned to mortuary duty in Operation Desert Storm (McCarroll, Ursano, Fullerton, & Lundy, 1993). The handling of the bodies of children appears to be the supreme stressor, particularly for rescue workers who have children of their own. In addition, the sheer "gruesomeness factor" of the remains and the overall death scene appears to strongly affect the level of traumatic stress experienced by the body handlers (McCarroll et al., 1995).

Dentists who were assigned the task of examining dental remains in order to identify the incinerated bodies of Branch Davidian cult members in Waco, Texas, were found to show significantly high levels of traumatic stress (McCarroll, Fullerton, Ursano, & Hermser, 1996). Examiners inexperienced at this type of forensic identification showed greater stress than more experienced examiners. Support from coworkers and family members helped mitigate the stress in the experienced dentists, but didn't seem to do much to ease the trauma of those who were new at this kind of job.

The stress of handling the dead can have vital physiological effects as well. Three groups of workers at the 1994 crash site of USAir Flight 427 were studied by Delahanty, Dougall, Craig, Jenkins, and Baum (1997). Workers who were unexpectedly exposed to human remains at the crash scene exhibited more intrusive stress symptomatology and had greater immunological activation (elevation of natural killer cell activity) than morgue workers who actually handled and examined greater numbers of bodies and body parts or workers who did not deal with the dead at all.

The seemingly paradoxical lower level of stress in the morgue workers, despite the higher sheer volume of death exposure, was interpreted in terms of the greater predictability and controllability of the death scene for these workers. They knew what they were in for, as opposed to the on-scene searchers who were apparently quite unpleasantly surprised by their grisly discoveries. Also, the morgue workers were in "home territory," while the searchers were out in the field. The authors recommend that rescue and recovery workers who may encounter bodies and human remains be fully briefed about this possibility ahead of time in order to avoid the highly stressful shock effect of unexpected encounters with fearsome death.

Dispatchers and Support Personnel

In addition to the on-line police officers, firefighters, and paramedics, a vital role in law enforcement and emergency services is played by the workers who operate "behind the scenes," namely, the dispatchers, complaint clerks, clerical personnel, crime and fire scene investigators, and other support personnel (Holt, 1989; Sewell & Crew, 1984). Although they are rarely directly exposed to actual danger or catastrophe (except where on-scene and off-scene personnel alternate shifts), several high-stress features characterize the job descriptions of these workers:

- *Multiple calls.* Much as with air traffic controllers, simultaneous peak traffic on the radio—"a million things going on at once"—is a particularly significant source of stress for dispatchers.

- *Required decisions.* The potential life-threatening nature of many calls and the sense of urgency connected with handling people's emergencies magnify the pressures created by multiple calls and constraints on time.
- *Low control.* Unlike on-scene personnel, who exert more discretion and control over their responses to requests for service and actions taken, communications personnel are limited in the flexibility of their response to demands from superiors, on-scene workers, and the public.
- *Citizen contact.* Intense stress can result from dealing with citizens who are experiencing life-threatening emergencies. The dispatcher must handle a wide range of human emotions with calm professionalism and attempt to impose some measure of order and control on a confusing and chaotic situation. The reactions are particularly complicated when citizens provide inaccurate or incomplete information to communications personnel.

The combination of high stress, low control, life-and-death decision-making in the absence of complete information, bearing the brunt of citizen outrage, and failure to enjoy the status and camaraderie of on-scene workers takes its toll on law enforcement and emergency services dispatchers and support personnel. After particularly difficult calls, dispatchers may show many of the classic posttraumatic reactions and symptoms, including numbed responsiveness, impaired memory for the event alternating with intrusive, disturbing images of the incident, irritability, hypervigilance, sleep disturbance, and interpersonal hypersensitivity.

In a number of stress debriefings that I have participated in, the dispatchers and clerical personnel have seemed genuinely surprised at being included, since they assumed that the on-scene workers would not take their ordeal seriously, as they were physically "removed" from the crisis. Happily, on-scene workers have often shown tremendous support for these desk and phone personnel. Perhaps part of this relates to the fact that in some departments personnel rotate desk and field assignments, so everyone gets a taste of both situations. Even where this is not the case, however, if the department overall is a cohesive one, a sometimes unexpected level of mutual support and validation emerges in dealing with aftermath of crises and critical incidents. But, of course, not always.

Delayed, Displaced, or Prolonged Reactions

In some cases, especially if no treatment or other appropriate support has been provided, the aftereffects of a traumatic incident may persist for many months or longer in the form of anger, hostility, irritability, problems with authority, fatigue, inability to concentrate, loss of self-confidence, or increased indulgence in food or mood-altering substances. Many of these long-term effects interfere with work performance and threaten the stability of close personal relationships. Ultimately, they may be responsible for early retirement, burnout, or suicide (Bohl, 1995).

In some cases, firefighters, police officers, paramedics, or other rescue personnel may appear to emerge from a dangerous situation or series of emergencies emotionally unscathed, only to later break down and develop a full-blown PTSD reaction following a relatively minor incident like a traffic accident (Davis & Breslau, 1994). The fender-bender, certainly far less traumatic than the dramatic scenes encountered in emergency work, seems to have symbolized vividly the personal risk, sense of human fragility, and existential uncertainty that their job-related activities entail but that they are unable to face directly if they are to maintain their necessary defenses and get the job done. The stifled affect may then be projected onto the minor incident, which is a "safer" target to blow up at.

Unfortunately, this may instigate a fear of losing control and going crazy, further propelling the vicious cycle of increased stress but greater reluctance to report it. Here, alert spouses and coworkers may be of help in urging the stricken crisis worker to get the help he or she needs.

In some cases, the delayed or prolonged stress reaction manifests itself in the form of "psychosomatic" physical complaints, such as headaches, chronic pain, or stomach, cardiac, respiratory, or musculoskeletal symptoms. Typically, physical symptoms are easier to justify as a cause of disability than "mental problems" for police officers, rescue workers, soldiers, and others who are invested in their sense of toughness and reslience (Benedikt & Kolb, 1986; Hall, 1986; McFarlane, Atchison, Rafalowicz, & Papay, 1994; Miller, 1995; Trimble, 1981).

This somatic presentation of PTSD is important to recognize, because PTSD often arises after an event that has also caused significant physical injuries. The significance of the physical symptoms is easy to miss, since the clinician is likely to assume that they relate to the injury. This can lead to prolonged and exaggerated physical disability as well as underdiagnosis of PTSD. While somatic expressions of anxiety, depression, and PTSD in emergency personnel may "mask" the emotional distress, just as commonly the emotional distress is experienced clearly, consciously, and severely. Nevertheless, emotional and psychiatric disturbances may go largely underdiagnosed in emergency rescue personnel, especially if clinical attention is limited to physical injuries (McFarlane et al., 1994).

INTERVENTION SERVICES AND
PSYCHOTHERAPEUTIC STRATEGIES

General Considerations

To avoid "shrinky" connotations, mental health intervention services with emergency service personnel are often conceptualized as *stress management, critical incident debriefing,* or other nonclinical-sounding terms (Belles & Norvell, 1990; Mitchell & Bray, 1990). In general, incident-specific, one-time interventions will be most appropriate for handling the effects of overwhelming trauma on otherwise normal, well-functioning personnel. Where posttraumatic sequelae persist, or where the psychological problems relate to a longer-term pattern of maladaptive functioning under relatively routine stresses, more extensive individual psychotherapeutic approaches are called for.

To have their greatest impact, intervention services should be part of an integrated program of services within the department and have full administrative commitment and support (Blau, 1994; Sewell, 1986). However, there is still a long way to go toward achieving this ideal in most departments. Over the last several decades, many police and firefighter administrators, particularly those of the "old school" invested in maintaining their tough guy image, have discouraged the utilization of psychological support services. Even where such utilization is officially sanctioned, the subtle negative attitudes of the departmental commanders inevitably filter down to the line personnel, who then take their cue as to what is acceptable and appropriate vs. what is shameful and stigmatizing. Things are changing, albeit slowly.

Critical Incident Stress Debriefing (CISD)

Although this approach has grown out of the general crisis intervention field and is an important element of all therapeutic work with traumatized patients, *critical incident stress debriefing,* or CISD, has been organizationally formalized for law enforcement and emergency services primarily by Jeff Mitchell and his colleagues (Mitchell, 1983, 1988; Mitchell & Bray, 1990; Mitchell & Everly, 1996). It is now implemented in public safety departments throughout the United States, Britain, and other parts of the world (Dyregrov, 1989), often subsumed under the broader umbrella category of *critical incident stress management* (CISM), which includes a range of crisis intervention strategies in addition to CISD.

CISD itself is a structured intervention designed to promote the emotional processing of traumatic events through the ventilation and normalization of reactions, as well as preparation for possible future experiences. Although CISD is designed for use in groups, other debriefing-type models have been used with individuals, couples, and families.

INDICATIONS FOR CISD.   The major classes of critical incident capable of causing distress for emergency personnel are: (1) a line-of-duty death; (2) a serious injury to emergency personnel; (3) a serious multiple-casualty incident; (4) the suicide of an emergency worker; (5) the traumatic death of children; (6) an event with excessive media interest; (7) a victim known to an emergency worker; or (8) any event that has an unusually powerful impact on the personnel.

There are a number of criteria by which peer support and command staff might decide to provide a CISD to personnel after a critical incident: (1) many individuals within a group appear to be distressed after a call; (2) the signs of stress appear to be quite severe; (3) personnel demonstrate significant behavioral changes; (4) personnel make significant errors on calls occurring after the critical incident; (5) personnel request help; (6) the event is extraordinary (Mitchell & Bray, 1990; Mitchell & Everly, 1996).

STRUCTURE OF THE DEBRIEFINGS.   A CISD debriefing is a peer-led, clinician-guided process. In addition to the actual law enforcement and emergency service workers being debriefed, the staffing of a CISD debriefing usually consists of one or more mental health professionals and one or more peer debriefers, i.e., fellow police officers, firefighters, or paramedics who have been trained in the CISD process and who usually have been through critical incidents and debriefings themselves. A typical debriefing takes place within 24 to 72 hours after the critical incident and consists of a single group meeting that lasts two to three hours, although shorter or longer meetings may be dictated by circumstances. Group size may range from a handful to a roomful, the deciding factor usually being how many people will have time to fully express themselves in the number of hours allotted for the debriefing. Where large numbers of workers are involved, such as in mass disaster rescues, several debriefings may be held successively over the course of days to accommodate all the personnel involved.

The CISD process consists of several phases (Mitchell & Everly, 1996):

- *Introduction.* The introduction phase of a debriefing is the time in which the team leader—either a mental health professional or peer debriefer, depending on the composition of the group—gradually introduces the CISD process, encourages participation by the group, and sets the ground rules by which the debriefing will operate. Generally, these involve confidentiality, attendance for the full session, nonforced participation in discussions, and the establishment of a noncritical atmosphere.

- *Fact phase.* During this phase, the group members are asked to describe briefly their job or role during the incident and, from their own perspective, some facts regarding what happened. The basic question is: "What did you do?"

- *Thought phase.* The CISD leader asks the group members to discuss their first and subsequent thoughts during the critical incident: "What went through your mind?"

- *Reaction phase.* This phase is designed to move the group participants from a predominantly cognitive and intellectual level of processing to a more cathartic, emotional level of processing: "What was the worst part of the incident for you?" Usually, it's at this point that the meeting gets hot, as members take their cue from one another and begin to vent their distress. Clinicians and peer-debriefers keep a keen eye out for any adverse reactions among the personnel.

- *Symptom phase.* This begins the movement back from the predominantly emotional-processing level toward the cognitive-processing level. Participants are asked to describe cognitive, physical, emotional, and behavioral signs and symptoms of distress that appeared (1) at the scene or within 24 hours of the incident, (2) a few days after the incident, and (3) continually, even at the time of the debriefing: "What have you been experiencing since the incident?"

- *Education phase.* Continuing the move back toward intellectual processing, information is exchanged about the nature of the stress response and the expected physiological and psychological reactions to critical incidents. This serves to normalize the stress and coping responses and provides a basis for questions and answers.

- *Reentry phase.* This is a wrap-up, during which any additional questions or statements are addressed, referral for individual follow-ups are made, and general group bonding is reinforced: "What have you learned?" "Is there anything positive that can come out of this experience that can help you grow personally or professionally?" "How can you help one another in the future?" "Anything we left out?"

This is not to suggest that these phases always follow one another in an unvarying, mechanical sequence. On the contrary, in practice I've found that once group participants feel comfortable with the whole process and start talking, the fact, thought, and reaction phases often blend together. Indeed, as Mitchell and Everly (1996) recognize, it would seem artificial and forced to abruptly interrupt someone expressing emotion just because it's not the "right phase." As long as the basic rationale and structure of the debriefing are maintained, the therapeutic effect will result. Indeed, on a number of occasions, previously silent members have spoken up at literally the last moment, when the group was all but getting up to leave. Team leaders typically have to step in only when emotional reactions become particularly intense, or where one or more members begin to blame or criticize others.

SPECIAL APPLICATIONS OF CISD TO LAW ENFORCEMENT.   Police officers tend to be clannish and reluctant to talk to outsiders. They may be more resistant to showing "weakness" in front of their own peers than other emergency personnel. Cops typically work alone or with a single partner, as opposed to firefighters and paramedics, who are trained to have more of a team mentality (Blau, 1994; Kirschman, 1997; Solomon, 1995). This has led to some special adaptations of the CISD approach for law enforcement.

To encourage participation and reduce fear of stigmatization, the administrative policy should strongly and unequivocally state that debriefings and other postincident mental health and peer-support interventions are confidential. The only exceptions to confidentiality are a clear and present danger to self or others and disclosure of a serious crime by the officer. Team members should be instructed to call the department psychologist or the team coordinator, if possible, when confidentiality cannot be honored (Solomon, 1995). Temporary administrative leave or light duty may be appropriate following high-impact situations, such as shootings (Solomon, 1990).

To keep the focus on the event itself and to reduce the singling-out stigmatization of individuals, many mental health and law enforcement professionals recommend that, following a critical incident, there be a policy of mandatory referral of all involved personnel to a debriefing or other appropriate mental health intervention (Horn, 1991; McMains, 1991; Mitchell, 1991; Reese, 1991; Solomon, 1988, 1995).

In cases where only one officer is involved (e.g., a shooting), or to supplement a formal debriefing, Solomon (1995) recommends that individual debriefings be conducted by a mental health professional. In an individual debriefing, the emotional impact of the incident is assessed and explored as thoughts, feelings, and reactions are discussed. An effective format for individual debriefing sessions is to go over the incident "frame by frame," with the officer verbalizing the moment-by-moment thoughts, perceptions, sensory details, feelings, and actions that occurred during the incident. This format helps the officer become aware of, sort out, and understand what happened.

Getting in touch with the perceptions and frame of mind experienced during the incident helps the officer understand why certain actions were taken or specific decisions were made. The frame-by-frame approach helps defuse inappropriate self-blaming by helping the officer to differentiate what was under his control from what was not, and what was known at the time from what was impossible to know then but may appear crystal clear in hindsight.

In cases of an officer-involved shooting, when there is an ongoing or impending investigation, Solomon (1995) recommends that the group debriefing be postponed until the initial investigation has been completed and formal statements have been taken by investigators. Otherwise, debriefing participants may be viewed as witnesses who are subject to questioning about what was said. For particularly sensitive or controversial situations or complicated investigations, it may be advisable not to hold a group debriefing until the investigation has been legally resolved. Individual debriefings can be provided for the involved officer(s) in the meantime, or a group debriefing may proceed with other, noninvolved personnel who may have been affected by the incident, especially where the response team was multidisciplinary (police, firefighters, paramedics, etc.).

In sensitive cases, Solomon (1988, 1995) suggests using a mental health professional who is bound by law to certain rules of confidentiality, rather than a peer, but it should be made clear that clinical confidentiality is not as inviolate as attorney-client privilege and that clinicians and their records may be subpoenaed. As always, a combination of legal protocol, departmental policy, sound clinical judgment, and common sense should guide decisions in sensitive individual cases.

Finally, as a follow-up measure, Solomon (1995) recommends what he terms a *critical incident peer support seminar*, which provides a retreat-like setting for the involved officers to come together for two or three days to revisit their experience several months following the critical incident. The seminar is facilitated by mental health professionals and peer support officers.

Sewell (1993, 1994) has endeavored to adapt a CISD-like stress management model to the particular needs of law enforcement officers, such as detectives who deal with the investigation of multiple murders and other violent crimes. The major objectives of this process are: (1) ventilation of intense emotions; (2) exploration of symbolic meanings; (3) group support under catastrophic conditions; (4) initiation of the grief process within a supportive environment; (5) reduction of the "fallacy of unique-

ness"; (6) reassurance that intense emotions under catastrophic conditions are normal; (7) preparation for the continuation of the grief and
stress process over the ensuing weeks and months; (8) preparing for the
possible development of emotional, cognitive, and physical symptoms
in the aftermath of a serious crisis; (9) education regarding normal and
abnormal stress response syndromes; and (10) encouragement of continued group support and/or professional assistance.

Sewell (1994) regards such interventions as appropriate for two specific
groups and at two specific times. First, the stress of the first responders
who dealt with the trauma of the original scene must be confronted
quickly and decisively. Second, the stress of involved investigators must
be handled regularly and as needed throughout the course of the crime's
investigation and prosecution. In the regular debriefing sessions, whether
for the first responders or case investigators, attendance should be mandatory and must be supported by the administration. Where an officer seeks
additional debriefing assistance, the visits should be administratively
encouraged and nonstigmatized.

The most extensive and comprehensive adaptation of the CISD process for law enforcement to date has been developed by Bohl (1995),
who explicitly compares and contrasts the steps or phases in her program
with the phases of the Mitchell CISD model.

In Bohl's (1995) program, the debriefing takes place as soon after the
critical incident as possible. A debriefing may involve a single officer
within the first 24 hours, later followed by a second, with a group debriefing taking place within one week to encourage bonding. This is to
address the above-noted lower team orientation of most police officers,
who may not express feelings easily even (or especially) in a group of
their fellow officers.

In the Bohl model, there is little meaningful distinction between the
cognitive and emotional phases of a debriefing. If an officer begins to
express emotion during the fact or cognitive phase, there is little point
in telling him to stifle it until later. To be fair, as noted above, the
Mitchell model certainly allows for flexibility and common sense in
structuring debriefings, and both formats recognize the importance of
responding empathically to the needs expressed by the individuals who
attend the debriefing, rather than following a rigid and arbitrary set
of rules.

In the emotion phase itself, what is important in the Bohl model is
not the mere act of venting, but rather the opportunity to validate feelings. Bohl does not ask what the "worst thing" was, since she finds that
the typical response is that "everything about it was the worst thing."
However, it often comes as a revelation to these law enforcement tough

guys that peers have had similar feelings. Nevertheless, some emotions may be difficult to validate. For example, guilt or remorse over actions or inactions may actually be appropriate, as when an officer's momentary hesitation or impulsive action resulted in someone getting hurt or killed. The question then becomes: "Okay, you feel guilty—what are you going to do with that guilt?" That is, "What can be learned from the experience to prevent something like this from happening again?"

The Bohl model inserts an additional phase, the *"unfinished business" phase*, which has no counterpart in the Mitchell model. Participants are asked, "What in the present situation reminds you of a past experience? Do you want to talk about that(those) other situation(s)?" This phase grew out of Bohl's observation that the incident that prompted the current debriefing often acts as a catalyst. Participants are reminded of prior critical incidents, which were probably not followed by formal debriefings. The questions give participants a chance to talk about incidents that may arouse strong and unresolved feelings. Bohl finds that such debriefing results in a greater sense of relief and closure than would otherwise be the case.

The education or teaching phase in the Bohl model resembles its Mitchell model counterpart, in that participants are schooled about normal and abnormal stress reactions, how to deal with coworkers and family members, and what to anticipate in the near future. For example, an officer's child may have heard that his or her parent shot and killed a suspect, and the child may be questioned or teased at school. How to deal with children's responses may therefore be an important part of this education phase.

Unlike the Mitchell model, the Bohl model does not ask whether anything positive, hopeful, or growth-promoting has arisen from the incident. Officers who have seen their partners shot or killed or who have had to deal with child abuse or other senseless brutality may find it difficult to see anything hopeful or positive in the experience, no matter how well they have handled the situation. Expecting them to extract a "growth experience" from such a situation may seem like a sick joke.

A final non-Mitchell phase of the debriefing added by the Bohl model is the *"round robin."* Each officer is invited to say anything that he or she wants. The remark can be addressed to anyone, but others cannot respond directly; this is supposed to give participants a feeling of safety. My own concern is that this may provide an opportunity for last-minute gratuitous sniping, which can chip away at the carefully crafted supportive atmosphere built up during the debriefing. Additionally, in practice, there doesn't seem to be anything particularly unique about this "round robin" phase to distinguish it from the standard reentry phase of the Mitchell model. Finally, adding more and more "phases" to the debriefing process may serve decrease the forthrightness and spontaneity of its implementation. Nevertheless, we should applaud efforts to extend and refine the critical incident debriefing model for individual target groups (see also Chapters 7, 9, and 11), while retaining its generic therapeutic components for all populations in crisis.

CRITIQUES OF CISD.   Despite the enthusiasm for this form of intervention, the CISD approach is not without its detractors, especially when it is used indiscriminately or regarded as the only necessary and sufficient form of intervention. Bisson and Deahl (1994) have reviewed the literature suggesting some of the limitations, pitfalls, and drawbacks of the CISD approach. They note that even Mitchell (1988) acknowledges that not everyone in every critical incident situation will benefit from a debriefing. In some cases, more extensive, individualized interventions may be called for.

In other cases, it's a matter of timing. There is a general consensus that debriefing is most effective if carried out sooner rather than later (Bordow & Porritt, 1979); in fact, my own clinical experience supports holding debriefing sessions toward the earlier end of the recommended 24-to-72-hour window. Working with Israeli soldiers suffering combat stress during the Lebanon war, Solomon and Benbenishty (1988) found that while early, brief intervention did not entirely eliminate posttraumatic stress reactions, it helped to reduce their intensity and duration.

There may be some negative side-effects of inappropriate CISD. In the Australian bushfire study, McFarlane (1988) found that while firefighters who received CISD shortly after the incident were less likely to develop acute posttraumatic stress reactions than nondebriefed workers, they were more likely to develop delayed PTSD. McFarlane (1989) expressed concern that overreliance on quick-fix, primary prevention methods might delay the diagnosis and effective treatment of workers who suffer more serious psychological sequelae and require more extensive follow-up interventions.

Griffiths and Watts (1992) examined relationships between stress debriefing and stress symptoms in 288 emergency personnel involved in rescue efforts at bus crashes. They found that those who attended debriefings had significantly higher levels of PTSD symptoms 12 months later than those who were not debriefed. Furthermore, there was no relationship between the perceived helpfulness of the debriefing and the symptoms. However, rescuers who experienced greater distress at the time of the crash were likely to have attended more debriefing sessions and to have perceived those sessions as more helpful.

Kenardy, Webster, Lewin, Carr, Hazell, & Carter (1996) studied the effect of stress debriefing on the recovery rate of 195 emergency service personnel and disaster workers following an earthquake in Newcastle, Australia. They found no evidence of an improved recovery rate among those helpers who were debriefed, even when levels of exposure and helping-related stress were taken into account.

Empirical studies are one thing, but recently the debate over CISD services has begun to turn personal. Some critics have accused CISD of having assumed cult-like status, with Jeff Mitchell being a shady operator and self-promoter, cashing in on what amounts to nothing more than a slick repackaging of the informal types of peer support that emergency workers have always used. Somewhat more high-toned are critiques that cite the frequent overuse of CISD, diluting both its effectiveness and its credibility, and asserting that there is no "objective" evidence of its efficacy.

Mitchell and Everly (1996, 1997) have responded to these critiques by (1) noting that many critical studies of CISD fail to use the true "Mitchell model"; (2) pointing out that the overuse or misuse of any technique doesn't mean that it's not effective when used properly; and (3) counterciting empirical studies supporting the efficacy of Mitchell-model CISD.

For example, Robinson and Mitchell (1993) conducted an exploratory, descriptive study of 172 emergency service, welfare, and hospital personnel who took part in 31 debriefings. Emergency service workers rated the debriefing as having considerable personal value. Most participants who experienced stress at the time of the incident attributed a reduction in stress symptoms, at least in part, to the debriefing. Similarly, Wee (1996) found that CISD significantly reduced stress symptoms in emergency services personnel operating during the 1992 Los Angeles riots.

Mitchell and Everly (1997) have called for an end to the "study wars" trying to demonstrate that CISD does or doesn't work, but I think empirical studies *should* continue to examine what types of CISD-type interventions work best with which populations under what circumstances. As is the case with any wholesale application of a promising psychological treatment modality, further research and clinical experience are likely to narrow and refine the appropriate therapeutic applications and identify certain limitations and even potentially harmful side-effects. This has been the case, for example, with cognitive rehabilitation (Hall & Cope, 1995; Miller, 1992), relaxation training (Lazarus & Mayne, 1990), biofeedback (Silver & Blanchard, 1978), EMDR (Allen &

Lewis, 1996; Shapiro, 1995), and various behavioral medicine modalities (Miller, 1994).

Excessive mandatory CISD can lead to passive participation and resentment among workers (Bisson & Deahl, 1994; Flannery, Fulton, & Tausch, 1991), and the CISD process may quickly become a boring routine if used indiscriminately after every incident, no matter how "critical." The danger here is that the therapeutic impact and credibility of CISD may then become diluted and fragmented, reducing its potential effectiveness in those situations where it really might have helped.

Overall, whether considering the strictly kosher Mitchell model or some variant thereof, there now exists substantial clinical, empirical, and anecdotal support to document the efficacy of CISD-type interventions in a wide variety of crisis situations and settings, from law enforcement to emergency rescue, school crises, disaster relief, workplace violence, and civilian crime victimization. I have personally utilized CISD-style approaches in these situations, and many of these topics are discussed throughout this book (see Chapters 7, 8, 9, and 11). For the most part, I find the overall CISD approach to be a valuable clinical tool in both preventive and responsive trauma therapy. Jeff Mitchell projects an impressive personal and professional commitment to CISD, and the attempt by detractors to dismiss the whole CISD approach as a shallow fad strikes me as ignorant and meanspirited.

While many law enforcement and emergency services critical incidents will not require any special intervention, and while the majority of those that do will be well served by a CISD approach, it is the responsibility of departmental administrators and the mental health professionals who advise them to ensure that debriefing modalities are used responsibly and that other forms of clinically appropriate psychotherapeutic intervention are available for those who need them.

Individual Psychotherapy

Crisis personnel, cops especially, have a reputation for shunning mental health services, often repudiating mental health practitioners as softies and bleeding hearts who help criminal dirtbags go free with overcomplicated psychobabble excuses. Other crisis personnel fear being "shrunk," having a Hollywood-type view of the psychotherapy experience as akin to brainwashing, a humiliating, infantilizing experience in which they lie on a couch and sob about their toilet training. More commonly, the idea of needing "mental help" implies weakness, cowardice, and lack of ability to do the job. In the environment of many departments, some workers realistically fear censure, stigmatization, ridicule, impaired career advancement, and alienation from coworkers if they are perceived as the type who "folds under pressure." Finally, others in the department who have something to hide may fear a colleague "spilling his guts" to the psychotherapist and blowing the malfeasor's cover.

ADMINISTRATIVE ISSUES.   There is some debate about whether psychological services, especially therapy services, should be provided by a psychotherapist within the department, even a psychologist who is a sworn officer or active-duty emergency services worker, or whether such matters are best handled by outside therapists who are less answerable to departmental politics and less likely to be in the gossip loop (Blau, 1994; Silva, 1991). A similar issue is faced by mental health clinicians who serve corporations (see Chapter 9) and also by clergy who serve the emergency services professions.

On the one hand, the departmental psychologist is likely to have more knowledge of and experience with the direct pressures faced by the personnel he serves; this is especially true if the psychologist is also a sworn officer or active-duty worker or has had formal training and ride-along experience. On the other hand, in addition to providing psychotherapy services, the departmental psychologist is likely to be involved in performing work-status and fitness-for-duty evaluations, as well as other assessment or legal tasks that may conflict with being an impartial psychotherapist. An outside therapist may have less direct experience with departmental roles and pressures but more therapeutic freedom of movement.

My own experience has been that the crisis workers who come for help—especially when they haven't been "forced" into treatment—are usually less concerned with the therapist's extensive technical knowledge of their job than with his demonstration of basic trust and a willingness to take the time and effort to understand the essential details of the worker's situation. They expect us mental health professionals to give "110 percent" in our own fields, just as they do in theirs. For the most part they don't want us to be another cop or firefighter; they want us to be skilled therapists—that's why they're talking to us and not their colleagues. Many are actually glad to find a haven outside the fishbowl atmosphere of the department and relieved that the therapeutic sessions provide a respite from shop talk. This is especially true where the referral problem has to do less with direct job-related issues than with outside pressures, such as family or alcohol problems that may secondarily impinge on job performance. Nevertheless, the therapist should have some basic understanding of the professional world in which the crisis worker operates.

Important referral issues relate to confidentiality and chain of command. Technically, the jurisdictional rules of confidentiality, privilege, and duty-to-warn apply to law enforcement and emergency services personnel just as they do to any other psychotherapy patient. Since "ground rules" and role boundaries are paramount issues with this group, it is important that the patient understand from the beginning the rules and protocols in the therapist's jurisdiction.

An additional issue for law enforcement and emergency services personnel is the knowledge of and/or attitude toward their treatment on the part of command staff and coworkers. Therapists often must be clear and firm with commanders and supervisors regarding what information is relevant to the patient's job role and work performance and what will remain confidential. In some cases, the therapeutic referral is concluded by a written summary that relates to fitness-for-duty or other job rating or qualification. It is crucial that the therapist phrase any such report in a way that honestly and succinctly presents his conclusions as they pertain to the job-fitness question, while not violating trust and confidentiality about the specific content of sessions. Admittedly, this is sometimes a delicate dance and may be one of the most challenging aspects of clinical work with this group (Blau, 1994; Silva, 1991).

TRUST AND THE THERAPEUTIC RELATIONSHIP.   As should be clear by this point, trust is a crucial element in doing effective psychotherapy with police officers (Silva, 1991), a lesson that can be applied to clinical work with all emergency services personnel. Difficulty with trust appears to be an occupational hazard for workers in public safety, who generally have a strong sense of self-sufficiency and insistence on solving their own problems. Therapists who work with crisis personnel may at first need to put up with a lot of testing on the part of their clientele: "Why are you doing this?" "What's in it for you?" "Who's going to get this information?" Workers may expose the therapist to mocking cynicism and criticism about the job, baiting the therapist to agree, and thereby hoping to expose the therapist's prejudices about the law enforcement and emergency services professions.

The development of trust during the establishment of the therapeutic alliance depends upon the therapist's skill in interpreting the patient's statements, thoughts, feelings, reactions, and nonverbal behavior. In the best case, the patient begins to feel at ease with therapist and finds comfort and a sense of predictability from the psychotherapy session. Silva (1991) outlines the following guidelines for the establishment of therapeutic mutual trust:

- *Accurate empathy*. The therapist conveys his understanding of the patient's background and experience (but beware of premature false familiarity and phony "bonding").
- *Genuineness*. The therapist is spontaneous yet tactful, flexible and creative, and communicates as directly and nondefensively as possible.
- *Availability*. The therapist is available, within reason, whenever needed and avoids making promises and commitments he cannot keep.
- *Respect*. The therapist is both tough-minded and gracious, and seeks to preserve the patient's sense of autonomy, control, and self-respect within the therapeutic relationship. Respect is shown by the therapist's overall attitude, language, and behavior, such as indicating regard for rank or job role by initially using formal departmental forms of address, such as "officer," "detective," "lieutenant," until trust and mutual respect allow the patient to ease formality. Here it is important to avoid the dual traps of overfamiliarity, patronizing, and talking down to the officer, on the one hand, and trying to "play cop" or force bogus camaraderie by assuming the role of a colleague or field commander, on the other.
- *Concreteness*. Whether performing a rescue or conducting an investigation, these workers are into action and results, and to the extent that it is clinically realistic, the therapeutic approach should emphasize active, goal-oriented, and problem-solving approaches (Silva, 1991).

THERAPEUTIC STRATEGIES AND TECHNIQUES.   Most law enforcement and emergency services personnel come under psychotherapeutic care in the context of some form of posttraumatic stress reaction (Blau, 1994; Fullerton et al., 1992). In general, the effectiveness of any intervention technique will be determined by the timeliness, tone, style, and intent of the intervention. Effective therapy with this group is brief, focuses on specific symptomatology or conflict issues, and involves direct operational efforts to resolve the conflict or to reach a satisfactory conclusion.

Blau (1994) recommends that the first meeting between the therapist and a police officer establish a safe and comfortable working atmosphere by the therapist's articulating: (1) a postitive regard for the officer's decision to seek help; (2) a clear description of the therapist's responsibilities and limitations with respect to confidentiality and privilege; and (3) an invitation to the officer to state his concerns. A straightforward, goal-directed, problem-solving approach for this patient group includes: (1) creating a sanctuary; (2) focusing on critical areas of concern; (3) identifying desired outcomes; (4) reviewing assets; (5) developing a general plan; (6) identifying practical initial implementations; (7) reviewing self-efficacy; and (8) setting appointments for review, reassurance, and further implementation.

Blau (1994) delineates a number of effective individual intervention strategies for police officers, which I have found adaptable to therapeutic work with most tough-job personnel. These include the following:

- *Attentive listening.* This includes good eye contact, an occasional nod, and genuine interest, without inappropriate comments or interruptions.
- *Being there with empathy.* This therapeutic attitude conveys availability, concern, and awareness of the turbulent emotions being experienced by the traumatized worker. It is also helpful to let the patient know, in a nonalarming manner, what he is likely to experience in the days and weeks ahead.
- *Reassurance.* This is valuable as long as it is reality-oriented. It should take the form of reassuring the patient that routine matters will be handled, premises and property will be secured, deferred responsibilities will be handled by others, and that organizational and command support will be provided.
- *Supportive counseling.* This includes effective listening, restatement of content, clarification of feelings, and reassurance, as well as community referral and networking with liaison agencies, as necessary.
- *Interpretive counseling.* This type of intervention should be used when the patient's emotional reaction is significantly greater than the circumstances of the critical incident seem to warrant. In appropriate cases, this therapeutic strategy can stimulate the patient to search for underlying emotional stresses that intensify a traumatic event. In some cases, this may lead to ongoing psychotherapy (Blau, 1994).

Not to be neglected is the use of humor. While humor has a place in many forms of psychotherapy (Fry & Salameh, 1987), it may be especially useful in working with law enforcement and emergency services personnel (Fullerton et al., 1992; Silva, 1991). In general, if the therapist and patient can laugh together, this may lead to the sharing of more intimate feelings. Humor serves to bring a sense of balance and proportion to a traumatically warped and twisted world. "Show me a man who knows what's funny," Mark Twain said, "and I'll show you a man who knows what's not."

Humor, even sarcastic or gross humor, may allow the venting of anger, frustration, and resentment and lead to constructive therapeutic work, as long as the therapist is able to keep a lid on destructive forms of self-mockery or inappropriate projective hostility in the form of sleazy, cynical, or meanspirited wisecracking. Also, remember that many traumatized patients may be quite "concrete" and suspicious at the outset of therapy, and so the constructive therapeutic use of humor may have to await the formation of a therapeutic relationship that allows some cognitive and emotional latitude.

Organizational and Departmental Responses

Following a department-wide critical incident, such as the death of a worker or a particularly stressful rescue event, the mental health consultant can advise and guide law enforcement and emergency service departments in encouraging and implementing several organizational response measures, gleaned from the available literature on individual and group coping strategies (Alexander, 1993; Alexander & Walker, 1994; Alexander & Wells, 1991; DeAngelis, 1995; Fullerton et al, 1992; Palmer, 1983; Ursano & Fullerton, 1990). Many of the following measures are applicable proactively, that is, as part of training before a disaster or critical incident occurs.

- Encourage mutual support among peers and supervisors. Peers commonly support one another, while supervisors may need some explicit encouragement to do so. Public safety workers often work as "partners" and find that shared decision-making and mutual reassurance actually enhance effective job performance.
- Utilize humor as a coping mechanism to facilitate emotional insulation, which forestalls excessive identification with victims, and group bonding, which encourages mutual group support via a shared language. Of course, as noted above, the line between adaptive gallows humor and maladaptive gratuitous nastiness should be monitored.
- Make use of appropriate rituals to give meaning and dignity to an otherwise existentially disorienting and overwhelming experience. This may include not only religious rites related to mourning, but also such things as a military-style honor guard to attend bodies before disposition and the formal acknowledgment of actions above and beyond the call of duty. Important here is the role of "grief leadership," i.e., the supervisor's or commanding officer's demonstrating by example that it's okay to grieve and mourn the death of fallen comrades or civilians with dignity and decorum, and that the appropriate, respectful expression of one's feelings about the incident will be supported, not denigrated.

Of equal importance is adequate training prior to a disaster or emergency, which is in itself an expression of organizational commitment (Fullerton et al., 1992). Emergency workers find that recall of training is important for keeping on task during a disaster or emergency event, performing successfully, and feeling active and in control during rescue work. When the ability to "go on automatic" and zero in on the technical aspects of the job is impaired, rescue workers are likely to feel isolated, guilty over poor performance, out of control, and victimized during and after a disaster. Training for disaster rescue work should include methods for maintaining communication, interaction, and involvement with co-workers and other social support networks. In addition, training should include improved interaction with the public, especially for law enforcement personnel, as this can serve the dual purpose of reducing officer stress and enhancing overall public relations (Cooper, 1997).

SIGNIFICANT OTHERS: FAMILY STRESSES AND FAMILY THERAPY

Considering the stresses and challenges of law enforcement and emergency services work, it may seem surprising that the marriages and family lives of these professionals do not differ dramatically from those of workers in other fields. However, there are a number of pressures and problems that are endemic to those who work in the fields of emergency services and public safety, and these must be addressed.

Family Stresses Among Crisis Personnel

Many of the marital stresses and strains experienced by police officers have been described by Blau (1994), Borum and Philpot (1993), and Kirschman (1997); their observations may be applied more generally to most crisis intervention and public safety professions.

Typically, the demands of the job and loyalties to the department compete with the marriage for time and commitment, as a crisis worker rarely keeps a steady 9-to-5 schedule; indeed, routine 72-hour shifts and 24-hour on-call status are common in many of these professions. Stereotypical "tough guy," macho values and attitudes— among both men and women—pervade the law enforcement and emergency services community. These include such behavioral and character traits as control, dominance, authority, and lack of sentimentality—traits that naturally conflict with the more cooperative, emotionally expressive, and relationship-oriented attitudes generally considered important in marriage.

Over 75 percent of spouses of police officers report stress from their mates' jobs. The most common cop referrals received by psychologists have to do with dissatisfaction between husband and wife regarding the work situation, finances, children, and unfulfilled promises. To mates, the crisis worker's job demands seem unfair, regardless of his rank, age, sex, or assignment. Children, especially adolescents, are often caught between feelings of loyalty and pride in their parent's work role and anxieties about peer rejection because of common pejorative attitudes toward "authority figures" such as police and other public safety personnel. Actually, this is a general problem for children of parents in any of the helping or service professions—the dilemma of the "cop's kid," "shrink's kid," or "preacher's kid."

On the job, public safety workers must maintain a keen sense of alertness, vigilance, and mental preparedness. For law enforcement, this includes an occupationally reinforced suspiciousness and general distrust of people's motives, statements, and actions. Carried over into the home, this back-to-the-wall, question-everything attitude often seems paranoid. The occupational cynicism heightens the spouse's feeling of being a perennial suspect under investigation ("Don't you ever trust me?") and puts a general damper on feelings of intimacy, as the officer "never lets down his guard." In extreme cases, pent-up anger and frustration from the job may spill over into verbal abuse or physical violence at home. The spouse may be reluctant to report the violence because of feared termination or censure of the officer by the department or because she concludes that "they'll all be on his side, anyway."

Law enforcement and emergency services systems facilitate departmental solidarity and boundary formation. Typically, the spouse feels excluded, often leading to jealousy as the worker seems to be more involved with the department than with his family. A vicious cycle may develop as the spouse's resentment further alienates the worker, who then spends even more time on the job or away from home, creating a higher risk for the development of extramarital affairs and substance abuse problems.

Many crisis workers well-meaningly try to create a "protective bubble" (Reese, 1987) around their families to shield them from the unsavory and distressing aspects of their work, as well as to make their home a separate haven from the pressures of the job. Thus, a worker may turn to his spouse for support during a particularly stressful time, then virtually the next moment clam up and refuse to discuss anything about the job. The resulting emotional roller-coaster takes its toll on the spouse and on the marriage (Alexander & Walker, 1994). A related problem is wider social isolation, as the worker's missed social engagements and immersion in the job drive friends away from the couple, making the spouse feel even more alone, and abetting the temptation toward dalliances of desperation on the other side of the relationship.

Occasionally, both partners work in law enforcement or emergency services, sometimes in the same department; perhaps that's where they met. An advantage of this arrangement is that each partner is able to truly understand the problems, pressures, and perspectives of the other; even if one is a cop and the other a paramedic or firefighter, many of the stresses are similar. In such cases, the carryover of the us-versus-them attitude from the department to the marriage may have a positive effect on connubial cohesion.

A disadvantage is the potential blurring of personal and professional roles, especially where one spouse holds a different rank in the same department. A related problem occurs where the spouse's role as protector interferes with his or her objectivity in perceiving the spouse as a work partner. However, even the most obtuse commander will usually have enough sense not to pair spouses as partners or shiftmates. Finally, in the fishbowl atmosphere of most departments, a married couple may be subject to meddling and harassment—some good-natured, some not—by coworkers (Blau, 1994; Borum & Philpot, 1993).

Family Therapy

Borum and Philpot (1993) have described a number of effective marital therapy goals and strategies with police couples, which may be applied to most public safety personnel. Goals include: (1) strengthening the boundary around the couple, relative to the departmental boundary; (2) reducing divided loyalties, triangulation, and jealousies between the job and the marriage; and (3) increasing intimacy and bonding between the couple. Therapeutic strategies to accomplish this include the following:

- Use the us-versus-them mentality as a metaphor for the police officer or emergency service worker to begin to understand the need to create an equivalent us/them atmosphere for the marital dyad. The goal of this should be inclusion and solidarity, not paranoia and isolation.
- Help the couple develop ways to create more time for each other. This may involve explicitly scheduling times for communication about non-job-related or generally non-problem matters. Assign "car-

ing days" homework, i.e., lists of nice things to do for each other. If practical, have the couple plan a "secret vacation" together, a romantic holiday that they reveal to only a few select people.

- Help the spouses gain insight into divided loyalties and triangulation and teach them to deal effectively with one another, instead of communicating with and through third parties. Teach them how to identify and appropriately express emotion to one another. Teach problem-solving, negotiation, and conflict-containment skills. Help the spouses expand their social world beyond the department and immediate families. It may also be useful to teach them to cognitively and emotionally compartmentalize in an adaptive way, so that they can turn on their "feeling channel" at home and turn it off at work. Many workers do this naturally.

- Identify, emphasize, and mobilize strengths that have thus far kept the marriage together. Have the spouses describe their early dating days, what attracted them to each other, old love letters, shared good times, private jokes, "our song," and so on. Ironically, the same characteristics that originally attracted the lovers to one another often become polarized and are now a source of friction. For example, the very logical, emotionally stilted police officer may have originally been attracted to his wife because of her open affection and warmth, which made it easier for him to get in touch with his own feelings. Now, as she looks to him for emotional nurturance, he becomes intimidated, turning into a superrational computeroid to "balance out" her emotionality. The therapist may use reframes to place the behavior of both spouses in a positive light (Borum & Philpot, 1993).

My only qualification regarding such approaches is that they be applied in the context of the therapist's thorough understanding of the couple's problems, within a trusting therapeutic relationship, and on the basis of a solid grounding in couples and family therapy strategies (Weeks & Treat, 1992)—not used as "therapy tricks" or cookbook-like, quick-fix "techniques," which may serve only to further alienate the couple from the therapy process.

The Ultimate Sacrifice: Police Spouse Survivors

When an officer is killed in the line of duty, his or her family must struggle on, and individual and family therapists have a crucial role to play in easing the pain of this very special form of bereavement.

Interaction within a cohesive group—a social network of trusted, close persons with similar characteristics, lifestyles, and attitudes—may decrease psychological discomfort resulting from the traumatic death of a loved one. Collegial and other social support facilitates trauma resolution in law enforcement and emergency service families by providing a "trauma membrane" that serves to protect them from further distress (Green, 1993; Lindy, Grace, & Green, 1981; Tyler & Gifford, 1991).

Despite the fact that police officers consistently rate the death of an officer as the most distressing event in their work (Violanti & Aron, 1994), there has been little research on the effects of line-of-duty deaths on surviving police spouses—even less, I might add, on the families of fallen firefighters and other rescuers. What previous studies exist have noted weight loss, sleep disturbances, apathy, depression, and suicidal thoughts in police widows (Danto, 1975). Lack of understanding by those outside the police profession contributes to problems experienced by surviving spouses of slain police officers (Niederhoffer & Niederhoffer, 1978). In another study (Stillman, 1987), over half of police spouse survivors met clinical criteria for PTSD and demonstrated heightened levels of depression, anxiety, hostility, and guilt. Such bereavements may be all the more stressful because of their high visibility and media scrutiny.

Police agencies have been criticized for abandoning the bereaved spouse after a line-of-duty death by failing to provide follow-up support services (Sawyer, 1988; Stillman, 1987). Officers and their wives may dislike interacting with the widow of a slain officer because it reminds them of their own vulnerability and mortality.

Violanti (1996) examined the impact of social interactions on the surviving spouse's psychological distress. The results provided modest evidence that police widows who participated in department-endorsed mutual support groups experienced lower levels of psychological distress and trauma symptomatology. Close police groups provided more meaningful support than outsiders (media, criminal justice system) to the widows and were more effective in reducing distress.

Psychotherapists can encourage the sharing of grief responses with others who have walked in the same shoes, as an adjunct to more formal psychotherapeutic grief work (Sprang & McNeil, 1995). Recently, a number of law enforcement family self-help support groups, such as *Concerns of Police Survivors (C.O.P.S.)* and others, have begun to spring up; survivors should be urged to consult their local directories (see Kirschman, 1997). Hopefully, this mutual support movement will spread to the families of other emergency services personnel.

In addition, therapists may play a more active clinical role in helping families cope with the loss of their fallen spouse and parent, using many of the techniques appropriate for traumatic bereavement in general (Sprang & McNeil, 1995; see also Chapters 2 and 8), such as (1) permitting appropriate venting; (2) helping the family identify physical and psychological symptoms of distress; (3) education about, and normalization of, the grief response process; (4) restoration of some control; (5) provision of basic psychological support; (6) reduction of self-blame; (7) training in physiological arousal regulation and symptom control; (8) fostering mastery over the trauma and integration of the traumatic experience; (9) dealing with inhibited awareness, arousal, or emotional expression; (10) restructuring family roles; (11) planning for the future; and (12) helping the family to "say goodbye" to the fallen family member. As in the case of crime victims (see Chapter 8), therapists may also play an important role in helping bereaved family members handle the stresses and challenges of the media and legal system.

Psychotherapy with law enforcement and emergency service personnel can be both doggedly challenging and supremely rewarding. In the best cases, the therapist will have the satisfaction of knowing that he or she has helped restore the productive career of a highly trained public servant who will go on to rescue and help untold numbers of people. Clinical work with these "tough guys" takes skill, dedication, and sometimes a strong stomach, but for therapists who are prepared to tough it out themselves this can be a fascinating and fulfilling area of clinical practice.

Chapter 11

HITTING HOME

Traumatized Psychotherapists and
the Stresses of Doing Therapy

All interest in disease and death is only another
expression of interest in life.

—Thomas Mann

Doing trauma psychotherapy is not for wimps; it's tough, grimy, demanding work that can take an exhausting toll on practitioners. Indeed, the issue of *compassion fatigue*—a special species of clinical burnout—is only now beginning to be addressed by our colleagues.

As if exhaustion and burnout weren't enough, psychotherapy can be a dangerous profession, especially when caseloads include severely disturbed, potentially violent patients, usually seen in institutional psychiatric and forensic settings but increasingly turning up in routine clinical practice. Therapists and other health care professionals are frequently assaulted, some are seriously injured, and a few of our colleagues have been killed.

In some cases, this direct traumatization occurs at the hands of the very patients we have worn ourselves out trying to help; it becomes the professional "last straw" that may propel us out of the field altogether. Such catastrophes force the most extreme stretches of the helping role and, as therapists, we owe it to ourselves and those we serve to get the best practical and moral support we can. This chapter discusses how.

THE STRESSES OF HELPING:
EFFECTS OF TRAUMA THERAPY ON
THE THERAPIST

Vulnerability of Trauma Therapists to Work Stress

The traumatic experiences and reactions of patients can "rub off" on therapists. For example, therapists who work with crime victims often begin to feel overly concerned about their own safety and seek greater security measures. Some authorities believe that the most effective therapists are also the most vulnerable to this "mirroring" or contagion effect, in that those who have enormous capacity for feeling and expressing empathy tend to be most at risk for compassion fatigue (Figley, 1995). However, I don't think heightened vulnerability to burnout is a necessary correlate of therapeutic empathy and skill. On the contrary, therapists who have the greatest degree of true empathy, autonomy, and personal resilience often make the most skilled helpers (Miller, 1993).

Nevertheless, therapists who work with traumatized patients on a regular basis may be subject to special stresses (Figley, 1995). Trauma workers are regularly surrounded by the extreme intensity of trauma-inducing events and their aftermaths. No matter how hard we try to resist it and how mature and resilient we may be, trauma workers are inevitably drawn into this vortex of emotional intensity.

Figley (1995) identifies several reasons why trauma therapists are especially vulnerable to compassion fatigue. First, empathy is a major resource for trauma workers to help the traumatized. While the process of empathizing with the trauma victim and family members helps us to understand their experience, in the process we may be traumatized ourselves. Second, many trauma therapists have experienced some traumatic event in their lives and this unresolved trauma may be activated by reports of similar traumas in patients. There is thus a danger of the trauma worker's overgeneralizing from her own experiences and methods of coping and overpromoting those methods with patients. Finally, special stresses are attendant to working with traumatized children.

The therapist's growing reputation as a "trauma specialist" commonly leads to greater and greater numbers of trauma referrals. As the cases mount, so does the therapist's growing burnout and compassion fatigue. The therapist may begin to lose her objectivity, overidentify with patients, and become depressed. The effects may spill over into the therapist's family, as she becomes more withdrawn and emotionally unavailable (Cerney, 1995). Other therapists may become "trauma junkies," increasingly reinforced by the lurid thrill of working with such dramatic cases (Yassen, 1995).

McCann and Pearlman (1990) coined the term *vicarious traumatization* to describe the transformation that occurs within the trauma therapist as the result of empathic engagement with patients' trauma experiences and their sequelae. These effects do not arise solely from one therapy relationship, but are cumulative across time and number of helping relationships. Research (Elliott & Guy, 1993; Follette, Polusny, & Milbeck, 1994) suggests that qualities of the therapist, such as age, sex, personal trauma history, and current personal stress, may interact with exposure to patient trauma material to contribute to trauma-related symptoms in the therapist.

Pearlman and Mac Ian (1995) examined vicarious traumatization in 188 self-identified trauma therapists. They found that, while most therapists generally function well, a subset experience significant psychological disturbance as a consequence of their work. The affected therapists tend to have a personal trauma history, to have been doing trauma work for a longer period of time, and to have larger numbers of traumatized patients in their caseloads.

The *burnout* literature (Ackerly, Burnell, Holder, & Kurdek, 1988; Deutsch, 1984; Gilliland & James, 1993; Rodolfa, Kraft, & Reilly, 1988) suggests that being younger or newer to trauma work is associated with the highest levels of burnout. In Pearlman and Mac Ian's (1995) study, the newest therapists in the personal trauma history group were experiencing the most difficulties. Unfortunately, these appeared to be the therapists who were receiving the least amount of supervision and were working in relatively high-stress hospital settings.

Some psychotherapists specialize in crisis intervention as well as trauma therapy; that is, they provide acute intervention to traumatized individuals, for example, crime victims (Gilliland & James, 1993). Talbot, Dutton, and Dunn (1995) describe some of the distinctive features that make trauma crisis work stressful for psychotherapists.

Typically, there is the urgency and immediacy of the response. The crisis response is usually of an outreach nature, which means that the therapist has no control over many aspects of the situation—when it happens, what the environment will be like, who will be there, and what services will be required in each instance. Often, there is no advance notice of such sudden events, little time to prepare, limited time for individual interventions, lack of space, and unfamiliar surroundings.

In a crisis, therapists need to be able to work speedily and effectively to stabilize the situation. The sheer volume of the work, both in terms of the number of people requiring attention in any one crisis and numerous successive crises, can have a debilitating effect. In addition, emotional intensity is high and victims are often in a regressed and decompensated state. Victims may perceive therapeutic interventions as intrusive and become hostile. Therapists accustomed to structured therapeutic interactions may find themselves feeling powerless when confronted by trauma victims whose needs are largely for basic empathy and containment. Often there is nothing to do but listen, and even this may be an extremely difficult task. Also, there is typically little or no history regarding the precrisis or premorbid functioning of the victims. The crisis often occurs within an organizational context, e.g., the criminal justice system, that makes particular demands on responders. The organization's expectations of the therapist are often high yet poorly defined, and these expectations may be in conflict with those of the victim or the therapist.

The stresses of crisis intervention can affect psychotherapists in a number of ways. In the aftermath of their interventions with victims of armed holdups, Talbot et al. (1995) often find themselves feeling isolated, angry, tense, confused, powerless, hopeless, anxious, emotionally exhausted, and overwhelmed with responsibility. Patients' problems seem alternately insurmountable or insignificant, and the therapists may begin to lose perspective and overidentify with them. Therapists may intellectualize, becoming overly rigid and inflexible in their thinking. Using denial as a protective strategy, therapists are often unaware of the way in which the work has affected them, and the recollection among different emergencies becomes blurred.

These therapists often feel exhausted, increase their alcohol use, suffer somatic symptoms such as headaches, gastrointestinal complaints, and sleep disturbances with nightmares, experience increased sensitivity to violence in general, and become emotionally demanding of family and friends. They become increasingly tense and distractible, expecting the phone to ring at any moment announcing yet another holdup or other emergency. They are suspicious and fearful on entering banks as customers. Indeed, I have experienced this latter reaction—thankfully temporary—following a number of bank holdup debriefings.

Effective Trauma Therapists: Qualities and Motivations

Therapists who are especially effective in their work with traumatized patients appear to possess a number of distinguishing characteristics, including: (1) more insight into their own feelings; (2) a greater capacity for empathy and understanding of their patients' emotional experience; (3) better ability to differentiate between the needs of self and patient;

(4) less overall anxiety with patients; and (5) greater skill at conceptualizing patient dynamics in both the patients' current and past contexts (Hayes, Gelso, Van Wagoner, & Diemer, 1991; Van Wagoner, Gelso, Hayes, & Diemer, 1991).

Those trauma therapists who are exposed to enormous emotional contagion and yet experience very little compassion fatigue and maintain considerable empathic ability and concern are able to avoid overidentifying with their patients and thus achieve a sense of satisfaction in helping the patients work through their traumas and easing their suffering (Figley, 1995).

Pearlman and Mac Ian (1995) found that more experienced therapists, who are often trauma survivors themselves, show less disrupted schemas and significantly less general distress than less experienced therapists. This may be due to self-selection, with less skilled and more distress-prone therapists leaving the field early. Or it may be that, as experience and competence develop, adverse stress reactions become fewer and less intense. More competent therapists are more likely to avail themselves of increased continuing education, training, and supervision. Also, perhaps by contributing to another person's healing and growth, trauma therapists additionally contribute to their own personal development. Some survivor therapists who enter this field in order to find meaning in their own traumas may actually accomplish this goal through their work, while others experience only unsatisfying retraumatization and leave the field early.

Transference and Countertransference

Therapeutic interactions with traumatized patients are by no means always appreciated or accepted, especially at the beginning of treatment. Well-intentioned therapists may be surprised to encounter patients' transferential perceptions of them as sadistic persecutors and torturers. In a countertransferential twist, therapists may experience disgust, revulsion, despair, terror, and helplessness as they now become the victims and their patients assume the roles of tormenters and persecutors, causing therapists to feel all the more inadequate and inept. In other cases, countertransference feelings can lead the therapist, under the guise of giving comfort, to repeat the trauma of the previous experience (Cerney, 1995). For example, the therapist may find herself taking an overly rigid or punitive stance or tone with certain patients.

Countertransference issues are of particular importance in crisis intervention because they tend to revolve about frightening aspects of one's life that are often unconscious and difficult to deal with, such as fears of violence, abandonment, death, helplessness, degradation, and maiming. Many traumatized patients are in such pain, and are so skilled at communicating it that therapists may accede in good faith to patients' inappropriate requests. In fact, what these patients are often really searching for is someone who can maintain appropriate boundaries and thereby prove that they, the patients, are not the perpetrators, and so are not responsible for their abuse, as they may have inferred or deliberately been led to believe (Cerney, 1995).

Cerney (1995) has delineated some of the transferential situations encountered in trauma therapy. In *projective identification*, the patient experiences feelings of being persecuted by the therapist. When these persecutory feelings become unbearable, the patient tends to project them outward, often with such intensity that the therapist internalizes the feelings to the point of identifying with them, and then acts accordingly, like a persecutor, even though that is not her usual style. The therapist may become rude, insulting, and cruel to the patient, often aware of this reaction, but bewilderingly unable to change it. Both parties suffer: the patient again undergoes the trauma of being victimized, and the therapist's self-perception of being a kind, understanding professional may be severely damaged (Catherall, 1991; Cerney, 1995).

Therapists may overidentify with the patient's pain, rage, and desire for revenge, especially when the therapist comes from a similar developmental, sociocultural, or experiential background as the patient. This therapist reaction may serve to intensify the patient's feelings rather than helping her to work through and beyond them, which is necessary for trauma resolution. On the other hand, if the patient comes from a different background, the therapist may tend to minimize, negate, or invalidate aspects of the patient's experience (Cerney, 1995).

The affront to the sense of self experienced by therapists of trauma victims can be so overwhelming that, despite their best efforts, therapists begin to exhibit the same characteristics as their patients. That is, they experience a change in their interactions with the world, themselves, and their families. They may begin to have intrusive thoughts, nightmares, and generalized anxiety. At this point, therapists themselves clearly need supervision and assistance in coping with their trauma (Cerney, 1995).

Therapists must remain vigilant for other specific patterns of transferential and countertransferential traumatic engagement that may work themselves out in the therapeutic process (Munroe, Shay, Fisher, Makary, Rapperport, & Zimering, 1995). One pattern is *exploiter/exploited*, in which the therapist is accused of being "just like all the others" who are abusing the patient or who have done so in the past. Variations of this pattern include the therapist "only being in it for the money," the patient being a "guinea pig," or the therapist "getting off on my suffering."

A second pattern is *allies/enemies*, most often observed in combat veterans; I've also encountered this pattern in police officers and in injured workers involved in legal or insurance claims against their employer. Here, the therapist is conscripted into the role of either an adversary who is out to "get something on" the patient or an idealized pal and confidant, "the only one who understands." The danger in both cases is that the therapist will fail to use appropriate therapeutic challenges and leverage, either to avoid confronting the patient in the "enemy" role or to avoid taking the shine off the idealized image in the "ally" role.

The *aggressor/aggressee* pattern is prominent in those patients who have grown up in a world of violence and intimidation. They have learned to use direct or implied threats to influence and manipulate people and may try this on the therapist. These patients may attempt to get the therapist to endorse violent revenge fantasies or to justify past acts of aggression based on their "victim" status. Such patients may often have serious personality disorders in the antisocial/narcissistic/borderline spectrum that underlie their trauma syndrome, and these need to be addressed early and forthrightly.

An unstable and potentially dangerous pattern is *rescuer/rescuee*, in which the patient shows up abruptly in breathless crisis, then drops out of sight until the next emergency. Therapists who play into this crisis cycle risk reinforcing the patient's view of the world as a hostile place where helping relationships occur only in emergencies and rescue relationships substitute for intimacy. In my view, the clinical challenge is for the therapist to provide a model of mature stability by being there when the patient needs him, while reinforcing the idea that dramatic displays are not necessary to elicit care and concern from others, and emphasizing the necessity for the patient to build up inner resources by maintaining carefully modulated therapeutic contact that will head off crises before they escalate.

Finally, a variant of the rescuer pattern is the *Lone Ranger*, the therapist who sets herself up as the sole sane voice, the only helper competent enough to protect the patient from the forces of evil pounding at the gate. While projecting a sense of therapeutic competence and hope is a necessary part of the therapeutic process, this exaggeratedly autonomous, "us-against-the-world" perspective may maladaptively reinforce the patient's traumatized view of the world as a hostile place where escape is possible only through an all-powerful rescuer who is stumbled upon by happenstance or beneficent fate (Munroe et al., 1995).

Training and Experience

The Hippocratic dictum, "primum no nocere" ("first, do no harm") applies no less to psychotherapy than to medicine. In the field of traumatology, we need to recognize that clinicians who have had little experience, training, or commitment to working with such patients can actually do them great harm (Figley, 1995). The cold facts are that some therapists may be better at working with some patients than others (Miller, 1993) and that some clinicians may not have the interpersonal skills to work with patients who elicit strong negative feelings (Maier & Van Rybroek, 1995).

I have colleagues who can't imagine how I put up with a steady therapeutic diet of brain-injured, chronic pain, toxic exposure, crime victim, PTSD, and tough-guy law enforcement and emergency personnel patients. At the same time, many of these colleagues have a flair for treating terminal cancer patients, suicidal borderlines, chronic substance abusers, convicted sex offenders, and other patients that I would consider equally, if not more, challenging. It's really a matter of what interests us clinically and the responsibility to afford ourselves the best possible education, training, supervision, experience, and ethical grounding to be maximally effective.

In this vein, research (Pearlman & Mac Ian, 1995) indicates the need for more training in trauma therapy and more supervision and support for trauma therapists who are out there practicing. Yassen (1995) notes that an important contribution of professional training is the provision of a theoretical framework that not only informs the kind of interventions to be made, but also offers intellectual containment in the face of violence and the powerlessness/helplessness it can engender. Theoretical understanding through training or scholarly perusal of the relevant professional literature can prepare the clinician for what may be encountered in the aftermath of trauma by providing structure and emotional distance as well as content knowledge.

IN HARM'S WAY: THERAPISTS AS
VICTIMS OF PATIENT VIOLENCE

Demographics and Causes

For those whose image of psychotherapy evokes pipe-puffing shrinks lolling in cushy recliner chairs, langorously taking in the dulcet sobs of hankie-wringing neurotics, it may come as a surprise that mental health professionals are quite frequently the victims of real violence. Many psychologically disordered patients are dangerous. Recent data suggest that injuries to mental health caregivers at times exceed rates of injury for construction workers, traditionally considered to be the most dangerous occupational category in the U.S. Especially at risk are health care providers who treat serious mental illness and emergency mental health services personnel who provide assistance during disasters. In recent years, disgruntled patients who have failed to find relief for their mental or physical pain, or who think they have been badly treated by the medical or mental health care systems, have come back to kill emergency room and mental health clinic personnel; many facilities now have metal detectors and other forms of security (Flannery, 1995; Simon, 1996; see also Chapter 9).

According to an American Psychiatric Association Task Force report, 40 percent of psychiatrists are assaulted by patients one or more times during their careers; other studies bump the figure up to 50 percent. Psychiatrists appear to be at higher risk than psychologists or social workers in inpatient settings, but not in outpatient ones. Nurses and rehabilitation staff are common targets in inpatient settings. Nearly three-fourths of assaults against all psychiatrists occur during the first meeting of the doctor and an unknown patient (Binder, 1995; Flannery, 1995; Miller, 1997; Simon, 1996; Tardiff, 1995).

At least three factors contribute to the increased number of violent patients currently in the mental health system (Appelbaum & Appelbaum, 1995). First, some categories of deviant behavior that were traditionally treated as crimes deserving of punishment have been reconceptualized and reclassified as indicators of mental illness suitable for psychiatric hospitalization and treatment. As a result, a higher percentage of patients with prior criminal histories are being diverted from the criminal justice system to mental health settings.

Second, the potential malpractice liability of mental health clinicians for a patient's violent acts expanded with the 1976 Tarasoff decision. Clinicians consequently may feel constrained to hospitalize and detain potentially dangerous patients in order to "cover themselves," regardless of whether the patients truly require inpatient treatment.

Third, the shift from "need for treatment" to a "dangerousness" criterion for civil commitment has further upped the number of dangerous persons in inpatient psychiatric settings. As resources diminish, there may simply not be enough room for nondangerous mentally ill persons who do not meet civil commitment criteria to be admitted to public sector facilities, already crowded with more violent commitable patients (Appelbaum & Appelbaum, 1995).

In other words, in an era of dwindling health care budgets, it's not enough to be crazy to get inpatient psychological treatment—you've got to be *dangerously* crazy. It is not uncommon in some urban areas for patients to work this system exquisitely to their advantage, menacingly harassing passersby or heaving a rock through a car window when they want to be hospitalized (they're hungry, the weather's getting cold, they want drugs), then acting sane and cooperative in order to get discharged when it suits them—a classic "revolving door."

Risk Factors for Patient-Therapist Assault

PATIENT RISK FACTORS.   Research and clinical experience have demonstrated a fairly consistent profile of the psychiatric patient prone to assault: a young, white male, with a psychotic disorder or neurological syndrome and a past history of violence and/or substance abuse, who is previously unknown to the clinician. The most common form of attack is being punched or kicked; less frequently, more serious forms of violence may occur (Fink, 1995; Flannery, 1995).

CLINICIAN RISK FACTORS.   In general, young and inexperienced clinicians are more likely to be the targets of psychiatric inpatient violence. Furthermore, assaulted clinicians are more likely to be perceived as irritable, to speak angrily, and to become confrontive in threatening situations (Fink, 1995; Tardiff, 1995). Perhaps not surprisingly, obnoxious therapists are more likely to tick off their patients and therefore more likely to be attacked.

SITUATIONAL RISK FACTORS.   Certain risk factors for violence that are generic for medical settings as a whole (Kinney, 1995) also apply more specifically to mental health settings. These include the presence of drug addicts, gang members, acutely disturbed patients and visitors, availability of weapons, shortage of staff, clinical settings situated in high crime areas, crowded emergency rooms and clinics, and nighttime operation.

The most common explanation given by clinicians for having been assaulted by a hospitalized psychiatric patient is that they denied or frustrated the patient in some way (Tardiff, 1995). In one study (Fink, 1995), the most common reasons for a patient assault or threat given by psychiatric residents were refusing to meet a patient's request (59 percent), setting a limit (44 percent), making an unfavorable comment (29 percent), not setting sufficient limits (14 percent), and forcing a patient to take medication (14 percent). Although most of the clinicians suggested that the aggressive incident was random and unpredictable, approximately half conceded that they had some inkling of the patient's dangerousness prior to the assault.

VIOLENCE TOWARD WOMEN IN MENTAL HEALTH CARE SETTINGS.   Violence toward women in mental health care settings is, in one sense, an extension of the larger problem of violence against women at work (see Chapter 9). In general, women feel more vulnerable to being attacked in mental health care settings because of the greater physical size and strength of potentially disturbed male patients (Binder, 1995). In addition, there are cultural expectations related to masculine authority; for example, male personnel have traditionally been employed to contain aggressive patients by a show of physical force (Levy & Harticollis, 1976).

A therapist's pregnancy may evoke in patients feelings of sibling rivalry, Oedipal conflicts, envy, rejection, or abandonment. Binder (1995) cites the case of a 38-year-old woman with breast cancer who was being treated by a woman therapist who became pregnant. As the pregnancy became noticeable, the patient showed tremendous anger and hostility. She saw the baby as a new life and contrasted this with her perception of her own impending death. To compound matters, the typical overt reaction of colleagues to a staff member's pregnancy is one of protectiveness and solicitiousness, which may evoke jealousy on the part of patients. In other instances, however, the therapist's pregnancy may exert a calming effect on patients (Binder, 1995).

Jealousy regarding female therapists may spill over into "clinically excusable" forms of sexual harassment within the facility, including intrusive intimacy, clinginess, and following the therapist around to an extent that might be classified as criminal stalking if it occurred outside facility walls. In fact, this pattern may continue after the patient is discharged. Although such dysfunctional attachments occur frequently in outpatient settings, the sheer level of psychological disturbance and potential for violence that characterizes many committed inpatients makes this phenomenon all the more disquieting and may itself lead to therapist burnout.

If female therapists are actually assaulted, they frequently develop classic symptoms of PTSD (as do many male clinicians). Unfortunately, the helper role may cause therapists to disregard their symptoms and delay or defer treatment. Assaults can also affect family members. For example, one woman noted that her children were upset after she was assaulted and continued to inquire if she was okay when she got home from work each day. After an assault, women clinicians are sometimes embarrassed by their reaction or are concerned that others may blame them for instigating the violence; this is similar to what is experienced by some rape victims. In addition, they may worry that the typically male-dominated staff structure will think they can't "cut it" in this type of work. Any or all of these factors may lead to underreporting of assaults and failure to seek appropriate treatment (Binder, 1995; Lanza, 1995, 1996).

Reducing Risks and Taking Action

Although at risk, mental health clinicians are not helpless in the face of potential patient violence. There are things we can do, measures we can take, but—and here's the key issue—as a group, we are notoriously prone to denial and minimization of the risks we're exposed to; hence, we typically fail to implement even those policies and procedures that could make our work safer for all concerned. The goal is hardly to maintain a fortress mentality and an adversarial relationship with every patient we treat. But knowing we are doing everything possible to establish a safe working environment may give us the security and confidence to apply our skills effectively.

SECURITY PRECAUTIONS AND TRAINING.   In mental health settings, security is often conspicuous by its absence. In one study (Tardiff, 1995), only 23 percent of psychiatrists attacked reported having taken any prior security precautions; of these, one-third failed to use the precautions already in place during the attack.

In mental health settings, training is often insufficient to deal with patient violence. In one Pennsylvania hospital system, typical training in managing patient violence consisted of two hours of classroom time and one and a half hours of practicum time. In contrast, residents reported an average of eight hours of didactic classroom time and seven hours of practicum time in the study of suicidal patients. That is, four times as many hours were spent in learning how to protect patients from themselves as in learning how to protect staff and other patients from in-house violence (Fink, 1995).

In trying to address these issues in my own work, I find that a typical source of such priority shuffling has little to do with concern for safety per se, but everything to do with institutional liability. If a patient kills himself, the relatives will probably sue for big bucks, hence the emphasis on prevention of patient suicide. But if a staff member is injured or killed, it may actually be far more difficult to press a case, unless gross negligence can be demonstrated, since the event took place in the course of normal job duties and expectations. I have treated several assaulted medical, mental health, and rehabilitation professionals whose physical injuries and psychological traumatization were handled as just another "Workers Comp injury," with clinical and administrative insensitivity leading to persistent retraumatization and entrenchment of disability (Miller, 1997).

When I consult with organizations, or just try to make the outpatient facilities where I work a little safer, my earnest appeals for improved precautions commonly fall on cost-conscious deaf ears—until I point out that a serious incident could cost the facility big money and bad publicity. Now they're listening. But even then, changes are slow, because, besides the money issue, the massive psychological denial of potential violence that occurs in all work settings (see Chapter 9) is a formidable impediment to progress in safety.

RISK FACTOR ASSESSMENT.   Tardiff (1989) provides a useful clinical profile that outlines risk factors for predicting short-term violence (days to a week). Factors include: (1) appearance of the patient (signs of substance abuse, anger, disorganized behavior, noncompliance); (2) detailed plan or threat of violence; (3) available means of inflicting injury (obtained or improvised weapons); (4) history of violence or other impulsive or antisocial behavior; (5) targets of past violence (women, authority figures); (6) degree of injury inflicted on past targets of violence; (7) circumstances and patterns of escalation of violence toward others; (8) history of childhood abuse or family violence; (9) current alcohol or drug abuse; (10) organic mental disorder; (11) paranoid or other psychotic symptomatology; (12) borderline or antisocial personality disorder; (13) demographic profile for violence (young, male, low socioeconomic status). (See also Chapter 9).

PRACTICAL AND SUPPORTIVE MEASURES.   Policies designed to effectively curb violence in medical, mental health, and rehabilitation settings include: (1) establishment of a violence task force; (2) criminalization of violent acts in emergency rooms and other health care settings; (3) injury prevention plans and procedures; (4) identification of security measures, such as lighting, access pathways, and alarm systems; and (5) staff training to deal with high risk patients and visitors (Kinney, 1995; Miller, 1997; see also Chapter 9).

In mental health care settings specifically, studies point to the need to have programs in which victims of violence can receive immediate peer support and the opportunity for longer term professional care to cope with the sequelae of violence. It is especially important that colleagues and supervisors who review assaults with clinicians not be perceived as blaming the victim when making suggestions about future precautions or discussing what might have been done differently (Binder, 1995; Tardiff, 1995).

DEALING WITH EMERGENCIES.   Several recommendations are offered for handling emergency situations (Caraulia & Steiger, 1997; Dubin, 1995; Eichelman, 1995; Flannery, 1995; Gilliland & James, 1993); these should be supplemented by appropriate training (also see Chapter 9). If a patient makes threats of violence and the clinician feels he will act on the threats, then security staff or, if appropriate, the local police should be notified. When a violent incident appears to be brewing, but the patient seems to still retain some emotional and behavioral control, first identify yourself as a clinician. This identification of medical authority may contribute to an enhanced sense of safety and control. Tell the patient that you are going for help. Paradoxically, this is often calming, especially with psychiatric patients who are feeling overwhelmed. The patient may welcome the presence of others who can help him to hold such feelings in check. But use your judgment if it seems that the patient may feel threatened by your going for "reinforcements."

Keep an appropriate physical distance. Individuals with an assaultive history have a larger "body buffer zone" than others. This zone is larger behind than in front of the individual, who may be paranoid about "sneak attacks." A general rule of thumb is to leave seven feet, or "two quick steps," between you and the patient—close enough to move in for quick restraint, if necessary, but far enough to avoid a sudden physical attack. To dissipate anxiety and anger, keep the patient talking about the perceived injustice or the perceived overwhelming medical or general life stress event. Violence often occurs when verbal communication fails. At the same time, avoid fanning the flames of outrage by encouraging venting that escalates into overt rage.

Although this advice may be hard to follow under extreme stress, talk with assaultive patients in a calm, easy, respectful style, as if speaking to a friend or peer, without necessarily compromising your legitimate authority. Let the patient know that his position is clearly understood and try to engage him in topics that will motivate his self-interest. Identify areas in which the patient's viewpoint is correct rather than trying to "argue him down." The alliance will be enhanced if you can identify similarities between yourself and the patient, but many disturbed patients are threatened by intimacy, so watch out for pathological projective identification or getting too "chummy."

If the patient attempts to flee from the room, by all means let him go and summon help from security and other staff. If the patient is assaultive, get yourself out of the room and to a place of safety as soon as possible.

Signal other staff for assistance, and check to see that other patients and staff are protected. If you cannot leave the room, call for assistance and use nonviolent self-defense procedures (Caraulia & Steiger, 1997; Gilliland & James, 1993; Wistedt & Freeman, 1994) until help arrives. While you're waiting, try to verbally engage the patient around the perceived injustice or threatening event—but without antagonizing or provoking him further. When order is restored, be sure the patient is back in personal control and provide any necessary medical treatment for the assault and the original medical or psychiatric presenting problem.

LEGAL ACTION AGAINST PATIENTS.   "What? Prosecute my patient? I'm supposed to *help* people!" Clinicians who react this way to the suggestion of legal action against assaultive patients do a grave disservice both to their own safety and to the profession as a whole. Yes, there are some people who, by virtue of their genetic priming, neurological impairment, or psychological disturbance have great difficulty controlling their violent and other impulsive acts. But with these rare exceptions, a civilized society generally holds people responsible for their behavior, and "mental patient" status should not automatically confer immunity from the consequences of one's actions (Baumeister, Tice, & Heatherton, 1995; Bidinotto, 1996; Etzioni, 1996; Kirwin, 1997; Miller, 1991; Simon, 1996; Slovenko, 1995; Szasz, 1987; Volavka, 1995; Wilson, 1993; Wilson & Herrnstein, 1985).

As reviewed by Appelbaum and Appelbaum (1995), prosecution of patients for violent behavior must rely on the same rationale and justification that govern the imposition of criminal sanctions on any other person. Unfortunately, the mental health community is typically unprepared to deal with assaultive behavior that is not associated with an underlying treatable mental illness. Not all violent behavior by patients can be attributed to their mental disturbance, and, as noted above, the status of being a patient should not be construed as a licence to offend with impunity. Prosecution may at times represent the only effective and justifiable means of protecting other patients and staff.

However, well-meaning but sometimes misguided efforts to protect patients' rights, along with (an often well-justified) law enforcement antipathy toward "mush-minded, criminal-coddling shrinks," may come back to haunt us when we seek the police's help in dealing with violent patients. Even when an arrest is made, the District Attorney's office may decline to pursue the charges, reasoning that being assaulted by patients "comes with the territory" of being a mental health professional. Even in those cases that receive a hearing, the judge may dismiss the charges and even admonish mental health staff for initiating a criminal process

against the poor patient, for whom "punishment" cannot be morally jus-
tified.

In other cases, the opposite may occur. Therapists who call the cops
on a patient "just to teach him a lesson" may then discover that the
prosecutor or judge decides to make a big deal of the case, putting
the therapist in the position of having to cooperate with or endorse an
unintendedly aggressive prosecution or harsh sentence for the patient
she was only trying to "scare straight." In addition to the stress of having
to "bust" patients we're supposed to treat, therapists may have to endure
legal abuse from law enforcement, defense attorneys, and judges for
"not cleaning up your own mess."

Still, lack of action only reinforces bad behavior, and responsible use
of the criminal justice system in dealing with mentally ill offenders is
presently considered the best approach (Appelbaum & Appelbaum,
1995). This is not to suggest that clinicians should go around "throwing
the book at" patients for each little infraction. Obviously, use your clinical
judgment and common sense, much as you would in deciding if a suicidal
patient is commitable, if a child-abusing parent is reportable, or if a duty-
to-warn exists when your patient speaks threateningly about a third party.
As in those cases, we may sometimes need to take decisive action in the
case of our patients who behave dangerously.

THERAPIST, HEAL THYSELF: HELP
FOR TRAUMA THERAPISTS

As discussed so far, trauma can affect therapists in two main ways. The
first involves the cumulatively demoralizing "rub-off" effect of dealing
daily with the outcomes of accidental and deliberate tragedy on the
human spirit. The second involves being assaulted, threatened, or otherwise traumatized by the very patients we are trying to help, forcing a
wrenching reconsideration of our professional role and sense of personal
safety. In addition to the practical risk assessment and follow-up measures
discussed above, this section discusses some of the more directly psychotherapeutic strategies that can be applied to personally or vicariously
traumatized therapists—often a difficult bunch to treat in any circumstance.

General Decompression and Self-Help Measures

All therapists should establish and maintain a balance between their
professional and personal lives, but for trauma therapists this is especially

important (Cerney, 1995). Some authorities recommend that a sense of civic responsibility expressed in social activism can be an outlet for frustration and serve to productively bind anxiety and focus energies (Comas-Diaz & Padilla, 1990; Yassen, 1995)—as long as such activism doesn't become an obsessional, self-destructive, dysfunctional "crusade." Letting the public know your views, beliefs, and ideals can be an antidote to the secretive and silencing nature of trauma. What may seem like small acts of activism can also combat powerlessness, the feeling that "with all I do, I don't make a dent."

Self-help occurs in the form of formal or informal support groups or incorporating stress-reduction activities and exercises in the therapist's daily life. A useful resource is Saakvitne and Pearlman's (1996) workbook for therapists dealing with vicarious traumatization, and many of the exercises in that manual can be adapted and expanded as needed.

Institutional Support for Traumatized Therapists

In cases where therapists have been directly traumatized, as when assaulted in psychiatric or criminal facilities, institutional leaders can take the following steps to ensure that traumatized workers are not ostracized by their colleagues (Catherall, 1995). First, leaders must recognize that other employees may have an emotional reaction to the traumatized worker. Second, leaders must create regular opportunities for the group to meet and talk about their exposure to traumatic stress. It is most effective if someone in a position of authority takes responsibility for normalizing the experience. Finally, leaders must actively encourage the group to see the individual traumatized worker's reaction as a common group problem and deal with it on that basis.

In dealing with countertransferential reactions to aggressive and violent patients, Maier and Van Rybroek (1995) describe the following institutional set of policies and procedures. In this model, staff are expected to identify and share feelings with their peers and supervisors in forums provided by the clinical administration. Should these feelings interfere with the ability to provide effective and humane treatment to a patient, staff are expected to address the relevant issues. The formal personnel process may be utilized to shape the required change, including referral to the employee assistance program. If, over time, the staff member is unable to keep feelings of fear and anger from affecting her work performance, a change in work area or assignment may be in order.

Maier and Van Rybroek (1995) describe an intervention called "*Me-Time*." Within this specially designated interval during the workday, the staff members are expected to verbalize negative feelings that could potentially affect their work with patients. The process of ventilation with group feedback and support helps identify defenses such as denial and projection and to develop effective coping strategies.

Typically, nursing and mental health staff victims of workplace violence such as assaults by patients experience intense emotional reactions (Lanza, 1995, 1996). They want to talk about their reactions but feel it is "unprofessional" to do so. Victims typically do not expect to receive support from hospital administrators, despite their history of loyal service to the institution, and this may produce further anger and demoralization.

A particularly useful intervention for assaulted staff is supportive counseling that focuses more on the victim's needs than on the administrative agenda of "improving performance." Lanza's (1995) study of one institution found that most of the staff sought counseling after being assaulted. Following the assault, victims reported feeling upset but then feeling better. They later sought counseling after experiencing unexpected delayed episodes of fearfulness and crying, which were especially distressing because they thought they had already coped with their feelings and put the incident behind them. Other reactions reported by victims were anger at the patient, humiliation at being criticized and not supported by coworkers, fear of returning to work, stress at having to cope with their families' concerns and pressures to leave their jobs, and anger at the amount of paperwork required to report the assault.

As we've seen in Chapter 2, blaming oneself is often a way of imputing at least some kind of meaning and controllability to a catastrophic event. Self-blame can be functional, if it involves attributions to one's specific behavior in a specific situation rather than to enduring personality characteristics, the oft-cited difference between *behavioral self-blame* and *characterological self-blame*. But behavioral self-blame is *not* helpful if victims feel that they used appropriate precautions, followed all the safety rules, and bad things happened anyway. Both administrators and clinicians can help assaulted staff sort out the realities of safe conduct from runaway catastrophic fears and fantasies.

Obviously, all of these supportive measures depend on a certain degree of trust and cooperation within an organization. This may not always be forthcoming, however, or it may not go far enough. In more complex cases, or those involving more severe trauma, good therapists may need good therapy.

Psychotherapy with Traumatized Therapists

Traumatized therapists who enter treatment require their own therapists to be accepting, nonjudgmental, and empathic, without becoming enmeshed or overawed—in other words, similar to the kind of therapist most effective in treating other traumatized patients. One of the most difficult issues traumatized therapists face is the assault on their perceptions of the world and its inhabitants (Cerney, 1995).

Cerney (1995) has treated a number of therapists suffering from secondary trauma or vicarious traumatization, using a suggestive imagery technique (Grove & Panzer, 1991) similar to the one used with primary trauma victims (see also Chapter 2). While there is no hypnotic induction per se, when patients are asked to form an image, they often spontaneously go into a suggestible trance state. When patients present a nightmare, flashback, or other type of intrusive thought or image, they are asked to redream the dream or go over the experience again. At the point at which the traumatic event is about to begin, the therapist suggests they freeze the scene so that they can program how the scenario is to proceed. They are then asked if they would like to enter the scene—be it dream, memory, or flashback—from the distance of a mature, safe perspective. Or they may bring anyone they wish into the scene with them and thereby restructure it in a less threatening and more empowering way.

CISD with Traumatized Psychotherapists

We have discussed *critical incident stress debriefing* (CISD) in Chapter 10 in connection with law enforcement and emergency service personnel, as well as its use in treating disaster-related trauma (Chapter 7) and workplace violence trauma (Chapter 9). The same kind of group crisis intervention and debriefing model ought to work well with mental health clinicians, with some modifications. Talbot et al. (1995) argue that psychotherapists, as distinct from other emergency responders, require *psychological* understanding and integration in order to intervene effectively. These authors' program has evolved largely through their work with the victims of armed holdups and the mental health clinicians who debrief them.

In this model, the aim of *psychological debriefing* for mental health clinicians is to help them deal with the stresses of this work via ventilation, catharsis, and sharing of experiences, in order to gain psychological mastery of the situation and prevent the development of more serious delayed stress syndromes (Raphael, 1986; Talbot et al., 1995). Particularly important for psychotherapists is the careful exploration of their identification with the victim's experience, which ordinarily enables them to properly assimilate the burden of empathy. Finally, the therapists are helped to integrate the traumatic experience and make a transition back to everyday life.

Psychotherapists need to know not only what happened, when, how, and where, but also *why*. That is, the debriefing must incorporate not just emotional ventilation, but an integrative intellectual understanding of the traumatic event and the therapist's role in dealing with victims in the aftermath. Consequently, the debriefing process employed by Manton and Talbot (1990) and Talbot et al. (1995) includes making psychological sense of what occurred to the victims and the psychotherapists both personally and professionally.

In this model, the debriefing of the therapist-debriefers is attended by two or more psychologists (here referred to as the "secondary debriefers") who were not part of the original civilian debriefing. The therapist debriefing is held away from the crisis scene as soon as is practicable for all involved therapists to attend.

The debriefing procedure incorporates the crisis event, the therapists' responses to that crisis, and the dynamic processes occurring in the current debriefing. The goal is to integrate and make sense of the crisis and the counseling to develop a clear, total picture of the event. The secondary debriefer is consequently dealing with a number of different levels of the crisis: the event itself, the victims' responses to the event, the therapists' responses to the event, the therapists' responses to the victims, and each therapist's personal and professional response to the events. Essentially, the secondary debriefer assumes a supervisory role to help each therapist reach an understanding of the interventions that she made, assess those that were useful, explore possible alternatives, and decide on future actions.

Secondary debriefers need to monitor and deal with the potential countertransference issues that may complicate the therapists' responses to the crisis and its victims. For example, the secondary debriefer needs to normalize feelings of fear and sadness that follow the traumatic event, as therapists internalize the experience of what the victims have experienced. Past unresolved issues may also come up, particularly if the therapist has experienced recent or past violence or abuse. Dealing comprehensively with countertransference issues is usually beyond the scope of a single debriefing, but these can be followed up if necessary.

The number of successive crises attended by psychotherapists may need to be addressed in the debriefing, as crises often come in clusters or waves. In one example cited by Talbot et al. (1995), a therapist had arrived on the posttrauma debriefing scene of a bank holdup already feeling overwhelmed by her workload of trauma therapy. Consequently, she developed a self-servingly defensive myth, encouraged by the bank's senior management, that this was not a "serious" holdup because no real threats of danger were involved. Because the psychologist felt she could not handle anymore, she conveniently bought into the consensual myth that the holdup "wasn't really so bad" and the victims "were really okay." Consequently, her work with this bank employee group felt unsatisfactory and was not particularly therapeutic for the victims, because they picked up on the therapist's downplaying of their distress in order to protect her own feelings.

To help make sense of the therapists' experiences in the original crisis and in the present debriefing, the secondary debriefer brings together his knowledge of the original crisis victims and the psychotherapists as individuals and as respective groups, and his understanding of psychological and group dynamics. Because greater psychological knowledge is often associated with more sophisticated defenses, the secondary debriefer may have to take a more confrontive stance with the debriefed therapists than clinicians typically take with civilian victims or, for that matter, than debriefers might take with other emergency responders, such as police officers or firefighter-paramedics. The aim ultimately is to tie in themes and personal issues, draw parallels, and put the experience into perspective.

Finally, as in a therapeutic session, the secondary debriefer needs to summarize, to contain, and to make sense of what occurred. Highly intellectual and verbal types such as psychotherapists should have little difficulty verbalizing what they have gained and learned from working in the crisis and from the victim debriefings. Talbot et al. (1995) emphasize that to continue to function and grow personally and professionally, psychotherapists need to maintain a sense of mastery, as well as the feeling of being valued, worthwhile, and grounded in their work. Cognitive understanding and adaptive self-insight give therapists mastery of the situation, objectivity, and a theoretical base for their interventions, which are essential in order for trauma therapists to continue to function effectively. The same recommendations apply to therapists in all fields. We serve best when we ourselves are well served.

Chapter 12

EGO AUTONOMY AND THE HEALTHY PERSONALITY

Cognitive Styles of Adaptive and Transcendent Coping

Quae nocent, docent.
[That which hurts, teaches]

—Ancient Roman Proverb

Forget your personal tragedy. We are all bitched
from the start and you especially have to hurt like
hell before you can write seriously. But when you
get the damned hurt use it—don't cheat with it.
—Ernest Hemingway

Of all the clinical stories I've accumulated in nearly 20 years of practice, this is pretty close to my favorite.

I first met Billy almost by accident when I was asked to fill in per diem at a local rehab hospital that was in the process of trying to hire a full-time psychologist. "This one's really depressed," the clinical staff told me. "See if there's anything you can do for him."

The record showed that Billy had been a plain, normal, nice guy of 22, who, happy with the simple satisfactions of a young man's life, seemed to have everything going for him. He was engaged to be married and had just started a landscaping business with his brother and father that was doing well. He and his fiancée were saving to buy a house. He'd just bought a new truck. Then, as he put it, "God must of had some sick sense of humor." Driving home from a job, he had just turned onto a main road when an elderly woman veered her Mercury into his path. The car clipped Billy's truck and, in an effort to avoid a more serious collision, he swerved hard, causing the truck to spin out of control and overturn. The woman walked away without a scratch. Billy didn't. He sustained what the medical record described as a traumatic lumbar spinal shear-crush injury with near-total cord transection, paralyzing him from the waist down. He'd never walk again.

When I first came into the room, Billy was lying in his bed, his face turned to the wall. He had no use for that overpleasant, clinical "Hi I'm Dr. Miller" lilt we sometimes use in our well-meaning attempts to lighten the somber hospital atmosphere. He basically told me where I could put my psychological crap, because unless I could make him walk again, he had nothing to say to me, and I was wasting his time and mine. Truthfully, what could I do for someone like Billy, someone who had had everything and lost it through no fault of his own, someone who by all accounts did indeed seem to be the victim of some cosmic sick sense of humor?

So I offered to check in with him once each day, listen if he wanted to talk, and get lost if he preferred to be alone. Sometimes you just have to let the patient know you're available, back off, and let the grief run its course.

Then one day he decided to talk to me, but it sure wasn't what I wanted to hear. "Doc, I got nothing to live for and you and all these other quacks can't help me. As soon as I get out of here, I'm gonna kill myself." Just in case I didn't get the point, he added, "So fuck you."

Yes, we referred him for a psychiatric consult, but before any decisive action could be taken, Billy was discharged. Attempts at home follow-up were fruitless, since he apparently had gone to stay with some relatives out of state and the family didn't want to be bothered. In my profession, no news is usually good news, but I couldn't help wondering if he had ever cashed in on his grim promise. I figured if anything happened I'd hear about it, so maybe no news *was* good news. Eventually the hospital hired its psychologist, I went back to my practice, and the whole incident receded from memory.

About three years later, I had just finished visiting one of my patients in that same rehab hospital and was trudging wearily down the hall after a long day, when from behind me came a shout, "Yo, doc!" I turned around to see a young man in a wheelchair grinning at me with an expression of recognition I couldn't reciprocate. There was something familiar about him; could this be—no, he was about 20 pounds heavier and now had a beard; also, he was wearing a baseball cap that obscured his features still further.

Then he started to laugh. "Don't you recognize me? I'm the guy who was gonna kill himself," he blurted loudly and exuberantly in a busy hospital hallway filled with people, some of whom were now turning and craning to stare. "Man," he chortled, "I thought you were gonna have a heart attack when I told you I was planning to do it. You know,

I felt sorry for you, the hard time I gave you." Tell me about it, I thought. Billy continued, "But I got over it."

Got over it? How does one "get over" a catastrophic crippling injury? How does one deal with the existential unfairness of a whole life turned upside down in an instant? I decided to find out. I asked Billy about the last three years, how he'd been doing, what kind of treatment he'd had, and so on. I gingerly skirted the main question, which essentially was, "How the hell can you be so happy, when the last time I saw you, you were inches from jumping out of the friggin' window?"

But I hedged. After all, if this were just some thin bubble of denial that Billy had spun around his pain, I didn't want it to be me, the great trauma psychologist, who pierced this fragile defensive membrane with my jagged, clumsily probing questions, sending his punctured, deflated psyche into a flailing, sputtering, suicidal spin. Especially right there in the hospital hallway, with everybody watching.

But the more we talked, the more I became convinced that Billy really *had* mastered and overcome his trauma, that he had wrested control of his life away from the forces of despair and truly made the best of what for most people would be the worst imaginable situation. He was employed again, he told me, having been retrained for some kind of electronics repair work. His original engagement had broken off after the accident ("No girl could've put up with me in the shape I was in then"), but now he had another girlfriend, he related happily. Most intriguingly, he had come back from the brink essentially on his own. No psychotherapy, a few brief counseling sessions with his church pastor, a reasonably cooperative insurance company, and a lot of support from his family—that was basically it.

He was here today for a biyearly checkup, and had to go to meet his ride. As he rolled away in his wheelchair, he suddenly spun around, and a serious look straightened his face. "You know, doc," he said. "If you had told me back then I'd be joking around with you one day, I'd have said you were more nuts than me. Look, I'm not happy this happened, but hey, it's not the worst thing. Stay outa trouble, doc." He caught my furrowed gawk: "Hey, lighten up." And he wheeled out of sight.

Not the worst thing? Here we go again. But the more I thought about our conversation, the more I had to conclude that this wasn't just denial, at least not all of it; this was *recovery.* Remarkable recovery, at that—I doubt that most therapists, me included, could pull ourselves out of that hole the way Billy did. Perhaps, I thought, all the fancy psychtalk we spout about the transcendent, healing potential of the human spirit is, at least for some catastrophically traumatized people, a workable reality. Maybe not all, maybe not most, maybe not even very many, but if it happens even once, it means its possible, right? If even one, real live human being can pull himself out of the hole, then it's the exception that *dis*proves the dour rule that traumatic disability inevitably must lead to despair, or at best, to an existentially lukewarm "acceptance" of a sadly limited life.

Billy had put his phenomenological money where our own therapeutic mouths had always claimed to be. And if he could do it, maybe more people could do it—or *learn* to do it. Imagine if we could harness this spontaneously recuperative, self-healing force and apply it therapeutically to the rest of our traumatized patients.

Even with less dramatically uplifting cases (recall the dangers of therapeutic rescue fantasies cited in Chapter 2), it's a sobering, refreshing splash in our collective clinical face to realize that, despite this book's emphasis on helping patients who develop severe traumatic disability syndromes in the wake of stress, pain, and injury, many affected people *don't* develop crippling posttraumatic illnesses. They appear to cope reasonably well, and a happy few like Billy appear to transcend and grow from their experience. Indeed, there is an emerging body of literature that suggests that a small group of people exposed to even the most terrifying or heartbreaking events may actually seize some good from their struggle with such tragedies, including rape, incest, bereavement, cancer, HIV infection, heart attacks, disasters, military combat, and the Holocaust (Tedeschi & Calhoun, 1995, 1996).

So why not study healthy, adaptive people? For one thing, they're hard to pin down. People usually come to clinical attention, and thereby find themselves as part of clinical studies, by reason of one or another kind of "bad" or "sick" or "maladaptive" behavior. They respond to adversity by drinking or drugging themselves to ruin, become immobilized by depression or compulsiveness, somaticize themselves from doctor to doctor, impulsively and self-destructively break the law and get caught, and thereby eventually get channeled through the legal or mental health system, perhaps eventually winding up as part of some ongoing behavioral research project or clinical study.

But when people are out there coping well and leading reasonably happy, productive lives, we clinicians have nothing to "treat." Due to practical and financial considerations (you can't bill someone for being healthy), the emphasis on deficit and maldevelopment in psychology has largely remained, following the example of medicine's emphasis on disease. But recently, there has been a movement in psychology to conceptualize human nature in terms of strengths and abilities as well as weaknesses and deficiencies (Aldwin, 1994; Anthony & Cohler, 1987;

Heath & Heath, 1991; Miller, 1988, 1990, 1991a, 1992a, 1992b, 1993; Tedeschi & Calhoun, 1995, 1996).

Far from limiting the need for mental health services, I think that paying more attention to adaptive coping can greatly amplify, deepen, and diversify the psychotherapeutic options available to serve our patients and improve society as a whole. Accordingly, this somewhat more theoretical chapter focuses on the psychological dimensions of ego autonomy and the healthy personality as they relate to our understanding of personality, and thereby to the clinical practice of trauma therapy and psychotherapy in general.

THE AUTONOMOUS EGO FUNCTIONS

It was Freud (1900, 1915, 1923) who originally proposed that the transformation of primitive instinctual impulses into consciously acceptable substitutive drive-derivatives involves the utilization of cognitive processes such as symbolization and language. The purpose of thinking, Freud believed, is to permit the ego to achieve a delay of motor discharge, to serve as a kind of experimental action that allows for the exploration of behavioral options with far less effort and painful consequence than would be required for the real-world testing of each separate alternative.

But Freud failed to elaborate on the roles of these cognitive processes in personality development, preferring to concentrate on the role of instinct. It remained for the later *ego-psychologists*, exemplified by Hartmann (1939), to stress the importance of such cognitive faculties as memory, perception, attention, and intelligence in comprising a core of adaptive psychological functioning that is relatively independent of instinctual conflict—what Hartmann called the *conflict-free ego sphere*. These cognitive apparatuses also influence how the individual characteristically handles conflict, that is, they are the prerequisites for, and the underpinnings of, the defense mechanisms.

Hartmann (1939) proposed that phylogenetic evolution and individual development both ideally should lead to increasing independence of the organism from its environment, so that reactions that originally occurred in relation to the external world are progressively displaced to a mental domain, where the person can think about consequences, anticipate outcomes, and create contingency plans of alternative means-end possibilities. Hartmann called this process *internalization*. Accordingly, he spoke of *ego autonomy* as involving the relative freedom of the ego or self from blind obedience to instinctual emotional and motivational de-

mands, as well as from dependence on immediate environmental reinforcement for each action and plan.

Consistent with his emphasis on the importance of cognition, Hartmann (1939) placed intelligence at the top of the list of the ego's regula-
tory faculties. Following Hartmann's lead, Rapaport (1967a, 1967b)
sought to develop a psychodynamic approach to the study of cognitive
processes, and he believed that intelligence tests could be used to system-
atize and quantify the various aspects of ego functioning. Partly because
of Rapaport's efforts, the rich diagnostic yield of intelligence tests came
to be widely appreciated, and the Wechsler IQ scales became a corner-
stone of the standard psychological test battery (Rapaport, Gill, &
Schafer, 1968).

The term *cognitive style* was introduced by Klein (1954, 1958) to refer
to the individual arrangement of cognitive control structures in each
person's psyche, which have a basis in the types of constitutional mental
capacities suggested by Hartmann (1939). The development of characterological differences in coping processes came to be understood as resulting from the interplay of relatively stable, constitutionally based cognitive
styles or control principles (Gardner, Holzman, Klein, Linton, & Spence,
1959; Klein, 1958) and variations in early nurturing experiences (Winnicott, 1965).

Shapiro (1965) subsequently used the term "style" in his conceptualization of *neurotic styles*, that is, lifelong maladaptive modes of functioning
that are built around each person's characterological pattern or style of
perception, thought, and action. Shapiro identified four main neurotic
styles, the *obsessive-compulsive*, the *paranoid*, the *hysterical*, and the *impulsive*.

Psychological symptoms or prominent pathological traits, said Shapiro,
are shaped by the intellectual, perceptual, cognitive, and attitudinal
endowments of each person, and thereby influence even social affiliations
and vocational paths. It's no accident, for example, that a person with
an obsessive style may become a scientist or accountant, a paranoid style
person may go into the surveillance and security industry, a person with
a hysterical style may choose fashion consulting or show biz, while an
impulsive person races cars or robs banks.

Accordingly, a psychopathological stress reaction is not simply the
result of instinctually driven, intrapsychic conflict superimposed on a
blank-slate personality; rather, the form that the stress reaction takes is
strongly determined by how the person perceives the world, thinks about
it, reacts emotionally to it, and behaves in it—that is, by how his own
set of constitutional cognitive traits is arrayed in the psyche. Under stress,
obsessives fret and ruminate, paranoids spin conspiracy theories and

plot revenge, hysterics emote histrionically or swoon with malaise, and impulsives take action—immediately, planlessly, and often disastrously (see Miller, 1990, 1991b, for a comprehensive neuropsychodynamic conceptualization of cognitive style and personality).

More recently, Shapiro (1989) has asserted that the neurotic person is "estranged from himself" to the extent that his maladaptive cognitive style contributes to the obfuscation of his own motivations and interpretations of external reality, thereby weakening his sense of self as an autonomous, self-determined being. One consequence of this self-estrangement and lack of measured reflection is a reversion to a pattern of egocentric reactiveness. In these circumstances, the ego flinches reflexively to dispel or forestall anxiety, and to protect against the threat to the brittle and fragile stability of the personality structure. Hence, there is also always a degree of distortion of self-awareness or a characteristic pattern of self-deception associated with such a personality. Internalizing types become depressed and fall ill, while externalizing types act-out and get in trouble. As we have seen, this lack of a broader perspective, or "constriction of the ego," occurs as a common mental state in the psychological reaction to traumatic disability syndromes, to a far greater degree in some persons than in others.

But the functions of the ego must go beyond passive or rigid defensiveness. Anthony (1987) points out that, when confronted with adversity, the ego does more than retreat, turtle-like; it often attempts to gain active mastery over the stimulus or situation. The ego often copes interactively with the environment, meeting challenges head-on and transforming situations rather than merely accepting them. True coping, in this view, employs many more ego skills than are required for purely defensive purposes. Coping mechanisms differ from defense mechanisms in being more flexible, purposive, selective, oriented toward present reality and future planning, involving largely conscious, reality-based thinking, and coordinating individual needs with external reality. While defense usually needs to be worked through in formal therapy, Anthony (1987) notes, coping is a learnable skill, which also means that parents and teachers, as well as therapists, can serve as appropriate models.

The autonomy of ego functioning, in this view, depends on the relative use of coping over defensive mechanisms, with the latter more typically involving the development of what we would regard as clinical symptoms, disorders of personality, or persistent traumatic disability syndromes. Only a personality with some flexible room to maneuver can effectively profit from any genuine method of therapy, education, or self-improvement. Without even a modicum of cognitive flexibility or ego autonomy to grab hold of, most attempts at formal psychotherapeutic intervention or lasting self-change strategies will quickly slip away like a carelessly thrown rappel on sheer frozen rock.

COGNITIVE STYLE, RESILIENCY, AND "INVULNERABILITY" TO TRAUMA

For most people, adversity, neglect, abuse, and other hard knocks are justifiably viewed as destructive life events that may prematurely clot and encrust the developing personality with lifelong cynicism and despair. Yet a few souls seem mysteriously able to slough off the effects of a truly rotten early life and to grow and thrive in defiance of their lot. Recent research has identified a class of individuals who, despite being raised under circumstances that range from the mildly dysfunctional to the twistedly cruel, seem to emerge as relatively well-functioning adolescents and adults—the so-called *invulnerable* or *resilient children*. The study of these survivors has important implications for the concept of ego autonomy and its development.

Anthony (1987) and Cohler (1987) have noted that, instead of breaking down in the face of adversity, "invulnerables" seem somehow to rise to their challenges and often perform better than ever. Their developmental histories are characterized by a certain temperamental robustness that is apparent even in infancy, coupled with strong "in-the-world" feelings and attitudes. They seem inherently endowed with a wide range of competencies, and their normal defenses, coping skills, and creativity grow with age. Their relationships are soundly based and enduring. They are interpersonally skillful, popular with other children and adults, well-regarded by themselves and others, assertive on their own behalf, have a strong sense of personal control, and take responsibility for their own actions. They are reflective, rather than impulsive, show a healthy creativity, and keep a good hold on their emotions, although they are capable of experiencing and expressing a full range of normal feelings. Their eagerness to learn, their curiosity, and their absorption with scholastic subjects endear them to teachers, so that school is often a place of refuge, support, and encouragement.

In dealing with stresses or potentially traumatic experiences, these resilient children demonstrate higher and better focused intelligence, use more divergent or creative thinking in approaching problems, show an increased capacity to select out the particular aspects of adversity required to be overcome, and make greater use of goal-oriented strategies to plan the necessary steps to solve the problem without becoming overwhelmed by the complexity or hopelessness of the situation. They also maintain good control over impulsive urges and feelings, with the capacity to plan ahead rather than to immediately act. They show increased persistence and a greater sense of mastery over their own lives. Of particular significance, these resilient children show an increased capacity for finding comfort and satisfaction in their own efforts at self-soothing and solace, rather than being overly dependent on others to provide such support.

In some cases, however, these traits of invulnerability or resilience are not without their downside. For example, a special group of invulnerables comprise those who have rebounded from particularly high-risk developmental histories. They frequently begin life as frail, weak, and ailing infants. Despite this fragility, as they mature, these children gradually develop a seemingly implacable resolve not to cave in under the pressures of their lives, and demonstrate an extraordinary degree of persistence in their continuous struggles with adversity. In the service of survival, they can display a high degree of creativity, which, however, tends to be inner-directed and often agonizingly expressed. These are the "tortured artists" whose creative capacity to transform intolerable reality through fantasy may ultimately gain attention and recognition by the outside world. This may relieve them of their overwhelming sense of vulnerability, but they remain susceptible to bouts of depression.

On a more pedestrian level, they may find a quiet but satisfying niche for themselves that fits their capacities and provides them with absorbing vocations. Many of these children develop interests in science and technology to the relative neglect of intimate human relationships. Successful in their studies and work, they may be less able to sustain the kind of close relationships that are important in coping with such important role transitions of adulthood as marriage and parenthood (Anthony, 1987; Cohler, 1987).

However, most adaptive, resilient children don't have to go it alone. Many are lucky enough to have a nurturing home environment that reinforces and texturizes their own strong character traits. Murphy and Moriarty (1976) note that many of the parents of children who cope well are good copers themselves and provide models of resilience to their children. Parents who cope well have a distinctive profile: they enjoy their children, provide them with a holding and facilitating environment without stepping on their autonomy, support their efforts to care for themselves, furnish a reassuring background, and are highly receptive to the ideas and creative expressions developed by their children.

Of course, not all parents provide such a psychologically salubrious environment for their offspring. Some parents are frankly crazy, and most of these raise disturbed and distressed children. Yet, despite growing up in the presence of major parental psychopathology, some resilient children defy the odds and emerge relatively healthy. According to Cohler (1987), a fortunate minority of the children of psychiatrically ill parents are better able to cope with the adversity of unreliable and often emotionally inaccessible caretakers because they have greater innate ego strength, creative abilities, and increased personal and physical attractiveness. Such traits enable these children to continue to reach out successfully to others inside and outside the family for support. To the extent that their parents are able to provide basic care and assistance, these resilient children appear to be successful in engaging the parents. When a disturbed parent is not accessible, these children are able to seek out alternative providers of adult care, turning to such available adults as relatives, teachers, and family friends.

Similarly, Rutter (1985) has observed that children reared by seriously mentally ill parents may cope by separating themselves emotionally from their homes and developing their ties elsewhere. Others become resilient by taking on responsibilities for coping with stress in the family situation and doing so successfully. Developing a philosophy of life or a religious outlook may also be highly effective in fostering and supporting resilience. Very often these children find some charismatic or inspirational person who helps "turn them on" and sustain them, and the positive effects of this nurturing influence may be long-lasting (Anthony, 1987). Finally, these children tend to have greater intelligence and come from families higher in social status; these characteristics may foster increased instrumental mastery of more highly-developed social skills (Cohler, 1987).

Dahlin, Cederblad, Antonovsky, and Hagnell (1990) studied 148 Swedish adoptees with high-risk childhood backgrounds, defined as three or more psychiatric risk factors. Almost half of the sample managed to overcome their difficult backgrounds and succeed in creating a reasonably successful and at least moderately healthy life. By setting narrow expectations, by learning to live with realistic limitations and not to complain about what "can't be helped," a person can apparently achieve what he feels to be a satisfying sense of productivity, health, social relatedness, and well-being. The authors stress that the resilience of such individuals is by no means independent of social-environmental and historical circumstances. The generation represented in this study matured as the modern, postwar Swedish welfare state came into being. It is in this enabling context that at least some persons were able to overcome the high risks imposed by adverse childhoods—perhaps an important lesson for our own society.

THE STRESS RESPONSE, TRAUMATIC
DISABILITY, AND PSYCHOTHERAPY

Why *do* some children and adults cope with trauma so well, while others are undone by even minor stresses and hassles? As we've seen previously (Chapters 1, 3, 4, and 5), it's important to consider the neurophysiological, as well as the cognitive and psychodynamic, sides of the person-stress-disability equation.

One intriguing psychobiological model of stress and coping has been presented by Dienstbier (1989), who describes the trait variable of *toughness* as a buffer against the health-debilitating effects of stressful life events. Toughness is defined as a distinct reaction pattern to stress—mental or physical—that characterizes animals and humans who cope effectively.

According to Dienstbier (1989), two main neurohormonal systems mediate the toughness response. The first consists of a pathway from the hypothalamus in the brain to the sympathetic branch of the autonomic nervous system, and from there to the adrenal medulla. The sympathetic nervous system (SNS) mediates the physiologically aroused "fight-or-flight" response that mobilizes the body to deal with threats or challenges. As part of this response, the adrenal gland releases its main hormone, adrenaline.

The second toughness system also begins in the hypothalamus but acts through the pituitary gland, which in turn stimulates the adrenal cortex to release cortisol, the chief "stress hormone" involved in Selye's (1956) now-famous General Adaptation Syndrome (GAS) stress model. Together, the pattern of SNS-adrenal medulla and pituitary-adrenal cortex responses to stressful challenges defines the nature of the toughness trait.

Animal and human research has shown that the bodily response of individuals high in the toughness trait differs dramatically from that of individuals low in toughness. In tough subjects, the normal, baseline activity in the two systems is relatively low, indicating that tough organisms are at relative ease under ordinary circumstances. When faced with a stressful challenge or threat, the SNS-adrenal medulla system springs into action quickly and efficiently, while the pituitary-adrenal cortex system remains relatively stable. As soon as the emergency is over, the adrenaline reponse abates quickly to baseline, while the cortisol response remains low. It is thus the smoothness and efficiency of the physiological arousal pattern that characterizes the toughness response. This graded reaction, says Dienstbier (1989), has the important effect of forestalling depletion of the brain's catecholamine neurotransmitters, which mediate mood, motivation, and activity level.

By contrast, the physiological reaction of nontoughs tends to be more exaggerated and long-lasting; further, this reaction occurs not just to dire emergencies but to everyday hassles. The adrenaline rush is greater and stays higher longer, while cortisol levels are also elevated. The result is greater, more disorganizing arousal, less effective coping, and faster depletion of brain catecholamines, which can lead to helplessness and depression. In a vicious cycle, each unsettling tribulation causes the nontoughs to overreact and then crash, rendering them unable to take constructive action and thus leaving them with little confidence in their own ability to cope in the future.

This is where Dienstbier's (1989) conceptualization leaves room for therapeutic intervention. According to the model, the physiological toughness response—or its absence—interacts with a person's psychological appraisal of his own ability to cope with challenge. This in turn contributes to the person's self-image as an effective master of adversity or, alternatively, as a helpless reactor. Completing the cycle, this self-assessment then influences later physiological responses to stress.

In this conceptualization, the most effective place to intervene would be at the psychological level. Learning effective coping skills can render the physiological reaction of the two systems to threat or challenge less intense and more automatic. Instead of being immobilized by uncertainty or panic, for example, the person can be stimulated by the nervous system's appraisal of threat to seek out adaptive solutions. Once the individual gets used to coping effectively and confidence grows in his ability to deal with a widening range of situations, the two physiological response systems waste less effort in the face of each new threat or challenge. In this now-positive cycle, more efficient physiological stress responses lead to better coping, reinforcing greater ego autonomy, which in turn makes for an even smoother psychobiological response pattern next time, and so on (Dubovsky, 1997). The result is the development of true toughness—the ability to handle adversity adaptively.

In fact, the idea that certain people naturally cope better with adversity than others, and thereby suffer fewer ill-health effects, has been articulated in a number of ways and supported by several lines of research. Kobasa (1979, 1982) and Maddi (1990; Maddi & Kobasa, 1984) have proposed the personality construct of *hardiness* as a moderator in the stress-illness relationship. Hardiness is comprised of three main beliefs about the self and the world: (1) *commitment*: thinking of yourself and your environment as interesting and worthwhile and being able to find something contructive and meaningful in whatever you're doing; (2) *control*: believing that your own efforts can have an effect on what goes on around you; and (3) *challenge*: believing that what improves your life is growth through learning rather than easy comfort and security. In contrast, low levels of hardiness favor regressive coping styles and lead to feelings of alienation, powerlessness, and compulsive striving for an elusive state of comfort, security, and gain without risk.

Similarly, Antonovsky (1979, 1987, 1990) has proposed a stress/health-mediating personality construct termed *sense of coherence,* or SOC, which is expressed in the form of three component orientations or beliefs: (1) *comprehensibility*: that the events deriving from your internal and external environments in the course of living are structured, predictable, and explicable; (2) *manageability*: that you possess the resources to meet the demands posed by these events; and (3) *meaningfulness*: that these demands are challenges that are worthy of your investment and engagement. The higher a person's SOC, the better able he will be to clarify the nature of a particular stressor, select the resources appropriate to the specific situation, and be open to feedback that allows the adaptive modification of behavior.

Obviously, what all these bright and burly-sounding models ("toughness," "hardiness," "coherence") have in common is a conceptualization of adaptive coping as an active, dynamic process that requires a certain combination of inner resource mobilization and purposeful effort in the environment, not just a passive cultivation of low-arousal states as is currently promulgated in many biofeedback and relaxation programs for "stress management." In many cases, the latter might be seen as a form of regressive withdrawal and thus contribute to overall negative health outcomes if used exclusively as a coping strategy, to the neglect of responses that involve more active engagement with the environment. How many times have we wanted to shout at our patients: "Don't just sit there, relaxing—*do* something!" Thus, the impetus and capacity for constructive action and problem-solving—both functions of the ego-autonomous cognitive style—appear to be important in modulating the effects of stress on physical and mental health.

GROWTH: TRANSCENDENT COPING WITH STRESS AND TRAUMA

Some individuals do more than cope; like Billy, even in the face of seemingly crushing traumas, they seem to rise above their experience, learn from it, and become better people for it. Recently, clinical research has begun to address the nature of *transcendent posttraumatic coping* in the kinds of people that manage to stay out of our clinics and therapy offices.

Benezra (1996) studied the biographies of 40 people who have coped successfully with traumatic experiences without professional help. For example, one man lived through the riots of Krystalnacht at the beginning of the Nazi persecution; one woman was raped and robbed at gunpoint in her apartment; another woman was threatened with execution as a child in an enemy-occupied foreign village; yet another woman lost her family in a concentration camp; one man was an air traffic controller who lost contact with a plane that later crashed, resulting in his having to endure profound shame and ostracism.

In analyzing the responses of these survivors who coped with trauma on their own, Benezra (1996) noted a number of key themes. Transcendent copers described a healthy, secure upbringing characterized by a supportive relationship with their families, friends, and others. After the incident, they were able to either freely express and cathartically talk out their trauma or, alternatively, suppress and deny the traumatic experience, simply putting it out of their minds and moving on. They typically enjoyed favorable, restorative circumstances following the trauma. They did not "dwell on" the trauma. They characteristically lived hardworking, productive lifestyles with self-determination and self-reliance. They were able to accept and learn from the traumatic experience and face life's future challenges. They found a way to do for themselves and/ or for others what was needed but lacking. They described personal religious or philosophical faith and hope. They were not embittered or cynical but kept a sense of humor. They showed what Benezra (1996) describes as "biological endurance, compensation, and regulation"— apparently similar to Dienstbier's (1989) concept of "toughness."

McMillen, Smith, and Fisher (1997) studied the responses of survivors of three separate mass traumas: (1) the 1988 Madison, Florida, tornado; (2) the 1987 Indianapolis Ramada Inn plane crash; and (3) the 1991 Luby's Cafeteria mass shooting in Killeen, Texas. Survivors of these three disasters were interviewed four to six weeks after the incident and again three years later. Those survivors who perceived a benefit from the disaster at the initial interview were found to show significantly better posttraumatic adjustment three years later. The types of benefits included increased personal closeness with others, increased cohesion of the overall community, greater sense of personal growth, increased efficacy, and material gain.

Subjects who thought they were going to die were more likely to report personal growth as a perceived benefit of the trauma. Additionally, those with a higher number of preincident mental health diagnoses were more likely to report perceived benefit at follow-up. The researchers speculate that those subjects who had greater problems before the disaster and those who faced life-and-death situations may have been more likely to regard the event as their existential wake-up call and thus to reassess the meaning and purpose of their lives in the wake of the disaster.

After studying the positive, adaptive, transcendent responses to traumas of diverse types, including bereavement, sexual assault, and life-threatening illness, Tedeschi and Calhoun (1996) identified three broad categories of subjective benefits. The first was *perceived positive changes in self,* described in terms of "emotional growth," the trauma making the survivor a "better person" or leaving her feeling "more experienced about life." For example, the most common positive change reported by cancer patients was feeling stronger and more self-assured. It appears that living through life traumas provides a great deal of information about one's own self-reliance. Sometimes people surprise themselves. A feeling of mastery and competence in difficult situations increases the likelihood that one will address future difficulties in an assertive fashion. Persons successfully coping with a traumatic event often draw the conclusion that they are stronger than they thought they were, a confidence that may generalize to all kinds of future situations, traumatic or mundane.

A second perceived benefit of trauma was a *changed sense of relationship with others.* Some rape victims, for example, learned from their experience that they must make certain important decisions on their own behalf, such as protecting themselves from abuse, leading to more positive and intimate relationships with family members. From a psychotherapeutic perspective, the increased self-disclosure that comes from reflective discussion of traumatic events may provide an opportunity to try out new behaviors and access help from appropriate persons in the support network. The recognition of one's vulnerability can lead to more emotional expressiveness, willingness to accept help, and therefore a greater willingness to utilize social supports that had previously been ignored. Part of the positive development of social relationships comes from an increased overall empathy and sensitivity to other people and efforts directed at improving relationships.

The third benefit was a *changed philosophy of life.* This included an increased appreciation of the subjects' own existence, a "better perspective on life," taking life easier and enjoying it more. While for some, tragedy may weaken spiritual beliefs and contribute to growing cynicism, the struggle for understanding may eventually lead many other trauma survivors to a strengthening of their beliefs. This range of responses to trauma was seen in the study of survivors of the World Trade Center bombing (Difede, Apfeldorf, Cloitre, Spielman, & Perry, 1997; see Chapter 7). A secure feeling of cosmic backup can in turn contribute to an increased sense of control, intimacy, and meaning. Indeed, recognizing meaning in the midst of trauma and its aftermath may allow a much-needed breath of existential relief and can lead to a new or changed philosophy of life. The particular benefits described may even be elements of a developing wisdom (Aldwin, 1994; Baumeister, 1991; Janoff-Bulman, 1992; Tedeschi & Calhoun, 1996).

Helping patients to become less dependent and more autonomous, less impulsive and more reflective, less reactive and more resilient, less passive and more assertive, less egocentric and more responsible, less cynical and more hopeful—isn't this what we try to do in psychotherapy every day? Is it then any wonder that the traits of good mental health that we strive to inculcate in our patients are also the traits that offer protection from, and facilitate the healing of, traumas of all types? Just as vicious cycles occur in the neurophysiological and psychodynamic responses to trauma, can our earnestly and empathically applied therapeutic ministrations effect *positive cycles*, a gradual, progressive "kindling" of ego-autonomy? Do certain variations and adaptations of therapeutic technique work best with individuals of certain temperamental and cognitive styles? Are hope and transcendence teachable traits? How can we create more "Billy"-type success stories in the everyday clinical practice of trauma therapy?

Although most of these principles have been covered throughout this book, I offer the following summary list of recommendations for successful, and in the best cases, transcendent trauma therapy:

1. Listen to your patient's story and let it emerge at its own pace. As with a sluggish vehicle, you may have to jump-start the disclosure process or give it a little extra gas at some points, but avoid flooding the emotional engine or grinding the mental gears by gunning the motor when you should just let the car coast. Guide and influence the therapeutic process but don't push it or it may stall.

2. People are different. Assess and respect your patient's strengths and weaknesses in the cognitive, emotional, temperamental, and relational spheres. For example, some patients may truly process traumatic material more effectively with an intellectual approach, while for others it may just be a defensive evasion of feelings. Other patients may spew and purge, session after session, but avoid any real understanding of, or commitment to, learning how to move forward.

3. Utilize therapeutic strategies that encourage the use of reflection, planning, and active problem-solving. Teach your patient how to take care of himself and exert some control over his circumstances, whether by learning to get through a panic attack by deep breathing or dealing with hostile legal cross-examination by cognitive-

behavioral role-playing. Train for efficacy and encourage its general-ization to as many areas of the patient's life as possible.

4. Encourage healthy human relationships, but also guide your patient away from relationships that may be damaging for any number of reasons. Some patients almost naturally accept healing nourishment from other people's support, while others may be intimidated or disturbed by such interactions. Know your patient's interpersonal strengths and weaknesses, and guide him accordingly in how to "dose" his human interactions at different stages of recovery.

5. Help your patient find some meaning in what's happened to him. Careful here: remember my warning about therapeutic rescue fanta-sies. You don't have to "save" a patient in order to help him to pick up one thread of philosophical, religious, personal, or historical meaning that will enable him to begin weaving some fabric of hope. But you, the therapist, have to believe it to encourage it. Even a "screw-the-whole-world" stance may be a patient's provisionally adaptive way of coming to grips with the unfaceable. For the time being, accept that, unless and until something better can be discov-ered. Again, let the meaning come from the patient and take shape as an autonomous existential project that you and he work on together.

As our experience in understanding and treating traumatic disability syndromes grows, no doubt we'll continue to seek more comprehensive, refined, and clinically useful models of health and behavior. For the sakes of both intellectual honesty and clinical utility, we must always carefully consider the interaction of innate temperament and cognitive style with developmental and current interpersonal relationships in deter-mining the complex personal matrix that underlies the trauma response and guides its effective treatment in individual cases.

We already understand a great deal about the basic elements of human personality and psychotherapy, both generally and as they directly relate to the treatment of traumatic disability. Now we are entering a new century beckoning with possibilities but fraught with dangers—some we can anticipate, others we can scarcely imagine. Today's challenge for skilled, knowledgeable, and ethical trauma therapists is to clearheadedly continue to find creative ways of answering the call of helping our fellow human beings transcend the unendurable. For when we do our jobs well, what we offer the world is nothing less than the precious gift of hope and the blessing of a second chance.

REFERENCES

CHAPTER 1. THE TRAUMA SYNDROME

Alarcon, R.D., Deering, C.G., Glover, S.G., Ready, D.J., & Eddleman, H.C. (1997). Should there be a clinical typology of posttraumatic stress disorder? *Australian and New Zealand Journal of Psychiatry, 31*, 159–167.

Aldwin, C.M. (1994). *Stress, coping, and development: An integrative perspective.* New York: Guilford.

American Psychiatric Association (1980). *Diagnostic and statistical manual of mental disorders* (3rd ed.). Washington DC: Author.

American Psychiatric Association (1987). *Diagnostic and statistical manual of mental disorders* (3rd ed.-rev.) Washington DC: Author.

American Psychiatric Association (1994). *Diagnostic and statistical manual of mental disorders* (4th ed.). Washington DC: Author.

Barrett, D.H., Green, M.L., Morris, M.A.R., Giles, W.H., & Croft, J.B. (1996). Cognitive functioning and posttraumatic stress disorder. *American Journal of Psychiatry, 153*, 1492–1494.

Brom, D., & Kleber, R.J. (1989). Prevention of posttraumatic stress disorders. *Journal of Traumatic Stress, 2*, 335–351.

Charcot, J.M. (1887). *Lecons sur les maladies du system nerveux* (Vol. 3). Paris: Progress Medical.

Charney, D.S., Deutsch, A.Y., Krystal, J.H., Southwick, S.M., & Davis, M. (1993). Psychobiologic mechanisms of posttraumatic stress disorder. *Archives of General Psychiatry, 50*, 294–305.

Dietz, J. (1992). Self-psychological approach to posttraumatic stress disorder: Neurobiological aspects of transmuting internalization. *Journal of the American Academy of Psychoanalysis, 20*, 277–293.

Eitinger, L. (1965). *Concentration camp survivors in Norway and Israel.* New York: Humanities Press.

Eitinger, L. (1971). Acute and chronic psychiatric and psychosomatic reactions in concentration camp survivors. In L. Levi (Ed.), *Society, stress, and disease, Vol 1: Psychosocial, environmental, and psychosomatic disease* (pp. 219–230). New York: Oxford University Press.

Evans, R.W. (1992). The postconcussion syndrome and the sequelae of mild head injury. *Neurologic Clinics, 10*, 815–847.

Everly, G.S., & Horton, A.M. (1989). Neuropsychology of posttraumatic stress disorder: A pilot study. *Perceptual and Motor Skills, 68*, 807–810.

Everstine, D.S., & Everstine, L. (1993). *The trauma response: Treatment for emotional injury.* New York: Norton.

Ferenczi, S., Abraham, K., & Simmel, E. (1921). *Psychoanalysis and the war neuroses.* Vienna: International Psycho-Analysis Press.

Frazier, F., & Wilson, R.M. (1918). The sympathetic nervous system and the "irritable heart of soldiers." *British Medical Journal, 2,* 27–29.

Freud, S. (1920). *Beyond the pleasure principle.* In J. Strachey (Ed. & Trans.), *The standard edition of the complete psychological works of Sigmund Freud* (Vol. XVIII, pp. 7–64). New York: Norton.

Gill, T., Calev, A., Greenberg, D., Kugelmas, S., & Lerer, B. (1990). Cognitive functioning in posttraumatic stress disorder. *Journal of Traumatic Stress, 3,* 29–45.

Green, B.L. (1995). Recent research findings on the diagnosis of posttraumatic stress disorder: Prevalence, course, comorbidity, and risk. In R.I. Simon (Ed.), *Posttraumatic stress disorder in litigation: Guidelines for forensic assessment* (pp. 13–29). Washington, DC: American Psychiatric Press, Inc.

Kardiner, A. (1941). *The traumatic neuroses of war.* Washington, DC: National Research Council.

Knight, J.A. (1997). Neuropsychological assessment of posttraumatic stress disorder. In J.P. Wilson & T.E. Keane (Eds.), *Assessing psychological trauma and PTSD* (pp. 448–492). New York: Guilford Press.

Kolb, L.C. (1987). A neuropsychological hypothesis explaining posttraumatic stress disorders. *American Journal of Psychiatry, 144,* 989–995.

Kretschmer, E. (1926). *Hysteria.* New York: Basic Books.

Kuch, K. (1989). Treatment of post-traumatic phobias and PTSD after car accidents. In R.A. Keller & S.R. Heyman (Eds.), *Innovations in clinical practice: A source book* (Vol. 8, pp, 263–271). Sarasota, FL: Professional Resource Exchange.

Ludwig, A.M. (1972). Hysteria: A neurobiological theory. *Archives of General Psychiatry, 27,* 771–777.

Matsakis, A. (1994). *Post-traumatic stress disorder: A complete treatment guide.* Oakland, CA: New Harbinger.

McCann, I.L., & Pearlman, L.A. (1990). *Psychological trauma and the adult survivor: Theory, therapy, and transformation.* New York: Brunner/Mazel.

Mearburg, J.C., & Wilson, R.M. (1918). The effect of certain sensory stimulations on respiratory and heart rate in cases of so-called "irritable heart." *Heart, 7,* 17–22.

Meek, C.L. (1990). Evaluation and assessment of post-traumatic and other stress-related disorders. In C.L. Meek (Ed.), *Post-traumatic stress disorder: Assessment, differential diagnosis, and forensic evaluation* (pp. 9–61). Sarasota, FL: Professional Resource Exchange.

Merskey, H. (1992). Psychiatric aspects of the neurology of trauma. *Neurologic Clinics, 10,* 895–905.

Miller, L. (1991). *Freud's brain: Neuropsychodynamic foundations of psychoanalysis.* New York: Guilford.

Miller, L. (1993a). Psychotherapeutic approaches to chronic pain. *Psychotherapy, 30,* 115–124.

Miller, L. (1993b). The "trauma" of head trauma: Clinical, neuropsychological, and forensic aspects of posttraumatic stress syndromes in brain injury. *Journal of Cognitive Rehabilitation, 11*(4), 18–29.

Miller, L. (1993c). Toxic torts: Clinical, neuropsychological, and forensic aspects of chemical and electrical injuries. *Journal of Cognitive Rehabilitation, 11*(1), 6–20.

Miller, L. (1994). Civilian posttraumatic stress disorder: Clinical syndromes and psychotherapeutic strategies. *Psychotherapy, 31,* 655–664.

Miller, L. (1995). Toxic trauma and chemical sensitivity: Clinical syndromes and psychotherapeutic strategies. *Psychotherapy, 32,* 648–656.

Miller, L. (1997). Neurosensitization: A pathophysiological model for traumatic disability syndromes. *Journal of Cognitive Rehabilitation, 15*(6), 2–19.

Modlin, H.C. (1983). Traumatic neurosis and other injuries. *Psychiatric Clinics of North America, 6,* 661–682.

Muran, E.M., & Motta, R.W. (1993). Cognitive distortions and irrational beliefs in post-traumatic stress, anxiety, and depressive disorders. *Journal of Clinical Psychiatry, 49*, 166–176.

Oppenheim, H. (1890). Tatsächliches und hypthothetisches über das wesen der hysterie. *Berlin Klinik Wschr, 27*, 553.

Parker, R.S. (1990). *Traumatic brain injury and neuropsychological impairment: Sensori-motor, cognitive, emotional, and adaptive problems in children and adults.* New York: Springer-Verlag.

Pavlov, I.P. (1927). *Conditioned reflexes: An investigation of the physiological activity of the cerebral cortex.* New York: Oxford University Press.

Rosen, G. (1975). Nostalgia: A forgotten psychological disorder. *Psychosomatic Medicine, 5*, 342–347.

Sapolsky, R.M., Krey, L.C., & McEwen, B.S. (1984). Glucocorticoid-sensitive hippo-campal neurons are involved in terminating the adrenocortical stress response. *Proceedings of the National Academy of Sciences, 81*, 6174–6177.

Shapiro, F. (1995). *Eye movement desensitization and reprocessing.* New York: Guilford.

Simon, R.I. (1995). Toward the development of guidelines in the forensic psychiatric examination of posttraumatic stress disorder. In R.I. Simon (Ed.), *Posttraumatic stress disorder in litigation* (pp. 31–84). Washington DC: American Psychiatric Press.

Southard, E. (1919). *Shell-shock and other neuropsychiatric problems.* Boston: Leonard.

Stein, M.B., Walker, J.R., Hazen, A.L., & Forde, D.R. (1997). Full and partial posttrau-matic stress disorder: Findings from a community survey. *American Journal of Psychiatry, 154*, 1114–1119.

Thompson, S.C. (1981). Will it hurt less if I can control it? A complex answer to a simple question. *Psychological Bulletin, 90*, 89–101.

Trimble, M.R. (1981). *Post-traumatic neurosis: From railway spine to whiplash.* New York: Wiley.

Weiner, H. (1992). *Perturbing the organism: The biology of stressful experience.* Chicago: University of Chicago Press.

Wilson, J.P. (1994). The historical evolution of PTSD diagnostic criteria: From Freud to DSM-IV. *Journal of Traumatic Stress, 7*, 681–698.

CHAPTER 2. PSYCHOTHERAPY OF PTSD

Allen, J.G., & Lewis, L. (1996). A conceptual framework for treating traumatic memo-ries and its application to EMDR. *Bulletin of the Menninger Clinic, 60*, 238–263.

Allen, S.N., & Bloom, S.L. (1994). Group and family treatment of post-traumatic stress disorder. *Psychiatric Clinics of North America, 17*, 425–437.

Bennett, T.L. (1988). Post-traumatic headaches: Subtypes and behavioral treatments. *Cognitive Rehabilitation, 6*(2), 34–39.

Brom, D., & Kleber, R.J. (1989). Prevention of posttraumatic stress disorders. *Journal of Traumatic Stress, 2*, 335–351.

Brom, D., Kleber, R.J., & Defares, P.B. (1989). Brief psychotherapy for posttraumatic stress disorder. *Journal of Consulting and Clinical Psychology, 57*, 607–612.

Cooper, N.A., & Clum, G.A. (1989). Imaginal flooding as a supplementary treatment for PTSD in combat veterans: A controlled study. *Behavior Therapy, 20*, 381–391.

Cowley, G., & Biddle, N.A. (1994). Waving away the pain. *Newsweek*, June 20, pp. 70–71.

Decker, L.R. (1993). The role of trauma in spiritual development. *Journal of Humanistic Psychology, 33*, 33–46.

Everly, G.S. (1990). PTSD as a disorder of arousal. *Psychology and Health: An Interna-tional Journal, 4*, 135–145.

Everly, G.S. (1993). Psychotraumatology: A two-factor formulation of posttraumatic stress. *Integrative Physiological and Behavioral Science, 28*, 270–278.

Everly, G.S. (1994). Short-term psychotherapy of acute adult onset post-traumatic stress. *Stress Medicine, 10,* 191–196.

Everly, G.S. (1995). The neurocognitive therapy of post-traumatic stress: A strategic metatherapeutic approach. In G.S. Everly & J.M. Lating (Eds.), *Psychotraumatology: Key papers and core concepts in post-traumatic stress* (pp. 159–169). New York: Plenum.

Everstine, D.S., & Everstine, L. (1993). *The trauma response: Treatment for emotional injury.* New York: Norton.

Figley, C.R. (1988). Post-traumatic family therapy. In F.M. Ochberg (Ed.), *Post-traumatic therapy and victims of violence* (pp. 83–109). New York: Brunner/Mazel.

Figley, C.R. (1989). *Helping traumatized families.* San Francisco: Jossey-Bass.

Gilliland, B.E., & James, R.K. (1993). *Crisis intervention strategies* (2nd ed.) Pacific Grove, CA: Brooks/Cole.

Horowitz, M.J. (1986). *Stress response syndromes* (2nd ed.). Northvale, NJ: Aronson.

Keane, T.M., Fairbank, J.A., Caddell, J.M., & Zimmerling, R.T. (1989). Implosive (flooding) therapy reduces symptoms of PTSD in Vietnam combat veterans: A controlled study. *Behavior Therapy, 20,* 245–260.

Lazarus, A.A., & Mayne, T.J. (1990). Relaxation: Some limitations, side effects, and proposed solutions. *Psychotherapy, 27,* 261–266.

Marano, H.E. (1994). Wave of the future. *Psychology Today,* August, pp. 22–25.

Matsakis, A. (1994). *Post-traumatic stress disorder: A complete treatment guide.* Oakland, CA: New Harbinger.

McCann, D.L. (1992). Post-traumatic stress disorder due to devastating burns overcome by a single session of eye movement desensitization. *Journal of Behavior Therapy and Experimental Psychiatry, 23,* 319–323.

McCann, I.L., & Pearlman, L.A. (1990). *Psychological trauma and the adult survivor: Theory, therapy, and transformation.* New York: Brunner/Mazel.

Meichenbaum, D. (1994). *A clinical handbook/practical therapist manual for assessing and treating adults with PTSD.* Waterloo: Author.

Miller, L. (1990). Chronic pain complicating head injury recovery: Recommendations for clinicians. *Cognitive Rehabilitation, 8*(5), 12–19.

Miller, L. (1993a). Who are the best psychotherapists? Qualities of the effective practitioner. *Psychotherapy in Private Practice, 12*(1), 1–18.

Miller, L. (1993b). *Psychotherapy of the brain-injured patient; Reclaiming the shattered self.* New York: Norton.

Miller, L. (1994a). Biofeedback and behavioral medicine: Treating the symptom, the syndrome, or the person? *Psychotherapy, 31,* 161–169.

Miller, L. (1994b). Civilian posttraumatic stress disorder: Clinical syndromes and psychotherapeutic strategies. *Psychotherapy, 31,* 655–664.

Modlin, H.C. (1983). Traumatic neurosis and other injuries. *Psychiatric Clinics of North America, 6,* 661–682.

Shalev, A.Y., Galai, T., & Eth, S. (1993a). Levels of trauma: A multidimensional approach to the treatment of PTSD. *Psychiatry, 56,* 166–177.

Shalev, A.Y., Schreiber, S., Galai, T., & Melmed, R.N. (1993b). Post-traumatic stress disorder following medical events. *British Journal of Clinical Psychology, 32,* 247–253.

Thompson, J. (1992). Stress theory and therapeutic practice. *Stress Medicine, 8,* 147–150.

Yalom, I.D. (1980). *Existential psychotherapy.* New York: Basic Books.

CHAPTER 3. THE POSTCONCUSSION SYNDROME

Andrasik, F., & Wincze, J.P. (1994). Emotional and psychosocial aspects of mild head injury. *Seminars in Neurology, 14,* 60–66.

Baumeister, R.F. (1991). *Meanings of life.* New York: Guilford.

Bennett, T.L. (1987). Neuropsychological counseling of the adult with minor head injury. *Cognitive Rehabilitation, 5*(1), 10–16.

Bennett, T.L. (1989). Individual psychotherapy and minor head injury. *Cognitive Rehabilitation, 7*, 20–25.

Ben-Yishay, Y., & Diller, L. (1983). Cognitive rehabilitation. In E.A. Griffith, M. Bond, & J. Miller (Eds.), *Rehabilitation of the head injured adult*. Philadelphia: F.A. Davis.

Binder, L.M. (1986). Persisting symptoms after mild head injury: A review of the postconcussive syndrome. *Journal of Clinical and Experimental Neuropsychology, 8*, 323–346.

Brooks, N. (1995). Comment. *Neurolaw Letter, 4*(9), 5.

Brooks, N., Campsie, L., & Symington, C. (1986). The five-year outcome of severe blunt head injury: A relative's view. *Journal of Neurology, Neurosurgery, and Psychiatry, 49*, 764–770.

Bryant, R.A. (1996). Posttraumatic stress disorder, flashbacks, and pseudomemories in closed-head injury. *Journal of Traumatic Stress, 9*, 621–629.

Bryant, R.A., & Harvey, A.G. (1995). Posttraumatic stress: A comparison of head-injured and non-head-injured patients. *Psychological Medicine, 25*, 869–874.

Cajal, S.R. (1928). *Degeneration and regeneration of the nervous system*. Oxford: Oxford University Press.

Carberry, H., & Burd, B. (1986). Individual psychotherapy with the brain-injured adult. *Cognitive Rehabilitation, 4*, 22–24.

Christman, C.W., Grady, M.S., Walker, S.A., Holloway, K.L., & Povlishock, J.T. (1994). Ultrastructural studies of diffuse axonal injury in humans. *Journal of Neurotrauma, 11*, 173–186.

Cicerone, K.D. (1989). Psychotherapeutic interventions with traumatically brain-injured patients. *Rehabilitation Psychology, 34*, 105–114.

Davidoff, D.A., Kessler, H.R., Laibstain, D.F., & Mark, V.R. (1988). Neurobehavioral sequelae of minor head injury: A consideration of post-concussive syndrome versus post-traumatic stress disorder. *Cognitive Rehabilitation, 6*(2), 8–13.

Elson, L.M., & Ward, C.C. (1994). Mechanisms and pathophysiology of mild head injury. *Seminars in Neurology, 14*, 8–18.

Erb, D.E., & Povlishock, J.T. (1991). Neuroplasticity following traumatic brain injury: A study of GABAergic terminal loss and recovery in the cat dorsal lateral vestibular nucleus. *Experimental Brain Research, 83*, 253–267.

Evans, R.W. (1992). The postconcussional syndrome and the sequelae of mild head injury. *Neurologic Clinics, 10*, 815–847.

Forrest, D.V. (1987). Psychosocial treatment in neuropsychiatry. In R.E. Hales & S.C. Yudofsky (Eds.), *American Psychiatric Press textbook of neuropsychiatry* (pp. 387–409). Washington, DC: American Psychiatric Press, Inc.

Gama, J.H.P. (1835). *Traite des plaies de tete et de l'encephalite*. Paris.

Gennarelli, T.A. (1993). Mechanisms of brain injury. *Journal of Emergency Medicine, 11*, 5–11.

Gouvier, W.D., Cubic, B., Jones, G., Brantly, P., & Cutlip, Q. (1992). Postconcussion symptoms and daily stress in normal and head-injured college populations. *Archives of Clinical Neuropsychology, 7*, 193–211.

Hayes, R.L., Povlishock, J.T., & Singhe, B. (1992). Pathophysiology of mild head injury. *Physical Medicine and Rehabilitation, 6*, 9–20.

Heilman, K.M., Bowers, D., Valenstein, E., & Watson, R.T. (1986). The right hemisphere: Neuropsychological functions. *Journal of Neurosurgery, 64*, 693–704.

Jeste, D.V., Lohr, J.B., & Goodwin, F.K. (1988). Neuroanatomical studies of major affective disorders: A review and suggestions for further research. *British Journal of Psychiatry, 153*, 444–459.

Kwentus, J., Hart, R., Peck, E., & Kornstein, S. (1985). Psychiatric complications of closed head trauma. *Psychosomatics, 26*, 8–17.

Layton, B.S., & Ward-Zonna, K. (1995). Posttraumatic stress disorder with neurogenic amnesia for the traumatic event. *Clinical Neuropsychologist, 9*, 2–10.

Levin, H.S. (1990). Pioneers in research on the behavioral sequelae of head injury. *Journal of Clinical and Experimental Neuropsychology, 13*, 1–22.

Lewis, L., & Rosenberg, S.J. (1990). Psychoanalytic psychotherapy with brain-injured adult psychiatric patients. *Journal of Nervous and Mental Disease, 178*, 69–77.

Lishman, W.A. (1973). The psychiatric sequelae of head injury: A review. *Psychological Medicine, 3*, 304–318.

MacMillan, T.M. (1991). Post-traumatic stress disorder and severe head injury. *British Journal of Psychiatry, 159*, 431–433.

Miller, L. (1990a). Neurobehavioral syndromes and the private practitioner: An introduction to evaluation and treatment. *Psychotherapy in Private Practice, 8*(3), 1–12.

Miller, L. (1990b). *Inner natures: Brain, self, and personality.* New York: St. Martin.

Miller, L. (1991a). Psychotherapy of the brain-injured patient: Principles and practices. *Journal of Cognitive Rehabilitation, 9*(2), 24–30.

Miller, L. (1991b). Significant others: Treating brain injury in the family context. *Journal of Cognitive Rehabilitation, 9*(3), 16–25.

Miller, L. (1991c). The "other" brain injuries: Psychotherapeutic issues with stroke and brain tumor patients. *Journal of Cognitive Rehabilitation, 9*(5), 10–16.

Miller, L. (1992a). The primitive personality and the organic personality: A neuropsychodynamic model for evaluation and treatment. *Psychoanalytic Psychology, 9*, 93–109.

Miller, L. (1992b). Cognitive rehabilitation, cognitive therapy, and cognitive style: Toward an integrative model of personality and psychotherapy. *Journal of Cognitive Rehabilitation, 10*(1), 18–29.

Miller, L. (1992c). Back to the future: Legal, vocational, and quality-of-life issues in the long-term adjustment of the brain-injured patient. *Journal of Cognitive Rehabilitation, 10*(5), 14–20.

Miller, L. (1992d). When the best help is self-help, or: Everything you always wanted to know about brain injury support groups. *Journal of Cognitive Rehabilitation, 10*(6), 14–17.

Miller, L. (1993a). Who are the best psychotherapists? Qualities of the effective practitioner. *Psychotherapy in Private Practice, 12*(1), 1–18.

Miller, L. (1993b). Family therapy of brain injury: Syndromes, strategies, and solutions. *American Journal of Family Therapy, 21*, 111–121.

Miller, L. (1993c). *Psychotherapy of the brain-injured patient: Reclaiming the shattered self.* New York: Norton.

Miller, L. (1993d). The "trauma" of head trauma: Clinical, neuropsychological, and forensic aspects of posttraumatic stress syndromes in brain injury. *Journal of Cognitive Rehabilitation, 11*(4), 18–29.

Miller, L. (1993e). Psychotherapeutic approaches to chronic pain. *Psychotherapy, 30*, 115–124.

Miller, L. (1994a). Sex and the brain-injured patient: Regaining love, pleasure, and intimacy. *Journal of Cognitive Rehabilitation, 12*(3), 12–20.

Miller, L. (1994b). Unusual head injury syndromes: Clinical, neuropsychological, and forensic considerations. *Journal of Cognitive Rehabilitation, 12*(6), 12–22.

Miller, L. (1996). Neuropsychology and pathophysiology of mild head injury and the postconcussion syndrome: Clinical and forensic considerations. *Journal of Cognitive Rehabilitation, 14*(1), 8–23.

Miller, L. (1997a, January). Typical and atypical postconcussion syndromes: Making clinical and forensic sense. *Neurolaw Letter*, 109–116.

Miller, L. (1997b). Neurosensitization: A pathophysiological model for traumatic disability syndromes. *Journal of Cognitive Rehabilitation, 15*(6), 2–19.

Miller, L. (1998). A conceptual history of psychotherapy with neuropsychologically impaired patients: Cognitive rehabilitation, psychodynamics, and cognitive style. In K.G. Langer, L. Laatsch & L. Lewis (Eds.), *Psychotherapy of the patient with neuropsychological impairment: A clinician's treatment resource.* New York: Psychosocial Press.

Nadell, J. (1991). Towards an existential psychotherapy with the traumatically brain-injured patient. *Journal of Cognitive Rehabilitation, 9*(6), 8–13.

Novack, T.A., Roth, D.L., & Boll, T.J. (1988). Treatment alternatives following mild head injury. *Rehabilitation Counseling Bulletin, 31,* 313–324.

Oppenheimer, D.R. (1968). Microscopic lesions in the brain following head injury. *Journal of Neurology, Neurosurgery, and Psychiatry, 31,* 299–306.

Packard, R.C. (1993). Mild head injury. *Headache Quarterly, 4,* 42–52.

Parente, R., & Herrmann, D. (1996). *Retraining cognition: Techniques and applications.* Gaithersburg, MD: Aspen.

Parker, R.S. (1990). *Traumatic brain injury and neuropsychological impairment: Sensorimotor, cognitive, emotional, and adaptive problems in children and adults.* New York: Springer-Verlag.

Pilowsky, I. (1985). Cryptotrauma and "accident neurosis." *British Journal of Psychiatry, 147,* 310–311.

Pilowsky, I. (1992). Minor accidents and major psychological trauma: A clinical perspective. *Stress Medicine, 8,* 77–78.

Povlishock, J.T. (1992). Traumatically induced axonal injury: Pathogenesis and pathological implications. *Brain Pathology, 2,* 1–12.

Prigatano, G.P., Fordyce, D.J., Zeiner, H.K., Roueche, J.R., Pepping, M., & Wood, B.C. (1986). *Neuropsychological rehabilitation after brain injury,* Baltimore: Johns Hopkins University Press.

Ranseen, J.D. (1990). Positive personality change following traumatic head injury: Four case studies. *Cognitive Rehabilitation, 8*(2), 8–12.

Sbordone, R.J. (1992). Distinguishing traumatic brain injury from posttraumatic stress disorder. *Neurolaw Letter, 1*(9), 3.

Shalev, A.Y. (1992). Post-traumatic stress disorder among injured survivors of a terrorist attack. *Journal of Mental Disease, 180,* 505–509.

Slagle, D.A. (1990). Psychiatric disorders following closed head injury: An overview of biopsychosocial factors in their etiology and management. *International Journal of Psychiatry in Medicine, 20,* 1–35.

Small, L. (1980). *Neuropsychodiagnosis in psychotherapy* (rev. ed.). New York: Brunner/Mazel.

Smith, L.M., & Godfrey, H.P.D. (1995). *Family support programs and rehabilitation: A cognitive-behavioral approach to traumatic brain injury.* New York: Plenum Press.

Strauss, I., & Savitsky, N. (1934). Head injury: Neurologic and psychiatric aspects. *Archives of Neurology and Psychiatry, 31,* 893–954.

Strich, S.J. (1956). Diffuse degeneration of the cerebral white matter in severe dementia following head injury. *Journal of Neurology, Neurosurgery, and Psychiatry, 19,* 163–185.

Strich, S.J. (1961). Shearing of nerve fibers as a cause of brain damage due to head injury. *Lancet, 2,* 443–448.

Stuss, D.T., & Benson, D.F. (1984). Neuropsychological studies of the frontal lobes. *Psychological Bulletin, 95,* 3–28.

Stuss, D.T., Gow, C.A., & Hetherington, C.R. (1992). "No longer Gage": Frontal lobe dysfunction and emotional changes. *Journal of Consulting and Clinical Psychology, 60,* 349–359.

Swinton, J. (1997). Restoring the image: Spirituality, faith, and cognitive disability. *Journal of Religion and Health, 36,* 21–27.

Taylor, J.S. (1996). Neurorehabilitation and neurolaw. *NeuroRehabilitation, 7,* 3–14.

Tyerman, A.D., & Humphrey, M. (1984). Changes in self-concept following severe head injury. *International Journal of Rehabilitation Research, 7,* 11–23.

Wright, J.C., & Telford, R. (1996). Psychological problems following minor head injury: A prospective study. *British Journal of Clinical Psychology, 35,* 399–412.

Yalom, I. (1980). *Existential Psychotherapy.* New York: Basic Books.

Zasler, N.D. (1995). Zasler comments. *Neurolaw Letter, 4*(10), 4.

CHAPTER 4. CHRONIC PAIN

Alarcon, R.D., Deering, C.G., Glover, S.G., Ready, D.J., & Eddleman, H.C. (1997). Should there be a clinical typology of posttraumatic stress disorder? *Australian and new Zealand Journal of Psychiatry, 31,* 159–167.

American Psychiatric Association (1980). *Diagnostic and Statistical Manual of Mental Disorders* (3rd ed.). Washington, DC: Author.

American Psychiatric Association (1987). *Diagnostic and Statistical Manual of Mental Disorders* (3rd ed.-rev.). Washington, DC: Author.

American Psychiatric Association (1994). *Diagnostic and Statistical Manual of Mental Disorders* (4th ed.). Washington, DC: Author.

Balla, J.I., & Moraitis, S. (1970). Knights in armour: A follow-up study of injuries after legal settlement. *Medical Journal of Australia, 2,* 355–361.

Benjamin, S. (1989). Psychological treatment of chronic pain: A selective review. *Journal of Psychosomatic Research, 33,* 121–131.

Benjamin, S., Barnes, D., Berger, S., Clarke, I., & Jeacock, J. (1988). The relationship of chronic pain, mental illness and organic disorder. *Pain, 32,* 185–195.

Blumer, D., & Heilbronn, M. (1981). The pain-prone disorder: A clinical and psychological profile. *Psychosomatics, 22,* 395–402.

Braha, R., & Catchlove, R. (1986). Pain and anger: Inadequate expression in chronic pain patients. *Pain Clinics, 1,* 125–129.

Breuer, J., & Freud, S. (1895). *Studies on hysteria.* In J. Strachey (Ed. & Trans.), *The standard edition of the complete psychological works of Sigmund Freud* (Vol. II). New York: Norton.

Butler, S. (1984). Present status of tricyclic antidepressants in chronic pain therapy. In C. Benedetti, C.R. Chapman, & G. Moricca (Eds.), *Advances in pain research and therapy* (Vol. 7, pp. 173–197). New York: Raven Press.

Coen, S.J., & Sarno, J.E. (1989). Psychosomatic avoidance of conflict in back pain. *Journal of the American Academy of Psychoanalysis, 17,* 359–376.

Coderre, T.J., Katz, J., Vaccarino, A.L., & Melzack, R. (1993). Contribution of central neuroplasticity to pathological pain: Review of clinical and experimental evidence. *Pain, 52,* 259–285.

Crook, J., Tunks, E., Kalaher, S., & Roberts, J. (1988). Coping with persistent pain: A comparison of persistent pain sufferers in a specialty pain clinic and in a family practice clinic. *Pain, 34,* 175–184.

Davis, G.C., & Breslau, N. (1994). Post-traumatic stress disorder in victims of civilian trauma and criminal assault. *Psychiatric Clinics of North America, 17,* 289–299.

Delapaine, R., Ifabamuyi, O.I., Merskey, H., & Zarfas, J. (1978). Significance of pain in psychiatric hospital patients. *Pain, 4,* 361–366.

Doleys, D.M., Crocker, M., & Patton, D. (1982). Response of patients with chronic pain to exercise quotas. *Physical Therapy, 62,* 1111–1114.

Dorsel, T.N. (1989). Chronic pain behavior pattern: A simple theoretical framework for healthcare providers. *Psychological Reports, 65,* 783–786.

Draspa, L.J. (1959). Psychological factors in muscular pain. *British Journal of Medical Psychology, 32,* 106–116.

Dufton, B.D. (1989). Cognitive failure and chronic pain. *International Journal of Psychiatry in Medicine, 19,* 291–297.

Encel, S., & Johnson, C.E. (1978). *Compensation and rehabilitation.* Kensington, Australia: New South Wales University Press.

Fernandez, E., & Turk, D.C. (1995). The scope and significance of anger in the experience of chronic pain. *Pain, 61,* 165–175.

Fishbain, D., Goldberg, M., Meagher, B.R., Steele, R., & Rosomoff, H. (1986). Male and female chronic pain patients categorized by DSM-III psychiatric diagnostic criteria. *Pain, 26,* 181–197.

Flor, H., Birbaumer, N., & Turk, D.C. (1990). The psychobiology of chronic pain. *Advances in Behavior Research and Therapy, 12,* 47–84.

Flor, H., Kerns, R.D., & Turk, D.C. (1987). The role of spouse reinforcement, perceived pain and activity levels of chronic pain patients. *Journal of Psychosomatic Research, 31,* 251–259.

Ford, C.V. (1977-78). A type of disability neurosis: The Humpty-Dumpty syndrome. *International Journal of Psychiatry in Medicine, 8,* 285–294.

Fordyce, W.E., Brockway, J.A., Bergman, J.A., & Spengler, D. (1986). Acute back pain: A control-group comparison of behavioral vs. traditional management methods. *Journal of Behavioral Medicine, 9,* 127–140.

Fordyce, W.E., Fowler, R.S., Lehman, J.F., Delateur, B.J., Sand, P.L., & Trieschmann, R.B. (1973). Operant conditioning in the treatment of chronic pain. *Archives of Physical Medicine and Rehabilitation, 54,* 399–408.

Fordyce, W.E., Roberts, A.H., & Sternbach, R.A. (1985). The behavioral management of chronic pain: A response to critics. *Pain, 22,* 113–125.

Funch, D.P., & Gale, E.N. (1986). Predicting treatment completion in a behavioral therapy program for chronic temporomandibular pain. *Journal of Psychosomatic Research, 30,* 57–62.

Gallagher, E.B. (1976). Lines of extension and reconstruction in the Parsonian sociology of illness. *Social Science and Medicine, 10,* 207–218.

Geisser, M.E., Gaskin, M.E., Robinson, M.E., & Greene, A.F. (1993). The relationship of depression and somatic focus to experimental and clinical pain in chronic pain patients. *Psychology and Health, 8,* 405–415.

Geisser, M.E., Roth, R.S., Bachman, J.E., & Eckert, T.A. (1996). The relationship between symptoms of post-traumatic stress disorder and pain, affective disturbance, and disability among patients with accident and non-accident related pain. *Pain, 66,* 207–214.

Gil, K.M., Keefe, F.J., Crisson, J.E., & Van Dalfsen, P.J. (1987). Social support and pain behavior. *Pain, 29,* 209–217.

Gotten, N. (1956). Survey of one hundred cases of whiplash injury after settlement of litigation. *Journal of the American Medical Association, 162,* 865–867.

Hanson, R.W., & Gerber, K.E. (1990). *Coping with chronic pain: A guide to patient self-management.* New York: Guilford.

Helzer, J.E., Robins, L.N., & McEnvoi, L. (1987). Post-traumatic stress disorder in the general population. *New England Journal of Medicine, 317,* 1630–1634.

Hendler, N. (1982). The anatomy and psychopharmacology of chronic pain. *Journal of Clinical Psychiatry, 43,* 15–20.

Heynemann, N.E., Fremouw, W.J., Gano, D., Kirkland, F., & Heiden, L. (1990). Individual differences and the effectiveness of different coping strategies for pain. *Cognitive Therapy and Research, 14,* 63–77.

Hohl, M. (1974). Soft-tissue injuries of the neck in automobile accidents. *Journal of Bone and Joint Surgery, 56A,* 1675–1682.

Hughes, A.M., Medley, I., Turner, G.N., & Bond, M.R. (1987). Psychogenic pain: A study in marital adjustment. *Acta Psychiatrica Scandinavica, 75,* 166–170.

Keefe, F.J., & Williams, D.A. (1989). New directions in pain assessment and treatment. *Clinical Psychology Review, 9,* 549–568.

Kellner, R. (1986). *Somatization and hypochondriasis.* New York: Praeger.

Kendall, P.C., & Watson, D. (1981). Psychological preparations for stressful medical procedures. In C.K. Prokop & L.A. Bradley (Eds.), *Medical psychology: Contributions to behavioral medicine.* New York: Academic Press.

Kerns, R.D., Rosenberg, R., & Jacob, M.C. (1994). Anger expression and chronic pain. *Journal of Behavioral Medicine, 17,* 57–67.

Kores, R., Murphy, W.D., Rosenthal, T., Elias, D., & Rosenthal, R. (1985). *Self-efficacy scale to predict outcome in chronic pain treatment.* Paper presented at the annual meeting of the Society of Behavioral Medicine, New Orleans, LA.

Kramlinger, K.G., Swanson, D.W., & Maruta, T. (1983). Are patients with chronic pain depressed? *American Journal of Psychiatry, 140,* 747–749.

Krishnan, R.R.K., France, R.D., Pelton, S., McCann, U.D., Davidson, J., & Urban, B.J. (1985). Chronic pain and depression. I. Classification of depression in chronic low back pain patients. *Pain, 22,* 279–287.

Kuch, K., Evans, R.J., Watson, P.C., & Bubela, C. (1991). Road vehicle accidents and phobias in 60 patients with fibromyalgia. *Journal of Anxiety Disorders, 5,* 273–280.

Lefebvre, M.F. (1981). Cognitive distortion and cognitive errors in depressed psychiatric and low back pain patients. *Journal of Consulting and Clinical Psychology, 49,* 517–525.

Lazarus, A.A., & Mayne, T.J. (1990). Relaxation: Some limitations, side effects, and proposed solutions. *Psychotherapy, 27,* 261–266.

Linton, S.J. (1982). A critical review of behavioral treatments for chronic benign pain other than headache. *British Journal of Clinical Psychology, 21,* 321–337.

Linton, S.J., & Gotestam, K.G. (1983). A clinical comparison of two pain scales: Correlation, remembering chronic pain and a measure of compliance. *Pain, 17,* 57–66.

Linton, S.J., Melin, L., & Stjernlof, K. (1985). The effects of applied relaxation and operant activity training on chronic pain. *Behavioral Psychotherapy, 13,* 87–100.

Matheson, L.N. (1988). Symptom magnification syndrome. In S.J. Isernhagen (Ed.), *Work injury: Management and prevention* (pp. 257–282). Gaithersburg, MD: Aspen.

McNab, I. (1964). Acceleration injuries of the cervical spine. *Journal of Joint and Bone Surgery, 46A,* 1797–1799.

Mechanic, D., & Angel, R.J. (1987). Some factors associated with the report and evaluation of back pain. *Journal of Health and Social Behavior, 28,* 131–139.

Mendelson, G. (1982). Not "cured by a verdict." Effect of legal settlement on compensation claimants. *Medical Journal of Australia, 2,* 132–134.

Merskey, H. (1980). The role of the psychiatrist in the investigation and treatment of pain. *Pain, 8,* 249–260.

Merskey, H., & Buhrich, N.A. (1975). Hysteria and organic brain disease. *British Journal of Medical Psychology, 48,* 359–366.

Miller, H. (1961a). Accident neurosis (lecture 1). *British Medical Journal, 1,* 919–925.

Miller, H. (1961b). Accident neurosis (lecture 2). *British Medical Journal, 1,* 992–998.

Miller, L. (1984). Neuropsychological concepts of somatoform disorders. *International Journal of Psychiatry in Medicine, 14,* 31–46.

Miller, L. (1990). Chronic pain complicating head injury recovery: Recommendations for clinicians. *Cognitive Rehabilitation, 8*(5), 12–19.

Miller, L. (1991a). Predicting relapse and recovery in alcoholism and addiction: Neuropsychology, personality, and cognitive style. *Journal of Substance Abuse Treatment, 8,* 277–291.

Miller, L. (1991b). Psychotherapy of the chronic pain patient: I. Clinical syndromes and sources. *Psychotherapy in Private Practice, 9*(4), 109–125.

Miller, L. (1992a). Psychotherapy of the chronic pain patient: II. Treatment principles and practices. *Psychotherapy in Private Practice, 11*(1), 69–82.

Miller, L. (1992b). Neuropsychology, personality, and substance abuse in the head injury case: Clinical and forensic issues. *International Journal of Law and Psychiatry, 15,* 303–316.

Miller, L. (1993a). Psychotherapeutic approaches to chronic pain. *Psychotherapy, 30,* 115–124.

Miller, L. (1993b). The "trauma" of head trauma: Clinical, neuropsychological, and forensic aspects of posttraumatic stress syndromes in brain injury. *Journal of Cognitive Rehabilitation, 11*(4), 18–29.

Miller, L. (1993c). Family therapy of brain injury: Syndromes, strategies, and solutions. *American Journal of Family Therapy, 21,* 111–121.

Miller, L. (1993d). *Psychotherapy of the brain-injured patient: Reclaiming the shattered self.* New York: Norton.

Miller, L. (1994). Biofeedback and behavioral medicine: Treating the symptom, the syndrome, or the person? *Psychotherapy, 31,* 161–169.

Miller, L. (1996a). Malingering in mild head injury and the postconcussion syndrome: Clinical, neuropsychological, and forensic considerations. *Journal of Cognitive Rehabilitation, 14*(4), 6–17.

Miller, L. (1996b, October). Malingering in mild brain injury: Toward a balanced view. *Neurolaw Letter,* 85–91.

Miller, L. (1998). Malingering in brain injury and toxic tort cases. In E. Pierson (Ed.), *1998 Wiley expert witness update: New developments in personal injury litigation* (pp. 225–289). New York: Wiley.

Miller, T.W., & Kraus, R.F. (1990). An overview of chronic pain. *Hospital and Community Psychiatry, 41,* 433–440.

Naliboff, B.D., Cohen, M.J., & Yellen, A.N. (1983). Frequency of MMPI profile types in three chronic illness populations. *Journal of Clinical Psychology, 39,* 843–847.

Oddy, M. (1984). Head injury and social adjustment. In N. Brooks (Ed.), *Closed head injury: Psychological, social, and family consequences* (pp. 108–122). New York: Oxford University Press.

Osterweis, M., Kleinman, A., & Mechanic, D. (1987). *Pain and disability: Clinical, behavioral and public policy perspectives.* Washington, DC: National Academy Press.

Phillips, H.C. (1988). *The psychological management of chronic pain: A treatment manual.* New York: Springer.

Pilowsky, I., Chapman, C.R., & Bonica, J.J. (1977). Pain, depression, and illness behavior in a pain clinic population. *Pain, 4,* 183–192.

Pitman, R.K., Orr, S.P., Forgue, D.F., de Jong, J.B., & Claiborn, J.M. (1989). Prevalence of posttraumatic stress disorder in wounded Vietnam veterans. *American Journal of Psychiatry, 146,* 667–669.

Reich, J. Tupin, J.P., & Abramowitz, S.I. (1983). Psychiatric diagnosis of chronic pain patients. *American Journal of Psychiatry, 140,* 1495–1498.

Roche, P.A., & Gijbers, K. (1986). A comparison of memory for induced ischemic pain and chronic rheumatoid pain. *Pain, 25,* 337–343.

Rosomoff, H.L. (1985). Do herniated disks produce pain? In H.L. Fields, R. Dubner, F. Cervero, & L.E. Jones (Eds.), *Advances in pain research and therapy* (Vol. 9, pp. 457–461). New York: Raven Press.

Roy, R. (1985). Family treatment for chronic pain: State of the art. *International Journal of Family Therapy, 7,* 297–309.

Schildkraut, J.J. (1965). The catecholamine hypothesis of affective disorders: A review of the evidence. *American Journal of Psychiatry, 122,* 509–522.

Schreiber, S., & Galai-Gat, T. (1993). Uncontrolled pain following physical injury as the core-trauma in post-traumatic stress disorder. *Pain, 54,* 107–110.

Schutt, C.H., & Dohan, F.C. (1968). Neck injury to women in auto accidents. *Journal of the American Medical Association, 206,* 2689–2692.

Shalev, A.Y., Schreiber, S., Galai, T., & Melmed, R.N. (1993). Post-traumatic stress disorder following medical events. *British Journal of Medical Psychology, 32,* 247–253.

Shaw, D.M., Camps, F., & Eccleston, E.G. (1967). 5-hydroxytryptamine in the hindbrain of depressive suicides. *British Journal of Psychiatry, 113,* 1407.

Shealy, C.N., & Cady, R.K. (1998). Multidisciplinary pain clinics. In R.S. Weiner (Ed.), *Pain management: A practical guide for clinicians* (pp. 35–44). Boca Raton, FL: St. Lucie Press.

Skinner, J.B., Erskine, A., Pearce, S., Rubenstein, M., Taylor, M., & Foster, C. (1990). The evaluation of a cognitive behavioural treatment programme in outpatients with chronic pain. *Journal of Psychosomatic Research, 34,* 13–19.

Smith, R.W., Follick, M.J., & Ahern, D.K. (1986). Cognitive distortion and disability in chronic low back pain. *Cognitive Therapy and Research, 10,* 201–210.

Smith, T.W., Peck, J.R., Milano, R., & Ward, J.R. (1986). Cognitive distortion in rheumatoid arthritis: Relationship to depression and disability. *Journal of Consulting and Clinical Psychology, 54,* 573–575.

Sperry, L. (1995). *Handbook of diagnosis and treatment of the DSM-IV personality disorders.* New York: Brunner/ Mazel.

Sternbach, R.A. (1974). *Pain patients*. New York: Academic Press, 1974.

Sternbach, R.A. (1986). Pain and "hassles" in the United States: Findings of the Nuprin Pain Report. *Pain, 27*, 69–80.

Swanson, D.W. (1984). Chronic pain as a third pathologic emotion. *American Journal of Psychiatry, 141*, 210–214.

Tan, S. (1982). Cognitive and cognitive-behavioral methods for pain control: A selective review. *Pain, 12*, 201–228.

Tarsh, M.J., & Royston, C. (1985). A follow-up study of accident neurosis. *British Journal of Psychiatry, 146*, 18–25.

Tunks, I. (1988). Behavioral interventions and their efficacy. In R. Dubner, G.F. Gebhart & M.R. Bond (Eds.), *Proceedings of the Fifth World Congress on Pain*. (298–309). Amsterdam: Elsevier.

Tunks, I. (1990). Is there a chronic pain syndrome? *Advances in Pain Research and Therapy, 13*, 257–266.

Turk, D.C., & Genest, M. (1979). Regulation of pain: The application of cognitive and behavioral techniques for prevention and remediation. In P.C. Kendall & S.D. Hollon (Eds.), *Cognitive-behavioral interventions: Therapy, research and practice* (pp. 287–318). New York: Academic Press.

Turk, D.C., Meichenbaum, D., & Genest, M. (1983). *Pain and behavioral medicine: A cognitive-behavioral perspective*. New York: Guilford Press.

Turk, D.C., & Rudy, T. (1990). Neglected factors in chronic pain treatment outcome studies: Referral patterns, failure to enter treatment, and attrition. *Pain, 43*, 7–25.

Turk, D.C., & Rudy, T.E. (1991). Neglected topics in the treatment of chronic pain patients: Relapse, noncompliance, and adherence enhancement. *Pain, 44*, 5–28.

Turner, J.A., & Chapman, C.R. (1982). Psychological intervention for chronic pain: A critical review. II. Operant conditioning, hypnosis and cognitive-behavioral therapy. *Pain, 12*, 23–46.

von Knorring, L. (1988). Affect and pain: Neurochemical mediators and therapeutic approaches. In R. Dubner, G.F. Gebhart, & M.R. Bond (Eds.), *Proceedings of the Fifth World Congress on Pain* (pp. 276–285). Amsterdam: Elsevier.

Ward, N.G., Bloom, V.L., & Friedel, R.O. (1979). The effectiveness of tricyclic antidepressants in the treatment of coexisting pain and depression. *Pain, 7*, 331–341.

Woodward, J.E. (1982). Diagnosis and prognosis in compensation claims. *Annals of the Royal College of Surgery, 64*, 192–194.

Ziegler, J.J., Imboden, J.B., & Meyer, E. (1960). Contemporary conversion reactions: A clinical study. *American Journal of Psychiatry, 116*, 901–910.

CHAPTER 5. TOXIC AND ELECTRICAL TRAUMA

Adler, T. (1994). Desert Storm's medical quandary. *Science News, 145*, 394–395.

Balla, J.L., & Moraitis, S. (1970). Knights in armour: A follow-up study of injured workers after legal settlement. *Medical Journal of Australia, 2*, 355–361.

Bell, I.R., Miller, C.S., & Schwartz, G.E. (1992). An olfactory-limbic model of multiple chemical sensitivity syndrome: Possible relationships to kindling and affective spectrum disorders. *Biological Psychiatry, 32*, 218–242.

Bell, I.R., Schwartz, G.E., Amend, D., Peterson, J.M., & Stini, W.A. (1994). Sensitization to early life stress and response to chemical odors in older adults. *Biological Psychiatry, 35*, 1–7.

Bell, I.R., Schwartz, G.E., Peterson, J.M., & Amend, D. (1993). Self-reported illness from chemical odors in young adults without clinical syndromes or occupational exposures. *Archives of Environmental Health, 48*, 6–13.

Boivin, M.J., & Giordani, B. (1995). A risk evaluation of the neuropsychological effects of childhood lead toxicity. *Developmental Neuropsychology, 11*, 157–180.

Bolla-Wilson, K., Wilson, R.J., & Bleeker, M.L. (1988). Conditioning of physical symptoms after neurotoxic exposure. *Journal of Occupational Medicine, 30*, 684–686.

Brodsky, C.M. (1983). "Allergic to everything": A medical subculture. *Psychosomatics, 24,* 731–742.

Brodsky, C.M. (1987). Multiple chemical sensitivities and other "environmental illness": A psychiatrist's view. *Occupational Medicine: State of the Art Reviews, 2,* 695–704.

Cone, J.E., Harrison, R., & Reiter, R. (1987). Patients with multiple chemical sensitivities: Clinical diagnostic subsets among an occupational health clinic population. *Occupational Medicine: State of the Art Reviews, 2,* 721–738.

Consumer's Union (1992). Is a dry-cleaned suit harmful? *Consumer Reports, 57,* 566.

Cullen, M.R. (1987). The worker with multiple chemical sensitivities: An overview. *Occupational Medicine: State of the Art Reviews, 2,* 655–661.

Eskenazi, B., & Maizlish, N.A. (1988). Effects of occupational exposure to chemicals on neurobehavioral functioning. In R.E. Tarter, D.H. Van Thiel, & K.L. Edwards (Eds.), *Medical neuropsychology: The impact of disease on behavior* (pp. 223–264). New York: Plenum.

Golos, N., O'Shea, J.F., Waickman, F.J., & Golbitz, F.G. (1987). *Environmental Medicine.* New Caanan, CT: Keats.

Gothe, C.J., Odont, C.M., & Nilsson, C.G. (1995). The environmental somatization syndrome. *Psychosomatics, 36,* 1–11.

Guglielmi, R.S., Cox, D.J., & Spyker, D.A. (1994). Behavioral treatment of phobic avoidance in multiple chemical sensitivity syndrome. *Journal of Behavior Therapy and Experimental Psychiatry, 25,* 197–209.

Haller, E. (1993). Successful management of patients with "multiple chemical sensitivities" on an inpatient psychiatric unit. *Journal of Clinical Psychiatry, 54,* 196–199.

Hartman, D.E. (1995). *Neuropsychological toxicology: Identification and assessment of human neurotoxic syndromes* (2nd ed.). New York: Plenum.

Hermann, S.L. (1992, March/April). Hazardous materials psychosomatic injuries. *9-1-1 Magazine,* pp. 38–39.

Hooshmand, H., Radfar, F., & Beckner, E. (1989). The neurophysiological aspects of electrical injuries. *Clinical Electroencephalography, 20,* 111–120.

Horowitz, M.J. (1986). *Stress response syndromes* (2nd ed.). Northvale, NJ: Jason Aronson.

Howes, C.T. (1994, July). Hazmat case study: The call to the mall. *Fire Chief,* pp. 50–53.

Hua, M.S., & Huang, C.C. (1991). Chronic occupational exposure to manganese and neurobehavioral function. *Journal of Clinical and Experimental Neuropsychology, 4,* 495–507.

Kilburn, K.H., Warsaw, R.H., & Shields, M.G. (1989). Neurobehavioral dysfunction in firemen exposed to polychlorinated biphenyls (PCBs): Possible improvement after detoxification. *Archives of Environmental Health, 44,* 345–350.

Koestner, A., & Norton, S. (1991). Nervous system. In *Handbook of toxicologic pathology* (pp. 625–674). New York: Academic Press.

Korgeski, G.P., & Leon, G. (1983). Correlates of self-reported and objectively determined exposure to Agent Orange. *American Journal of Psychiatry, 140,* 1443–1449.

Lees-Haley, P.R., & Williams, C.W. (1997). Neurotoxicity of chronic low-dose exposure to organic solvents: A skeptical review. *Journal of Clinical Psychology, 53,* 699–712.

Levin, A.S., & Byers, V.S. (1987). Environmental illness: A disorder of immune regulation. *Occupational Medicine: State of the Art Reviews, 2,* 669–681.

Levy, C.J. (1988). Agent Orange exposure and posttraumatic stress disorder. *Journal of Nervous and Mental Disease, 176,* 242–245.

McLellan, R.K. (1987). Biologic interventions in the treatment of patients with multiple chemical sensitivities. *Occupational Medicine: State of the Art Reviews, 2,* 755–777.

Miller, L. (1992). When the best help is self-help, or: Everything you always wanted to know about brain injury support groups. *Journal of Cognitive Rehabilitation, 10*(6), 14–17.

Miller, L. (1993a). Family therapy of brain injury: Syndromes, strategies, and solutions. *American Journal of Family Therapy, 21,* 111–121.

Miller, L. (1993b). Toxic torts: Clinical, neuropsychological, and forensic aspects of chemical and electrical injuries. *Journal of Cognitive Rehabilitation, 11*(1), 6–20.

Miller, L. (1993c). *Psychotherapy of the brain-injured patient: Reclaiming the shattered self.* New York: Norton.

Miller, L. (1994). Sex and the brain-injured patient: Regaining love, pleasure, and intimacy. *Journal of Cognitive Rehabilitation, 12*(3), 12–20.

Miller, L. (1995). Toxic trauma and chemical sensitivity: Clinical syndromes and psychotherapeutic strategies. *Psychotherapy, 32*, 648–656.

Miller, L. (1997a). Neuropsychology of the toxic tort: Making the case for chemical injury. *Neurolaw Letter*, March, pp. 123–126.

Miller, L. (1997b). Neurosensitization: A pathophysiological model for traumatic disability syndromes. *Journal of Cognitive Rehabilitation, 15*(6), 2–19.

Miller, L. (1998). Malingering in brain injury and toxic tort cases. In E. Pierson (Ed.), *1998 Wiley expert witness update: New developments in personal injury litigation* (pp. 225–289). New York: Wiley.

Milner, I.B., Axelrod, B.N., Pasquantonio, J., & Sillanpaa, M. (1994). Is there a Gulf War syndrome? *Journal of the American Medical Association, 271*, 661.

Morrow, L.A., Ryan, C.M., Goldstein, G., & Hodgson, M.J. (1989). A distinct pattern of personality disturbance following exposure to mixtures of organic solvents. *Journal of Occupational Medicine, 31*, 743–746.

Morrow, L.A., Ryan, C.M., Hodgson, M.J., & Robin, N. (1990). Alterations in cognitive and psychological functioning after organic solvent exposure. *Journal of Occupational Medicine, 32*, 444–450.

Morrow, L.A., Ryan, C.M., Hodgson, M.J., & Robin, N. (1991). Risk factors associated with persistence of neuropsychological deficits in persons with organic solvent exposure. *Journal of Nervous and Mental Disease, 179*, 540–545.

Mowrer, O.H. (1947). On the dual nature of learning: A reinterpretation of "conditioning" and "problem-solving." *Harvard Educational Review, 17*, 102–150.

Nemiah, J.C. (1963). Psychological complications in industrial injuries. *Archives of Environmental Health, 7*, 481–486.

Patten, B.M. (1992). Lightning and electrical injuries. *Neurologic Clinics, 10*, 1047–1058.

Persian Gulf Veterans Coordinating Board (1995). Unexplained illnesses among Desert Storm veterans: A search for causes, treatment, and cooperation. *Archives of Internal Medicine, 13*, 262–268.

Primeau, M., Engelstatter, G.H., & Bares, K.K. (1995). Behavioral consequences of lightning and electrical injury. *Seminars in Neurology, 15*, 279–285.

Reidy, T.J., Bowler, R.M., Rauch, S.S., & Pedroza, G.I. (1992). Pesticide exposure and neuropsychological impairment in migrant farm workers. *Archives of General Psychiatry, 7*, 85–95.

Ryan, C.M., Morrow, L.A., & Hodgson, M. (1988). Cacosmia and neurobehavioral dysfunction associated with occupational exposure to mixtures of organic solvents. *American Journal of Psychiatry, 145*, 1442–1445.

Schottenfeld, R.S. (1987). Workers with multiple chemical sensitivities: A psychiatric approach to diagnosis and treatment. *Occupational Medicine: State of the Art Reviews, 2*, 739–753.

Schottenfeld, R.S., & Cullen, M.R. (1985). Occupation-induced posttraumatic stress disorders. *American Journal of Psychiatry, 142*, 198–202.

Schottenfeld, R.S., & Cullen, M.R. (1986). Recognition of occupation-induced posttraumatic stress disorders. *Journal of Occupational Medicine, 28*, 365–369.

Shusterman, D., Balmes, J., & Cone, J. (1988). Behavioral sensitization to irritants/odorants after acute overexposure. *Journal of Occupational Medicine, 30*, 565–567.

Simon, G.E., Katon, W.J., & Sparks, P.J. (1990). Allergic to life: Psychological factors in environmental illness. *American Journal of Psychiatry, 147*, 901–906.

Spyker, D.A. (1995). Multiple chemical sensitivities: Syndrome and solution. *Clinical Toxicology, 33*, 95–99.

Stewart, D.E., & Raskin, J. (1985). Psychiatric assessment of patients with "20th century disease" ("total allergy syndrome"). *Canadian Medical Association Journal, 133,* 1001–1006.

Terr, A.I. (1986). Environmental illness: A clinical review of 50 cases. *Archives of Internal Medicine, 246,* 731–742.

Terr, A.I. (1987). "Multiple chemical sensitivities": Immunologic critique of clinical ecology theories and practice. *Occupational Medicine: State of the Art Reviews, 2,* 683–694.

Tvedt, B., Skyberg, K., Aaserud, O, Hobbesland, A., & Mathiesen, T. (1991). Brain damage caused by hydrogen sulfide: A follow-up study of six patients. *American Journal of Industrial Medicine, 20,* 91–101.

Valciukas, J.A. (1991). *Foundations of environmental and occupational neurotoxicology.* New York: Van Nostrand Reinhold.

Weinstein, M. (1978). The concept of the disability process. *Psychosomatics, 19,* 94–97.

Wilson, J.P. (1990). Post-traumatic stress disorder (PTSD) and experienced anomalous trauma (EAT): Similarities in reported UFO abductions and exposure to invisible toxic contaminants. *Journal of UFO Studies, 2,* 1–17.

Wu, C. (1997). A green clean: New detergents dissolve obstacles to pollution-free solvents. *Science News, 152,* 108–109.

CHAPTER 6. TRANSPORTATION ACCIDENTS

Albrecht, S. (1996). *Crisis management for corporate self-defense.* New York: Amacom.

Baum, A., Fleming, R., & Singer, J. (1983). Coping and victimization by technological disaster. *Journal of Social Issues, 39,* 117–138.

Best, C.L., & Ribbe, D.P. (1995). Accidental injury: Approaches to assessment and treatment. In J.R. Freedy & Stevan E. Hobfoll (Eds.), *Traumatic stress: From theory to practice* (pp. 315–337). New York: Plenum.

Blanchard, E.B., Hickling, E.J., Taylor, A.E., & Loos, W.R. (1995a). Psychiatric morbidity associated with motor vehicle accidents. *Journal of Nervous and Mental Disease, 183,* 495–504.

Blanchard, E.B., Hickling, E.J., Taylor, A.E., Loos, W.R., & Gerardi, R.J. (1994). Psychological morbidity associated with motor vehicle accidents. *Behavior Research and Therapy, 3,* 283–290.

Blanchard, E.B., Hickling, E.J., Vollmer, A.J., Loos, W.R., Buckley, T.C., & Jaccard, J. (1995b). Short-term follow-up of post-traumatic stress symptoms in motor vehicle accident victims. *Behavior Research and Therapy, 33,* 369–377.

Foeckler, M.M., Garrard, F.H., Williams, C.C., Thomas, A.M., & Jones, T.J. (1978). Vehicle drivers and fatal accidents. *Suicide and Life-Threatening Behavior, 8,* 174–182.

Hodge, J.R. (1971). The whiplash neurosis. *Psychosomatics, 12,* 245–249.

Karlehagen, S., Malt, U.F., Hoff, H., Tibell, E., Herrstromer, U., Hildingson, K., & Leymann, H. (1993). The effect of major railway accidents on the psychological health of train drivers—II. A longitudinal study of the one-year outcome after the accident. *Journal of Psychosomatic Research, 37,* 807–817.

Kilpatrick, D.G., Saunders, B.E., Amick-McMullan, A.E., Best, C.L., Veronen, L.J., & Resnick, H.S. (1989). Victim and crime factors associated with the development of crime-related post-traumatic stress disorder. *Behavior Therapy, 20,* 199–214.

Kuch, K. (1987). Treatment of posttraumatic stress disorder following automobile accidents. *Behavior Therapy, 10,* 224–225.

Kuch, K. (1989). A treatment for post-traumatic phobias and PTSD after car accidents. In P.A. Keller & S.R. Heyman (Eds.), *Innovations in clinical practice: A source book* (Vol. 8, pp. 263–271). Sarasota, FL: Professional Resource Exchange.

Kuch, K., Cox, B.J., Evans, R., & Shulman, I. (1994). Phobias, panic, and pain in 55 survivors of road vehicle accidents. *Journal of Anxiety Disorders, 8,* 181–187.

Kuch, K., Evans, R.J., & Mueller-Busch, H.C. (1993). Accidents, anxiety, and chronic pain. *The Pain Clinic, 6,* 3–7.

Kuch, K., Evans, R., & Watson, C.P. (1991a). Accidents and chronic myofascial pain. *Pain Clinics, 4,* 79–86.

Kuch, K., Evans, R., Watson, C.P., Bubela, C., & Cox, B.J. (1991b). Road vehicle accidents and phobias in 60 patients with fibromyalgia. *Journal of Anxiety Disorders, 5,* 273–280.

Kuch, K., & Swinson, R.P. (1985). Post-traumatic stress disorder after car accidents. *Canadian Journal of Psychiatry, 30,* 426–427.

Lazarus, A.A., & Mayne, T.J. (1990). Relaxation: Some limitations, side effects, and proposed solutions. *Psychotherapy, 27,* 261–266.

Malt, U.F., Hoivik, B., & Blikra, G. (1993). Psychosocial consequences of road accidents. *European Psychiatry, 8,* 227–228.

Marks, M., Yule, W., & de Silva, P. (1995, March). Posttraumatic stress disorder in airplane cabin crew attendants. *Aviation, Space, and Environmental Medicine,* pp. 264–268.

Miller, L. (1994). Biofeedback and behavioral medicine: Treating the symptom, the syndrome, or the person? *Psychotherapy, 31,* 161–169.

Munjack, D.J. (1984). The onset of driving phobias. *Journal of Behavior Therapy and Experimental Psychiatry, 15,* 305–308.

Parker, N. (1977). Accident litigants with neurotic symptoms. *Australian Medical Journal, 2,* 318–322.

Parker, R.S. (1996). The spectrum of emotional distress and personality changes after minor head injury incurred in a motor vehicle accident. *Brain Injury, 10,* 287–302.

Susskind, L., & Field, P. (1996). *Dealing with an angry public: The mutual gains approach to resolving disputes.* New York: Free Press.

Watts, R. (1995). Posttraumatic stress disorder after a bus accident. *Australian and New Zealand Journal of Psychiatry, 29,* 75–83.

Winje, D., & Ulvik, A. (1995). Confrontations with reality: Crisis intervention services for traumatized families after a school bus accident in Norway. *Journal of Traumatic Stress, 8,* 429–444.

Wolpe, J. (1973). *The practice of behavior therapy.* New York: Pergamon.

CHAPTER 7. DISASTERS

Adams, P.R. & Adams, L.R. (1984). Mount Saint Helen's ashfall: Evidence for a disaster stress reaction. *American Psychologist, 34,* 252–260.

Abueg, F.R., Drescher, K.D., & Kubany, E.S. (1994). Natural disasters. In F.M. Dattilio & A. Freeman (Eds.), *Cognitive-behavioral strategies in crisis intervention* (pp. 238–257). New York: Guilford.

Aldwin, C.M. (1994). *Stress, coping, and development: An integrative perspective.* New York: Guilford.

Baum, A. (1987). Toxins, technology, and natural disasters. In G.R. VandenBos & B.K. Bryant (Eds.), *Cataclysms, crises, and catastrophes* (pp. 5–53). Washington, DC: American Psychological Association.

Baum, A., & Fleming, I. (1993). Implications of psychological research on stress and technological accidents. *American Psychologist, 48,* 665–672.

Baum, A., Fleming, R., & Singer, J.E. (1983). Coping with victimization by technical disaster. *Journal of Social Issues, 39,* 117–138.

Cohen, R., Culp, C., & Genser, S. (1987). *Human problems in major disasters: A training curriculum for emergency medical personnel.* Washington, DC: U.S. Government Printing Office.

Difede, J., Apfeldorf, W.J., Cloitre, M., Spielman, L.A., & Perry, S.W. (1997). Acute psychiatric responses to the explosion at the World Trade Center: A case series. *Journal of Nervous and Mental Disease, 186,* 519–522.

Eranen, L., & Liebkind, K. (1993). Coping with disaster: The helping behavior of communities and individuals. In J.P. Wilson & B. Raphael (Eds.), *International handbook of traumatic stress syndromes* (pp. 957–964). New York: Plenum.

Freedy, J.R., Shaw, D., Jarrell, M.P., & Masters, C. (1992). Towards an understanding of the psychological impact of natural disaster: An application of the conservation resources stress model. *Journal of Traumatic Stress, 5,* 441–454.

Green, B.L. (1991). Evaluating the effects of disasters. *Psychological Assessment, 3,* 538–546.

Green, B.L., Lindy, J.D., Grace, M.C., & Leonard, A.L. (1992). Chronic PTSD and diagnostic comorbidity in a disaster sample. *Journal of Nervous and Mental Disease, 18,* 760–766.

Hanson, R.F., Kilpatrick, D.G., Freedy, J.R., & Saunders, B.E. (1995). Los Angeles County after the 1992 civil disturbances: Degree of exposure and impact on mental health. *Journal of Consulting and Clinical Psychology, 63,* 987–996.

Harris, C. (1991). A family crisis-intervention model of treatment of post-traumatic stress reaction. *Journal of Traumatic Stress, 4,* 195–207.

Hobfoll, S. (1989). Conservation of resources: A new attempt at conceptualizing stress. *American Psychologist, 44,* 513–524.

Janoff-Bulman, R.J., & Wortman, C.B. (1977). Attributions of blame and coping in the "real world": Severe accident victims react to their lot. *Journal of Personality and Social Psychology, 35,* 351–363.

Johnson, K. (1989). *Trauma in the lives of children: Crisis and stress management techniques for counselors and other professionals.* Alameda, CA: Hunter House.

Kiecolt-Glaser, J.K., & Williams, D.A. (1987). Self-blame compliance and distress among burn patients. *Journal of Personality and Social Psychology, 53,* 187–193.

Kinston, W., & Rosser, R. (1974). Disaster: Effects on mental and physical state. *Journal of Psychosomatic Research, 18,* 437–456.

Lindemann, E. (1944). Symptomatology and management of acute grief. *American Journal of Psychiatry, 101,* 141–148.

Lindy, J.D., Grace, M.C., & Green, B.L. (1981). Survivors: Outreach to a reluctant population. *American Journal of Orthopsychiatry, 51,* 468–478.

Maslow, A.H. (1968). *Toward a psychology of being.* Princeton: Van Nostrand.

McCarroll, J.E., Ursano, R.J., & Fullerton, C.S. (1993). Traumatic responses to the recovery of war dead in Operation Desert Storm. *American Journal of Psychiatry, 150,* 1875–1877.

McCarroll, J.E., Ursano, R.J., & Fullerton, C.S. (1995). Symptoms of PTSD following recovery of war dead: 13–15 month follow-up. *American Journal of Psychiatry, 152,* 939–941.

Miller, L. (1993a). The "trauma" of head trauma: Clinical, neuropsychological, and forensic aspects of posttraumatic stress syndromes in brain injury. *Journal of Cognitive Rehabilitation, 11*(4), 18–29.

Miller, L. (1993b). Toxic torts: Clinical, neuropsychological, and forensic aspects of chemical and electrical injuries. *Journal of Cognitive Rehabilitation, 11*(1), 6–20.

Miller, L. (1995). Toxic trauma and chemical sensitivity: Clinical syndromes and psychotherapeutic strategies. *Psychotherapy, 32,* 648–656.

Mitchell, J.T. (1988). Development and functions of a critical incident stress debriefing team. *Journal of Emergency Medical Services, 13,* 43–46.

Mitchell, J.T., & Everly, G.S. (1996). *Critical incident stress debriefing: An operations manual for the prevention of traumatic stress among emergency services and disaster workers.* Ellicott City, MD: Chevron.

Murphy, S.A. (1984). Stress levels and health status of victims of a natural disaster. *Research in Nursing and Health, 7,* 205–215.

Nader, K., & Pynoos, R. (1992). School disaster: Planning and initial interventions. *Journal of Social Behavior and Personality, 8,* 1–21.

Pitcher, G.D., & Poland, S. (1992). *Crisis intervention in the schools.* New York: Guilford.

Pynoos, R., & Nader, K. (1988). Psychological first aid and treatment approaches to children exposed to community violence: Research implications. *Journal of Traumatic Stress, 1*, 445–473.

Raphael, B. (1986). *When disaster strikes: How individuals and communities cope with catastrophe.* New York: Basic Books.

Ritter, R. (1994). Critical incident stress debriefing teams and schools. In R.G. Stevenson (Ed.), *What will we do? Preparing a school community to cope with crises* (pp. 169–174). Amityville: Baywood.

Sattler, D.N., Sattler, J.M., Kaiser, C., Hamby, B.A., Adams, M.G., Love, L., Winkler, J., Abu-Ukkaz, C., Watts, B., & Beatty, A. (1995). Hurricane Andrew: Psychological distress among shelter victims. *International Journal of Stress Management, 2*, 133–143.

Singh, B., & Raphael, B. (1981). Postdisaster morbidity of the bereaved: A possible role for preventive psychiatry. *Journal of Nervous and Mental Disease, 169*, 203–212.

Solomon, M.J., & Thompson, J. (1995). Anger and blame in three technological disasters. *Stress Medicine, 11*, 199–206.

Stewart, J.S., Hardin, S.B., Weinrich, S., McGeorge, S., Lopez, J., & Pesut, D. (1992). Group protocol to mitigate disaster stress and enhance social support in adolescents exposed to Hurricane Hugo. *Issues in Mental Health Nursing, 13*, 105–109.

Underwood, A., & Liv, M. (1996, August 12). "Why are you doing this?" *Newsweek*, 46–47.

Ursano, R.J., Fullerton, C.S., Bhartiya, V., & Kao, T.C. (1995). Longitudinal assessment of posttraumatic stress disorder and depression after exposure to traumatic death. *Journal of Nervous and Mental Disease, 183*, 36–42.

Ursano, R.J., Fullerton, C.S., & Norwood, A.E. (1995). Psychiatric dimensions of disaster: Patient care, community consultation, and preventive medicine. *Harvard Review of Psychiatry, 3*, 196–209.

Ursano, R.J., Kao, T.C., & Fullerton, C.S. (1992). Posttraumatic stress disorder and meaning: structuring human chaos. *Journal of Nervous and Mental Disease, 180*, 756–759.

Ursano, R.J., & McCarroll, J.E. (1990). The nature of the traumatic stressor: Handling dead bodies. *Journal of Nervous and Mental Disease, 178*, 396–398.

Vernberg, E.M., & Vogel, J.M. (1993). Interventions with children after disasters. *Journal of Clinical Child Psychology, 22*, 485–498.

Walster, E. (1966). Assignment of responsibility for accident. *Journal of Personality and Social Psychology, 3*, 73–79.

Weinberg, R.B. (1990). Serving large numbers of adolescent victim-survivors: Group interventions following trauma at school. *Professional Psychology: Research and Practice, 21*, 271–278.

Weiner, H. (1992). *Perturbing the organism: The biology of stressful experience.* Chicago: University of Chicago Press.

CHAPTER 8. CRIME VICTIM TRAUMA

American Psychiatric Association (1994). *Diagnostic and statistical manual of mental disorders* (4th ed.). Washington, DC: Author.

Bidinotto, R.J. (Ed.) (1996). *Criminal justice? The legal system vs. individual responsibility.* New York: Foundation for Economic Education.

Breslau, N., Davis, G.C., Andreski, P., & Peterson, E. (1991). Traumatic events and posttraumatic stress disorder in an urban population of young adults. *Archives of General Psychiatry, 48*, 216–222.

Breslau, N., & Davis, G.C. (1992). Posttraumatic stress disorder in an urban population of young adults: Risk factors for chronicity. *American Journal of Psychiatry, 149*, 671–675.

Brown, C.G. (1993). *First get mad, then get justice: The handbook for crime victims*. New York: Birch Lane Press.

Budiansky, S., Gregory, S., Schmidt, K.F., & Bierck, R. (1996, March 4). Local TV: Mayhem central. *U.S. News and World Report*, pp. 63–64.

Bureau of Justice Statistics (1993). *Criminal Victimization in the United States, 1992*. Washington, DC: US Department of Justice.

Clark, S. (1988, March). The violated victim: Prehospital psychological care for the crime victim. *Journal of Emergency Medical Services*, pp. 48–51.

Echeburua, E., de Corral, P., Zubizarreta, I., & Sarasua, B. (1997). Psychological treatment of chronic posttraumatic stress disorder in victims of sexual aggression. *Behavior Modification, 21*, 433–456.

Falsetti, S.A., & Resnick, H.S. (1995). Helping the victims of violent crime. In J.R. Freedy & S.E. Hobfoll (Eds.), *Traumatic stress: From theory to practice* (pp. 263–285). New York: Plenum.

Foa, E.B., Hearst-Ikeda, D., & Perry, K.J. (1995). Evaluation of a brief cognitive-behavioral program for the prevention of chronic PTSD in recent assault victims. *Journal of Consulting and Clinical Psychology, 63*, 948–955.

Foa, E.B., & Kozak, M.J. (1986). Emotional processing of fear: Exposure to corrective information. *Psychological Bulletin, 99*, 20–35.

Foa, E.B., & Riggs, D.S. (1993). Posttraumatic stress disorder and rape. In J. Oldham, M.B. Riba, & A. Tasman (Eds.), *American Psychiatric Press review of psychiatry* (Vol. 12, pp. 273–303). Washington, DC: American Psychiatric Press, Inc.

Foa, E.B., Rothbaum, B.O., Riggs, D.S., & Murdoch, T.B. (1991). Treatment of posttraumatic stress disorder in rape victims: A comparison between cognitive-behavioral procedures and counseling. *Journal of Consulting and Clinical Psychology, 59*, 715–723.

Frank, E., & Stewart, B.D. (1984). Depressive symptoms in rape victims: A revisit. *Journal of Affective Disorders, 7*, 77–85.

Frederick, C.J. (1994). The psychology of terrorism and torture in war and peace: Diagnosis and treatment of victims. In R.P. Liberman & J. Yager (Eds.), *Stress in psychiatric disorders* (pp. 140–158). New York: Springer.

Freedy, J.R., Resnick, H.S., Kilpatrick, D.G., Dansky, B.S., & Tidwell, R.P. (1994). The psychological adjustment of recent crime victims in the criminal justice system. *Journal of Interpersonal Violence, 9*, 450–468.

Gilliland, B.E., & James, R.K. (1993). *Crisis intervention strategies* (2nd ed.). Pacific Grove, CA: Brooks/Cole.

Hough, M. (1985). The impact of victimization: Findings from the British Crime Survey. *Victimology, 10*, 498–511.

James, B. (1989). *Treating traumatized children: New insights and creative interventions*. New York: Free Press.

Kirwin, B.R. (1997). *The mad, the bad, and the innocent: The criminal mind on trial—Tales of a forensic psychologist*. Boston: Little, Brown.

Kleinknecht, R.A., & Morgan, M.P. (1992). Treatment of posttraumatic stress disorder with eye movement desensitization. *Journal of Behavior Therapy and Experimental Psychiatry, 23*, 43–49.

Miller, L. (1987). Neuropsychology of the aggressive psychopath: An integrative review. *Aggressive Behavior, 13*, 119–140.

Miller, L. (1988). Neuropsychological perspectives on delinquency. *Behavioral Sciences and the Law, 6*, 409–428.

Miller, L. (1989). Neuropsychology, personality, and substance abuse: Implications for head injury rehabilitation. *Cognitive Rehabilitation, 7*(5), 26–31.

Miller, L. (1990). Major syndromes of aggressive behavior following head injury. *Cognitive Rehabilitation, 8*(6), 14–19.

Miller, L. (1992a). Neuropsychology, personality, and substance abuse in the head injury case: Clinical and forensic issues. *International Journal of Law and Psychiatry, 1992, 15*, 303–316.

Miller, L. (1992b). When the best help is self-help, or: Everything you always wanted to know about brain injury support groups. *Journal of Cognitive Rehabilitation*, *10*(6), 14–17.

Miller, L. (1994a). Alcohol and drug abuse in traumatic brain injury. In A.T. DiKengil, S. Morganstein, M.C. Smith, & M.C. Thut (Eds.), *Family articles about traumatic brain injury* (pp. 167–168). Tucson, AZ: Communication Skill Builders.

Miller, L. (1994b). Traumatic brain injury and aggression. In M. Hillbrand & N.J. Pallone (Eds.), *The psychobiology of aggression: Engines, measurement, control* (pp. 91–103). New York: Haworth.

Miller, L. (1994c). Unusual head injury syndromes: Clinical, neuropsychological, and forensic considerations. *Journal of Cognitive Rehabilitation*, *12*,(6), 12–22.

Miller, L. (1997a, May). Traumatic brain injury, substance abuse, and personality: Facing the challenges to neuropsychological testimony. *Neurolaw Letter*, pp. 137–141.

Miller, L. (1997b). Workplace violence in the rehabilitation setting: How to prepare, respond, and survive. *Florida State Association of Rehabilitation Nurses Newsletter*, *7*, 4–6.

Norris, F.H. (1992). Epidemiology of trauma: Frequency and impact of different potentially traumatic events on different demographic groups. *Journal of Consulting and Clinical Psychology*, *60*, 409–418.

Pitman, R.K., Altman, B., Greenwald, E., Longpre, R.E., Macklin, M.L., Poire, R.E., & Steketee, G.S. (1991). Psychiatric complications during flooding therapy for post-traumatic stress disorder. *Journal of Clinical Psychiatry*, *52*, 17–20.

Resnick, H.S., Kilpatrick, D.G., Dansky, B.S., Saunders, B.E., & Best, C.L. (1993). Prevalence of civilian trauma and posttraumatic stress disorder in a representative national sample of women. *Journal of Consulting and Clinical Psychology*, *61*, 984–991.

Rosenberg, T. (1997, December 28). To hell and back. *New York Times Magazine*, pp. 32–36.

Rothbaum, B.O., Foa, E.B., Riggs, D.S., Murdock, T., & Walsh, W. (1992). A prospective examination of posttraumatic stress disorder on rape victims. *Journal of Traumatic Stress*, *5*, 455–475.

Rynearson, E.K. (1988). The homicide of a child. In F.M. Ochberg (Ed.), *Post-traumatic therapy and victims of violence* (pp. 213–224). New York: Brunner/Mazel.

Rynearson, E.K. (1994). Psychotherapy of bereavement after homicide. *Journal of Psychotherapy Practice and Research*, *3*, 341–347.

Rynearson, E.K. (1996). Psychotherapy of bereavement after homicide: Be offensive. *In Session: Psychotherapy in Practice*, *2*, 47–57.

Rynearson, E.K., & McCreery, J.M. (1993). Bereavement after homicide: A synergism of trauma and loss. *American Journal of Psychiatry*, *150*, 258–261.

Saunders, B.E., Kilpatrick, D.G., Resnick, H.S., & Tidwell, R.P. (1989). Brief Screening for lifetime history of criminal victimization at mental health intake: A preliminary study. *Journal of Interpersonal Violence*, *4*, 267–277.

Schlosser, E. (1997). A grief like no other. *Atlantic Monthly*, September, pp. 37–76.

Temple, S. (1997). Treating inner-city families of homicide victims: A contextually oriented approach. *Family Process*, *36*, 133–149.

Uhde, T.W., Boulenger, J.P., Roy-Byrne, P.P., Geraci, M.P., Vittone, B.J., & Post, R.M. (1985). Longitudinal course of panic disorder: Clinical and biological considerations. *Progress in Neuropsychopharmacology and Biological Psychiatry*, *9*, 39–51.

Young, M.A. (1988). Support services for victims. In F.M. Ochberg (Ed.), *Post-traumatic therapy and victims of violence* (pp. 330–351). New York: Brunner/Mazel.

CHAPTER 9. WORKPLACE VIOLENCE

Albrecht, S. (1996). *Crisis management for corporate self-defense.* New York: Amacom.

Brom, D., & Kleber, R.J. (1989). Prevention of posttraumatic stress disorders. *Journal of Traumatic Stress, 2,* 335–351.

Brownell, P. (1996). Domestic violence in the workplace: An emergent issue. *Crisis Intervention, 3,* 129–141.

Caraulia, A.P., & Steiger, L.K. (1997). *Nonviolent crisis intervention: Learning to defuse explosive behavior.* Brookfield, MA: CPI Publishing.

Crawley, J. (1992). *Constructive conflict management: Managing to make a difference.* London: Nicholas Brealey.

Dubin, W.R. (1995). Assaults with weapons. In B.S. Eichelman & A.C. Hartwig (Eds.), *Patient violence and the clinician* (pp. 53–72). Washington, DC: American Psychiatric Press, Inc.

Everstine, D.S., & Everstine, L. (1993). *The trauma response: Treatment for emotional injury.* New York: Norton.

Flannery, R.B. (1995). *Violence in the workplace.* New York: Crossroad.

Flannery, R.B., Fulton, P., Tausch, J., & DeLoffi, A. (1991). A program to help staff cope with psychological sequelae of assaults by patients. *Hospital and Community Psychiatry, 42,* 935–942.

Flannery, R.B., Penk, W.E., Hanson, M.A., & Flannery, G.J. (1996). The Assaulted Staff Action Program: Guidelines for fielding a team. In G.R. VandenBos & E.Q. Bulatao (Eds.), *Violence on the job: Identifying risks and developing solutions* (pp. 327–341). Washington, DC: American Psychological Association.

Friedman, L.N., Tucker, S.B., Neville, P.R., & Imperial, M. (1996). The impact of domestic violence on the workplace. In G.R. VandenBos & E.Q. Bulatao (Eds.), *Violence on the job: Identifying risks and developing solutions* (pp. 153–161). Washington, DC: American Psychological Association.

Gilliland, B.E., & James, R.K. (1993). *Crisis intervention strategies* (2nd ed.). Pacific Grove, CA: Brooks/Cole.

Grote, D. (1995). *Discipline without punishment: The proven strategy that turns problem employees into superior performers.* New York: Amacom.

Grote, D., & Harvey, E.L. (1983). *Discipline without punishment.* New York: McGraw-Hill.

Hamberger, L.K., & Holtzworth-Munroe, A. (1994). Partner violence. In F.M. Dattilio & A. Freeman (Eds.), *Cognitive-behavioral strategies in crisis intervention* (pp. 302–324). New York: Guilford.

Kinney, J.A. (1995). *Violence at work: How to make your company safer for employees and customers.* Englewood Cliffs, NJ: Prentice-Hall.

Labig, C.E. (1995). *Preventing violence in the workplace.* New York: Amacom.

Lowman, R.L. (1993). *Counseling and psychotherapy of work dysfunctions.* Washington DC: American Psychological Association.

Mantell, M., & Albrecht, S. (1994). *Ticking bombs: Defusing violence in the workplace.* New York: Irwin.

Meloy, J.R. (1997). The clinical risk management of stalking: "Someone is watching over me." *American Journal of Psychotherapy, 51,* 174–184.

Miller, L. (1997). Workplace violence in the rehabilitation setting: How to prepare, respond, and survive. *Florida State Association of Rehabilitation Nurses Newsletter, 7,* 4–6.

Mitchell, J.T., & Everly, G.S. (1993). *Critical incident stress debriefing (CISD): An operations manual for the prevention of traumatic stress among emergency services and disaster workers.* Ellicott City, MD: Chevron.

Mitchell, J.T., & Everly, G.S. (1996). *Critical incident stress debriefing: An operations manual for the prevention of traumatic stress among emergency services and disaster workers.* Ellicott City, MD: Chevron.

O'Brien, P. (1992). *Positive management: Assertiveness for managers.* London: Nicholas Brealy.

Pierce, C.A., & Aguinis, H. (1997). The incubator: Bridging the gap between romantic relationships and sexual harassment in organizations. *Journal of Organizational Behavior, 18,* 197–200.

Schouten, R. (1996). Sexual harassment and the role of psychiatry. *Harvard Review of Psychiatry, 3,* 296–298.

Simon, R.I. (1996). *Bad men do what good men dream: A forensic psychiatrist illuminates the darker side of human behavior.* Washington, DC: American Psychiatric Press, Inc.

Slaikeu, K.A. (1996). *When push comes to shove: A practical guide to mediating disputes.* San Francisco: Jossey-Bass.

Sperry, L. (1996). *Corporate therapy and consulting.* New York: Brunner/Mazel.

Stout, N.A., Jenkins, E.L., & Pizatella, T.J. (1996). Occupational injury mortality rates in the United States: Changes from 1980 to 1989. *American Journal of Public Health, 86,* 73–77.

Susskind, L., & Field, P. (1996). *Dealing with an angry public: The mutual gains approach to resolving disputes.* New York: Free Press.

Walker, L.A.E. (1994). *Abused women and survivor therapy: A practical guide for the psychotherapist.* Washington, DC: American Psychological Association.

White, R.K., McDuff, D.R., Schwartz, R.P., Tiegel, S.A., & Judge, C.P. (1996). New developments in employee assistance programs. *Psychiatric Services, 47,* 387–391.

Yandrick, R.M. (1996). *Behavioral risk management: How to avoid preventable losses from mental health problems in the workplace.* San Francisco: Jossey-Bass.

CHAPTER 10. POLICE AND EMERGENCY SERVICES

Alexander, D.A. (1993). Stress among body handlers: A long-term follow-up. *British Journal of Psychiatry, 163,* 806–808.

Alexander, D.A., & Walker, L.G. (1994). A study of methods used by Scottish police officers to cope with work-related stress. *Stress Medicine, 10,* 131–138.

Alexander, D.A., & Wells, A. (1991). Reactions of police officers to body-handling after a major disaster: A before-and-after comparison. *British Journal of Psychiatry, 159,* 547–555.

Allen, J.G., & Lewis, L. (1996). A conceptual framework for treating traumatic memories and its application to EMDR. *Bulletin of the Menninger Clinic, 60,* 238–263.

Becknell, J.M. (1995, March). Tough stuff: Learning to seize the opportunities. *Journal of Emergency Medical Services,* 52–59.

Belles, D., & Norvell, N. (1990). *Stress management workbook for law enforcement officers.* Sarasota, FL: Professional Resource Exchange.

Benedikt, R.A., & Kolb, L.C. (1986). Preliminary findings on chronic pain and post-traumatic stress disorder. *American Journal of Psychiatry, 143,* 908–910.

Bisson, J.I., & Deahl, M.P. (1994). Psychological debriefing and prevention of post-traumatic stress: More research is needed. *British Journal of Psychiatry, 165,* 717–720.

Blau, T.H. (1994). *Psychological services for law enforcement.* New York: Wiley.

Bohl, N. (1995). Professionally administered critical incident debriefing for police officers. In M.I. Kunke & E.M. Scrivner (Eds.), *Police psychology into the 21st century* (pp. 169–188). Hillsdale, NJ: Erlbaum.

Bordow, S., & Porritt, D. (1979). An experimental evaluation of crisis intervention. *Psychological Bulletin, 84,* 1189–1217.

Borum, R., & Philpot, C. (1993). Therapy with law enforcement couples: Clinical management of the "high-risk lifestyle." *American Journal of Family Therapy, 21,* 122–135.

Cooper, C. (1997). Patrol officer conflict resolution processes. *Journal of Criminal Justice, 25,* 87–101.

Danto, B.L. (1975). Bereavement and the widows of slain police officers. In E. Schoenberg (Ed.), *Bereavement: Its psychological aspects* (pp. 150–163). New York: Columbia University Press.

Davis, G.C., & Breslau, N. (1994). Post-traumatic stress disorder in victims of civilian and criminal violence. *Psychiatric Clinics of North America, 17,* 289–299.

DeAngelis, T. (1995). Firefighters' PTSD at dangerous levels. *APA Monitor,* February, pp. 36–37.

Delahanty, D.L., Dougall, A.L., Craig, K.J., Jenkins, F.J., & Baum, A. (1997). Chronic stress and natural killer cell activity after exposure to traumatic death. *Psychosomatic Medicine, 59,* 467–476.

Dyregrov, A. (1989). Caring for helpers in disaster situations: Psychological debriefing. *Disaster Management, 2,* 25–30.

Evans, B.J., Coman, G.J., Stanley, R.O., & Burrows, G.D. (1993). Police officers' coping strategies: An Australian police survey. *Stress Medicine, 9,* 237–246.

Flannery, R.B., Fulton, P., & Tausch, J. (1991). A program to help staff cope with psychological sequelae of assaults by patients. *Hospital and Community Psychiatry, 42,* 935–938.

Fry, W.F., & Salameh, W.A. (Eds.), (1987). *Handbook of humor and psychotherapy.* Sarasota: Professional Resource Exchange.

Fullerton, C.S., McCarroll, J.E., Ursano, R.J., & Wright, K.M. (1992). Psychological responses of rescue workers: Firefighters and trauma. *American Journal of Orthopsychiatry, 62,* 371–378.

Green, B.L. (1993). Identifying survivors at risk. In J.P. Wilson & H. Raphael (Eds.), *International handbook of traumatic stress syndromes* (pp. 135–144). New York: Plenum.

Griffiths, J.A., & Watts, R. (1992). *The Kempsey and Grafton bus crashes: The aftermath.* East Lismore: Instructional Design Solutions.

Hall, K.M., & Cope, D.N. (1995). The benefit of rehabilitation in traumatic brain injury: A literature review. *Journal of Head Trauma Rehabilitation, 10,* 1–13.

Hall, W. (1986). The Agent Orange controversy after the Evatt Royal Commission. *Medical Journal of Australia, 145,* 219–255.

Hays, T. (1994, September 28). Daily horrors take heavy toll on New York City police officers. *Boca Raton News,* September 28, pp. 2A–3A.

Hildebrand, J.F. (1984a). Stress research: A perspective of need, a study of feasibility. *Fire Command, 51,* 20–21.

Hildebrand, J.F. (1984b). Stress research (part 2). *Fire Command, 51,* 55–58.

Holt, F.X. (1989, November). Dispatchers' hidden critical incidents. *Fire Engineering,* pp. 53–55.

Horn, J.M. (1991). Critical incidents for law enforcement officers. In J.T. Reese, J.M. Horn, & C. Dunning (Eds.), *Critical Incidents in Policing* (rev. ed., pp. 143–148). Washington, DC: U.S. Government Printing Office.

Jones, D.R. (1985). Secondary disaster victims: The emotional effects of recovering and identifying human remains. *American Journal of Psychiatry, 142,* 303–307.

Kenardy, J.A., Webster, R.A., Lewin, T.J., Carr, V.J., Hazell, P.L., & Carter, G.L. (1996). Stress debriefing and patterns of recovery following a natural disaster. *Journal of Traumatic Stress, 9,* 37–49.

Kirschman, E. (1997). *I love a cop: What police families need to know.* New York: Guilford.

Lazarus, A.A., & Mayne, T.J. (1990). Relaxation: Some limitations, side effects, and proposed solutions. *Psychotherapy, 27,* 261–266.

Lindy, J.D., Grace, M.C., & Green, B.L. (1981). Survivors: Outreach to a reluctant population. *American Journal of Orthopsychiatry, 51,* 468–479.

MacLeod, A.D. (1995). Undercover policing: A psychiatrist's perspective. *International Journal of Law and Psychiatry, 18,* 239–247.

McCafferty, R.L., McCafferty, E., & McCafferty, M.A. (1992). Stress and suicide in police officers: Paradigm of occupational stress. *Southern Medical Journal, 85,* 233.

McCarroll, J.E., Fullerton, C.S., Ursano, R.J., & Hermser, J.M. (1996). Posttraumatic stress symptoms following forensic dental identification: Mt. Carmel, Waco, Texas. *American Journal of Psychiatry, 153,* 778–782.

McCarroll, J.E., Ursano, R.J., Fullerton, C.S., & Lundy, A.C. (1993). Traumatic stress of a wartime mortuary. *Journal of Nervous and Mental Disease, 181,* 545–551.

McCarroll, J.E., Ursano, R.J., Fullerton, C.S., Oates, G.L., Ventis, W.L., Friedman, H., Shean, G.L., & Wright, K.M. (1995). Gruesomeness, emotional attachment, and personal threat: Dimensions of the anticipated stress of body recovery. *Journal of Traumatic Stress, 8,* 343–349.

McFarlane, A.C. (1988). The longitudinal course of post-traumatic morbidity: The range of outcomes and their predictors. *Journal of Nervous and Mental Disease, 176,* 30–39.

McFarlane, A.C. (1989). The treatment of post-traumatic stress disorder. *British Journal of Medical Psychology, 62,* 81–90.

McFarlane, A.C., Atchison, M., Rafalowicz, E., & Papay, P. (1994). Physical symptoms in post-traumatic stress disorder. *Journal of Psychosomatic Research, 38,* 715–726.

McMains, M.J. (1991). The management and treatment of postshooting trauma. In J.T. Reese, J.M. Horn, & C. Dunning (Eds.), *Critical incidents in policing* (rev. ed., pp. 191–198). Washington, DC: U.S. Government Printing Office.

Miller, L. (1992). Cognitive rehabilitation, cognitive therapy, and cognitive style: Toward an integrative model of personality and psychotherapy. *Journal of Cognitive Rehabilitation, 10*(1), 18–29.

Miller, L. (1994). Behavioral medicine: Treating the symptom, the syndrome, or the person? *Psychotherapy, 31,* 161–169.

Miller, L. (1995). Tough guys: Psychotherapeutic strategies with law enforcement and emergency services personnel. *Psychotherapy, 32,* 592–600.

Mitchell, J.T. (1983). When disaster strikes: The critical incident stress process. *Journal of the Emergency Medical Services, 8,* 36–39.

Mitchell, J.T. (1987). By their own hand. *Chief Fire Executive,* January/February, pp. 48–52, 65, 72.

Mitchell, J.T. (1988). The history, status and future of critical incident stress debriefings. *Journal of the Emergency Medical Services, 13,* 47–52.

Mitchell, J.T. (1991). Law enforcement applications for critical incident stress teams. In J.T. Reese, J.M. Horn, & C. Dunning (Eds.), *Critical incidents in policing* (rev. ed., pp. 201–212). Washington DC: U.S. Government Printing Office.

Mitchell, J.T., & Bray, G.P. (1990). *Emergency services stress: Guidelines for preserving the health and careers of emergency services personnel.* Englewood Cliffs, NJ: Prentice-Hall.

Mitchell, J.T., & Everly, G.S. (1996). *Critical incident stress debriefing: An operations manual for the prevention of traumatic stress among emergency services and disaster workers* (rev. ed.). Ellicott City, MD: Chevron.

Mitchell, J.T., & Everly, G.S. (1997, January). The scientific evidence for critical incident stress management. *Journal of the Emergency Medical Services,* 86–93.

Niederhoffer, A., & Niederhoffer, E. (1978). *The police family: From station house to ranch house.* Lexington: Heath.

Palmer, C.E. (1983). A note about paramedics' strategies for dealing with death and dying. *Journal of Occupational Psychology, 56,* 83–86.

Raphael, B. (1986). *When disaster strikes.* London: Hutchinson.

Reese, J.T. (1987). Coping with stress: It's your job. In J.T. Reese (Ed.), *Behavioral science in law enforcement* (pp. 75–79). Washington, DC: FBI.

Reese, J.T. (1991). Justifications for mandating critical incident aftercare. In J.T. Reese, J.M. Horn, & C. Dunning (Eds.), *Critical incidents in policing* (rev. ed., pp. 213–220). Washington DC: U.S. Government Printing Office.

Robinson, R.C., & Mitchell, J.T. (1993). Evaluation of psychological debriefings. *Journal of Traumatic Stress, 6,* 387–392.

Sawyer, S. (1988). *Support services to surviving families of line-of-duty death.* Maryland: COPS, Inc.

Seligmann, J., Holt, D., Chinni, D., & Roberts, E. (1994, September 26). Cops who kill—themselves. *Newsweek*, p. 58.

Sewell, J.D. (1986). Administrative concerns in law enforcement stress management. *Police Studies: The International Review of Police Development, 9,* 153–159.

Sewell, J.D. (1993). Traumatic stress of multiple murder investigations. *Journal of Traumatic Stress, 6,* 103–118.

Sewell, J.D. (1994). The stress of homicide investigations. *Death Studies, 18,* 565–582.

Sewell, J.D., & Crew, L. (1984, March). The forgotten victim: Stress and the police dispatcher. *FBI Law Enforcement Bulletin,* March, pp. 7–11.

Sewell, J.D., Ellison, K.W., & Hurrell, J.J. (1988, October). Stress management in law enforcement: Where do we go from here? *The Police Chief,* October, pp. 94–98.

Shapiro, F. (1995). *Eye movement desensitization and reprocessing: Basic principles, protocols, and procedures.* New York: Guilford.

Silva, M.N. (1991). The delivery of mental health services to law enforcement officers. In J.T. Reese, J.M. Horn, & C. Dunning (Eds.), *Critical incidents in policing* (rev. ed., pp. 335–341). Washington, DC: U.S. Government Printing Office.

Silver, B.V., & Blanchard, E.B. (1978). Biofeedback and relaxation training in the treatment of psychophysiologic disorders: Or, are the machines really necessary? *Journal of Behavioral Medicine, 1,* 217–239.

Solomon, R.M. (1988, October). Post-shooting trauma. *The Police Chief,* pp. 40–44.

Solomon, R.M. (1990, February). Administrative guidelines for dealing with officers involved in on-duty shooting situations. *Police Chief,* p. 40.

Solomon, R.M. (1995). Critical incident stress management in law enforcement. In G.S. Everly (Ed.), *Innovations in disaster and trauma psychology: Applications in emergency services and disaster response* (pp. 123–157). Baltimore: Chevron.

Solomon, R.M., & Horn, J.M. (1986). Post-shooting traumatic reactions: A pilot study. In J.T. Reese & H.A. Goldstein (Eds.), *Critical incidents in policing* (rev. ed., pp. 383–394). Washington DC: U.S. Government Printing Office.

Solomon, Z., & Benbenishty, R. (1988). The role of proximity, immediacy, and expectance in frontline treatment of combat stress reactions among Israelis in the Lebanon War. *American Journal of Psychiatry, 143,* 613–617.

Sprang, G., & McNeil, J. (1995). *The many faces of bereavement: The nature and treatment of natural, traumatic, and stigmatized grief.* New York: Brunner/Mazel.

Stillman, F.A. (1987). *Line-of-Duty Deaths: Survivor and Departmental Responses.* Washington DC: National Institute of Justice.

Trimble, M.R. (1981). *Post-traumatic neurosis: From railway spine to whiplash.* New York: Wiley.

Tyler, M.P. & Gifford, R.K. (1991). Field training accidents: The military unit as a recovery context. *Journal of Traumatic Stress, 4,* 233–249.

Ursano, R.J., & Fullerton, C.S. (1990). Cognitive and behavioral responses to trauma. *Journal of Applied Psychology, 20,* 1766–1775.

Ursano, R.J., & McCarroll, J.E. (1990). The nature of a traumatic stressor: Handling dead bodies. *Journal of Nervous and Mental Disease, 178,* 396–398.

Violanti, J.M. (1996). The impact of cohesive groups in the trauma recovery context: Police spouse survivors and duty-related death. *Journal of Traumatic Stress, 9,* 379–386.

Violanti, J.M., & Aron, F. (1994). Ranking police stressors. *Psychological Reports, 75,* 824–826.

Wee, D. (1996). Research in critical incident stress management: How effective is this? *Life Net, 7,* 4–5.

Weeks, G.R., & Treat, S. (1992). *Couples in treatment: Techniques and approaches for effective practice.* New York: Brunner/Mazel.

CHAPTER 11. THERAPIST STRESS

Ackerley, G.D., Burnell, J., Holder, D.C., & Kurdek, L.A. (1988). Burnout among licensed psychologists. *Professional Psychology: Research and Practice, 19,* 624–631.

Appelbaum, K.L., & Appelbaum, P.S. (1995). Prosecution as a response to violence by psychiatric patients. In B.S. Eichelman & A.C. Hartwig (Eds.), *Patient violence and the clinician* (pp. 155–175). Washington, DC: American Psychiatric Press, Inc.

Baumeister, R.F., Tice, D.M., & Heatherton, T.F. (1995). *Losing control: How and why people fail at self-regulation.* New York: Academic Press.

Bidinotto, R.J. (Ed.) (1996). *Criminal justice? The legal system vs. individual responsibility.* New York: Foundation for Economic Education.

Binder, R.L. (1995). Women clinicians and patient assaults. In B.S. Eichelman, & A.C. Hartwig (Eds.), *Patient violence and the clinician* (pp. 21–32). Washington, DC: American Psychiatric Press.

Caraulia, A.P., & Steiger, L.K. (1997). *Nonviolent crisis intervention: Learning to defuse explosive behavior.* Brookfield, MA: Crisis Prevention Institute.

Catherall, D.R. (1991). Aggression and projective identification in the treatment of victims. *Psychotherapy, 28,* 145–149.

Catherall, D.R. (1995). Preventing institutional secondary traumatic stress disorder. In C.R. Figley (Ed.), *Compassion fatigue: Coping with secondary traumatic stress disorder in those who treat the traumatized* (pp. 232–247). New York: Brunner/Mazel.

Cerney, M.S. (1995). Treating the "heroic treaters." In C.R. Figley (Ed.), *Compassion fatigue: Coping with secondary traumatic stress disorder in those who treat the traumatized* (pp. 131–149). New York: Brunner/Mazel.

Comas-Diaz, L., & Padilla, A. (1990). Countertransference in working with victims of political repression. *American Journal of Orthopsychiatry, 60,* 125–134.

Deutsch, C.J. (1984). Self-reported sources of stress among psychotherapists. *Professional Psychology: Research and Practice, 15,* 833–845.

Dubin, W.R. (1995). Assaults with weapons. In B.S. Eichelman & A.C. Hartwig (Eds.), *Patient violence and the clinician* (pp. 53–72). Washington, DC: American Psychiatric Press.

Eichelman, B.S. (1995). Strategies for clinician safety. In B.S. Eichelman & A.C. Hartwig (Eds.), *Patient violence and the clinician* (pp. 139–154). Washington, DC: American Psychiatric Press.

Elliott, D.M., & Guy, J.D. (1993). Mental health professionals versus non-mental health professionals: Childhood trauma and adult functioning. *Professional Psychology: Research and Practice, 24,* 83–90.

Etzioni, A. (1996). *The new golden rule: Community and morality in a democratic society.* New York: Basic Books.

Figley, C.R. (1995). Compassion fatigue as secondary traumatic stress disorder: An overview. In C.R. Figley (Ed.), *Compassion fatigue: Coping with secondary traumatic stress disorder in those who treat the traumatized* (pp. 1–20). New York: Brunner/Mazel.

Fink, D. (1995). Violence and psychiatric residency. In B.S. Eichelman & A.C. Hartwig (Eds.), *Patient violence and the clinician* (pp. 33–41). Washington, DC: American Psychiatric Press.

Flannery, R.B. (1995). *Violence in the workplace.* New York: Crossroad.

Follette, V.M., Polusny, M.M., & Milbeck, K. (1994). Mental health and law enforcement professionals: Trauma history, psychological symptoms, and impact of providing services to child sexual abuse survivors. *Professional Psychology: Research and Practice, 25,* 275–282.

Gilliland, B.E., & James, R.K. (1993). *Crisis intervention strategies* (2nd ed.). Pacific Grove, CA: Brooks/Cole.

Grove, D.J. & Panzer, B.I. (1991). *Resolving traumatic memories: Metaphors and symbols in psychotherapy.* New York: Irvington.

Hayes, J.A., Gelso, C.J., Van Wagoner, S.L., & Diemer, R.A. (1991). Managing countertransference: What the experts think. *Psychological Reports, 69,* 138–148.

Kinney, J.A. (1995). *Violence at work: How to make your company safer for employees and customers.* Englewood Cliffs: Prentice Hall.

Kirwin, B.R. (1997). *The mad, the bad, and the innocent: The criminal mind on trial— Tales of a forensic psychologist.* Boston: Little Brown.

Lanza, M.L. (1995). Nursing staff as victims of patient assault. In B.S. Eichelman & A.C. Hartwig (Eds.), *Patient violence and the clinician* (pp. 105–124). Washington, DC: American Psychiatric Press, Inc.

Lanza, M.L. (1996). Violence against nurses in hospitals. In G.R. VandenBos & E.Q. Bulatao (Eds.), *Violence on the job: Identifying risks and developing solutions* (pp. 189–198). Washington, DC: American Psychological Association.

Levy, P., & Harticollis, P. (1976). Nursing aides and patient violence. *American Journal of Psychiatry, 133*, 429–431.

Lion, J.R. (1995). Verbal threats against clinicians. In B.S. Eichelman & A.C. Hartwig (Eds.), *Patient violence and the clinician* (pp. 43–52). Washington, DC: American Psychiatric Press, Inc.

Maier, G.J., & Van Rybroek, G.J. (1995). Managing countertransference reactions to aggressive patients. In B.S. Eichelman & A.C. Hartwig (Eds.), *Patient violence and the clinician* (pp. 73–104). Washington, DC: American Psychiatric Press, Inc.

Manton, M., & Talbot, A. (1990). Crisis intervention after an armed hold-up: Guidelines for counselors. *Journal of Traumatic Stress, 3*, 507–522.

McCann, I.L., & Pearlman, L.A. (1990). *Psychological trauma and the adult survivor: Theory, therapy, and transformation.* New York: Brunner/Mazel.

Miller, L. (1991). *Inner natures: Brain, self, and personality.* New York: St. Martin's.

Miller, L. (1993). Who are the best psychotherapists? Qualities of the effective practitioner. *Psychotherapy in Private Practice, 12*, 1–18.

Miller, L. (1997). Workplace violence in the rehabilitation setting: How to prepare, respond, and survive. *Florida State Association of Rehabilitation Nurses Newsletter, 7*, 4–6.

Munroe, J.F., Shay, J., Fisher, L., Makary, C., Rapperport, K., & Zimering, R. (1995). Preventing compassion fatigue: A team treatment model. In C.R. Figley (Ed.), *Compassion fatigue: Coping with secondary traumatic stress disorder in those who treat the traumatized* (pp. 209–231). New York: Brunner/Mazel.

Pearlman, L.A., & Mac Ian, P.S. (1995). Vicarious traumatization: An empirical study of the effects of trauma work on trauma therapists. *Professional Psychology: Research and Practice, 26*, 558–565.

Raphael, B. (1986). *When disaster strikes.* London: Hutchinson.

Rodolfa, E.R., Kraft, W.A., & Reilley, R.R. (1988). Stressors of professionals and trainees at APA-approved counseling and VA medical center internship sites. *Professional Psychology: Research and Practice, 19*, 43–49.

Saakvitne, K.W., & Pearlman, L.A. (1996). *Transforming the pain: A workbook on vicarious traumatization.* New York: Norton.

Simon, R.I. (1996). *Bad men do what good men dream: A forensic psychiatrist illuminates the darker side of human behavior.* Washington, DC: American Psychiatric Press, Inc.

Slovenko, R. (1995). *Psychiatry and criminal responsibility.* New York: Wiley.

Szasz, T. (1987). *Insanity: The idea and its consequences.* New York: Wiley.

Talbot, A., Dutton, M., & Dunn, P. (1995). Debriefing the debriefers: An intervention strategy to assist psychologists after a crisis. In G.S. Everly & J.M. Lating (Eds.), *Psychotraumatology: Key papers and core concepts in post-traumatic stress* (pp. 281–298). New York: Plenum.

Tardiff, K. (1989). *Assessment and management of violent patients.* Washington, DC: American Psychiatric Press, Inc.

Tardiff, K. (1995). The risk of being attacked by patients: Who, how often, and where? In B.S. Eichelman & A.C. Hartwig (Eds.), *Patient violence and the clinician* (pp. 13–20). Washington, DC: American Psychiatric Press, Inc.

Van Wagoner, S.L., Gelso, C.J., Hayes, J.A., & Diemer, R.A. (1991). Countertransference and the reputedly excellent therapist. *Psychotherapy: Theory, Research, and Practice, 28*, 411–421.

Volavka, J. (1995). *Neurobiology of violence.* Washington, DC: American Psychiatric Press, Inc.

Wilson, J.Q. (1993). *The moral sense.* New York: Free Press.
Wilson, J.Q., & Herrnstein, R.J. (1985). *Crime and human nature.* New York: Simon & Schuster.
Wistedt, B., & Freeman, A. (1994). Aggressive patients. In F.M. Dattilio & A. Freeman (Eds.), *Cognitive-behavioral strategies in crisis intervention* (pp. 345–361). New York: Guilford.
Yassen, J. (1995). Preventing secondary traumatic stess disorder. In C.R. Figley (Ed.), *Compassion fatigue: Coping with secondary traumatic stress disorder in those who treat the traumatized* (pp. 178–208). New York: Brunner/Mazel.

CHAPTER 12. THE HEALTHY PERSONALITY

Aldwin, C.M. (1994). *Stress, coping, and development.* New York: Guilford.
Anthony, E.J. (1987). Risk, vulnerability, and resilience: An overview. In E.J. Anthony & B.J. Cohler (Eds.), *The invulnerable child* (pp. 3–48). New York: Guilford.
Anthony, E.J., & Cohler, B.J. (Eds.) (1987). *The invulnerable child.* New York: Guilford.
Antonovsky, A. (1979). *Health, stress, and coping.* San Francisco: Jossey-Bass.
Antonovsky, A. (1987). *Unraveling the mystery of health.* San Francisco: Jossey-Bass.
Antonovsky, A. (1990). Personality and health: Testing the sense of coherence model. In H.S. Friedman (Ed.), *Personality and disease* (pp. 155–177). New York: Wiley.
Baumeister, R.F. (1991). *Meanings of life.* New York: Guilford.
Benezra, E.E. (1996). Personality factors of individuals who survive traumatic experiences without professional help. *International Journal of Stress Management, 3,* 147–153.
Cohler, B.J. (1987). Adversity, resilience, and the study of lives. In E.J. Anthony & B.J. Cohler (Eds.), *The invulnerable child* (pp. 363–424). New York: Guilford.
Dahlin, L., Cederblad, M., Anotovsky, A., & Hagnell, O. (1990). Childhood vulnerability and adult invincibility. *Acta Psychiatrica Scandinavica, 82,* 228–232.
Dienstbier, R.A. (1989). Arousal and physiological toughness: Implications for mental and physical health. *Psychological Review, 96,* 84–100.
Difede, J., Apfeldorf, W.J., Cloitre, M., Spielman, L.A., & Perry, S.W. (1997). Acute psychiatric responses to the explosion at the World Trade Center: A case series. *Journal of Nervous and Mental Disease, 186,* 519–522.
Dubovsky, S.L. (1997). *Mind-body deceptions: The psychosomatics of everyday life.* New York: Norton.
Freud, S. (1900). *The interpretation of dreams.* In J. Strachey (Ed. and Trans.), *The standard edition of the complete psychological works of Sigmund Freud* (Vol. IV & V). New York: Norton.
Freud, S. (1915). The unconscious. In J. Strachey (Ed. and Trans.), *The standard edition of the complete works of Sigmund Freud* (Vol. XIV, pp. 161–215). New York, Norton.
Freud, S. (1923). *The ego and the id.* In J. Strachey (Ed. and Trans.), *The standard edition of the complete psychological works of Sigmund Freud* (Vol. XIX). New York: Norton.
Gardner, R.W., Holzman, P.S., Klein, G.S., Linton, H.B., & Spence, D.P. (1959). Cognitive control: A study of individual consistencies in cognitive behavior. *Psychological Issues, 1,* 1–185.
Hartmann, H. (1939/1958). *Ego psychology and problem of adaptation.* New York: International Universities Press.
Heath, D.H., & Heath, H.E. (1991). *Fulfilling lives: Paths to maturity and success.* San Francisco: Jossey-Bass.
Janoff-Bulman, R. (1992). *Shattered assumptions.* New York: Free Press.
Klein, G.S. (1954). Need and regulation. In M.R. Jones (Ed.), *Nebraska symposium on motivation.* Lincoln: University of Nebraska Press.
Klein, G.S. (1958). Cognitive control and motivation. In G. Lindzey (Ed.), *Assessment of human motives.* New York: Rinehart.

Kobasa, S.C. (1979). Stressful life events, personality, and health: An inquiry into hardiness. *Journal of Personality and Social Psychology, 37*, 1–11.

Kobasa, S.C. (1982). The hardy personality: Toward a social psychology of stress and illness. In G. Sanders & J. Suls (Eds.), *Social psychology of health and illness* (pp. 3–32). Hillsdale, NJ: Erlbaum.

Maddi, S.R. (1990). Issues and interventions in stress mastery. In H.S. Friedman (Ed.), *Personality and disease* (pp. 121–154). New York: Wiley.

Maddi, S.R., & Kobasa, S.C. (1984). *The hardy executive: Health under stress.* Homewood, IL: Dow Jones-Irwin.

McMillen, J.C., Smith, E.M., & Fisher, R.H. (1997). Perceived benefit and mental health after three types of disaster. *Journal of Consulting and Clinical Psychology, 65*, 733–739.

Miller, L. (1988). Ego autonomy, creativity, and cognitive style: A neuropsychodynamic approach. *Psychiatric Clinics of North America, 11*, 383–397.

Miller, L. (1990). *Inner natures: Brain, self, and personality.* New York: St. Martin.

Miller, L. (1991a). Brain and self: Toward a neuropsychodynamic model of ego autonomy and personality. *Journal of the American Academy of Psychoanalysis, 19*, 213–234.

Miller, L. (1991b). *Freud's brain: Neuropsychodynamic foundations of psychoanalysis.* New York: Guilford.

Miller, L. (1992a). The primitive personality and the organic personality: A neuropsychodynamic model for evaluation and treatment. *Psychoanalytic Psychology, 9*, 93–109.

Miller, L. (1992b). Cognitive rehabilitation, cognitive therapy, and cognitive style: Toward an integrative model of personality and psychotherapy. *Journal of Cognitive Rehabilitation, 10*(1), 18–29.

Miller, L. (1993). Who are the best psychotherapists? Qualities of the effective practitioner. *Psychotherapy in Private Practice, 12*(1), 1–18.

Miller, L. (1997). Freud and consciousness: The first one hundred years of neuropsychodynamics in theory and clinical practice. *Seminars in Neurology, 17*, 171–177.

Murphy, L.B., & Moriarty, A.E. (1976). *Vulnerability, coping, and growth.* New Haven: Yale University Press.

Rapaport, D. (1967a). Psychological testing: Its practical and heuristic significance. In M. Gill (Ed.), *The collected papers of David Rapaport* (pp. 261–275). New York: Basic Books.

Rapaport, D. (1967b). The autonomy of the ego. In M. Gill (Ed.), *The collected papers of David Rapaport* (pp. 357–367). New York: Basic Books.

Rapaport, D., Gill, M., & Schafer, R. (1968). *Diagnostic psychological testing* (rev. ed.). New York: International Universities Press.

Rutter, M. (1985). Resilience in the face of adversity: Protective factors and resistance to psychiatric disorder. *British Journal of Psychiatry, 147*, 598–611.

Selye, H. (1956). *The stress of life.* New York: McGraw-Hill.

Shapiro, D. (1965). *Neurotic styles.* New York: Basic Books.

Shapiro, D. (1989). *Psychotherapy of neurotic character.* New York: Basic Books.

Tedeschi, R.G., & Calhoun, L.G. (1995). *Trauma and transformation: Growing in the aftermath of suffering.* Newburry Park, CA: Sage.

Tedeschi, R.G., & Calhoun, L.G. (1996). The Posttraumatic Growth Inventory: Measuring the positive legacy of trauma. *Journal of Traumatic Stress, 9*, 455–471.

Winnicott, D.W. (1965). *The motivational process and the facilitating environment.* New York: International Universities Press.

INDEX

316

prevalence of, and involvement in the criminal
   justice system, 164
somatomorphic type of, 86
subtypes of, 10
in therapists after assault by patients, 259
after traffic accidents, 122, 124
and traumatic brain injury, 52–58
treatment for, 2
   imaginal exposure therapy, 169
wartime, ix–x
and workplace violence, 191–92, 204
Povlishock, J. T., 52
pregnancy, therapist's, patients' reactions to, 259
prevention, of workplace violence, 195–99
Prigatano, G. P., 59, 61, 65
Primeau, M., 116, 119
projective identification, in trauma therapy, 254
protective bubble, around families of crisis
   workers, 244–45
psychobiology, of posttraumatic stress disorder,
   15–19
psychodynamics, of chronic pain, 83–84
psychodynamic therapy
   for multiple chemical sensitivity, 112–14
   posttraumatic, 32–40
psychoeducation, after workplace violence, 209
psychological hypersensitivity, in response to
   trauma, 21
psychological theories
   of multiple chemical sensitivity, 106–9
   of the trauma response, 13–15
psychological treatment, of chronic pain, 86–92
psychologist
   departmental, potential conflicting roles of, 238
   role of
      in workplace termination, 198
      in workplace violence prevention, 197
      in workplace violence response, 205–6
   see also therapist
psychology, of chronic pain, 76–84
psychophysiology, of chronic pain, 85–86
psychosocial factors
   in postconcussion problems, 47–50
   in workplace violence, 186–89
psychotherapy
   of crime victims, 165–78
   after disaster, with children and families, 153–56
   of disaster victims, 151–53
   of electric shock trauma, 119–20
   existential, of the brain-injured patient, 64–67
   expressive, 175
   individual, for crisis personnel, 237–42
   of the postconcussion/posttraumatic patient,
      58–67
   specific recommendations, for crime victims,
      168–78
   of toxic trauma and chemical sensitivity, 109–15
      individual approaches, 110–14
   of traffic accident posttraumatic stress disorder,
      127–33
   of traumatized therapists, 266–67
   see also therapy; treatment
psychotic-like subtype, posttraumatic stress
   disorder, 10
psychotropic medication, during sleep recovery,
   29–30
Putnam, R., 162

qualifications, of practitioners in Employee
   Assistance Programs, 184

Radfar, F., 116, 117
Rafalowicz, E., 227
rage
   after head injury, 49
   in police officers, 218
railway accidents, 135–37
railway spine, defined, 4
Ranseen, J. D., 49
Rapaport, D., 275
Raphael, B., 143, 148, 154, 223, 267
Rapperport, K., 254, 255
Raskin, J., 107
rational-emotive therapy, for traffic accident
   survivors, 130
Rauch, S. S., 98
Ready, D. J., 10–11, 86
reafferentation, in brain injury, 52
realism, in treating traumatic disability syndrome,
   xii–xiii
reality, concept of, in acute trauma, 23–24
reasons, for workplace violence, 182–83
reassurance, in therapy with tough-job personnel,
   241
recovery from workplace violence, 203–11
   reconstruction of equilibrium, 204
Reese, J. T., 231, 244
referral, mandatory, of law enforcement personnel
   to debriefing, 231
reframing, in family therapy, 42
regression
   behavioral, after brain damage, 60
   in response to danger, 13–14
Reich, J., 77, 79
Reidy, T. J., 98
Reilley, R. R., 251
reintegration
   of brain injured patients, 66
   of a shattered self, 56–57
Reiter, R., 102, 111
relationships with others
   changed sense of, after trauma, 284
   encouraging in therapy, 285–86
relaxation therapy
   for crime victims, 170
   for disaster victims, 152
   in posttraumatic stress disorder, 25–26
request for restitution, at sentencing, 165
rescuer/rescuee pattern, in therapy, 255
resilient children, 277–79
Resnick, H. S., 125, 157, 158, 159, 163–64, 166, 169
respect
   aspect of treatment for posttraumatic stress
      disorder, 23, 92
   of the therapist for patients, 240
responsibility, and severity of posttraumatic stress,
   38–40
rheumatoid arthritis, cognitive distortion associated
   with, 80–81
Ribbe, D. P., 127–29, 130, 132
Riggs, D. S., 159, 169–70, 171, 172
rights, for crime victims, 163, 164–65
riots, response to, 144–45
risk factors
   clinical profile of targets for patient violence,
      258–60